# *DNP Education, Practice, and Policy*

**Stephanie W. Ahmed, DNP, FNP-BC, DPNAP,** currently holds a dual role as the nursing director at Brigham and Women's/Massachusetts General Hospital Health Care Center in Foxboro, MA, and an expanded role of nursing director across the ambulatory enterprise of Brigham and Women's Hospital, in Boston. In this capacity, she has a key role as clinical leader of the discipline of nursing and is actively engaged in the organization's care redesign initiatives. She coordinated the complex care of the nation's first partial face transplant patient at Brigham and Women's Hospital, Boston, and recognizing the value of the DNP to expand the leadership skills of the advanced practice nurse, she received a DNP in administration. She is an assistant professor of nursing at the University of Massachusetts Graduate School of Nursing, in Worcester, MA, where she has taught Trends in Nursing and further provided instruction and oversight for the DNP residency program. She has served in both faculty and lecturer roles in various Boston-based nursing programs including the Massachusetts General Hospital (MGH) Institute of Health Professions, where she taught an Adult Primary Care seminar and Professional Issues in Nursing, and also at Simmons College, where she serves as faculty for Leadership and Management in the Clinical Setting. Dr. Ahmed has been intimately involved in leadership roles with several professional societies, including STTI (Chapter Secretary for the Upsilon Lambda Chapter), Massachusetts Coalition of Nurse Practitioners (Legislative Committee president-elect), and the Institute for Nursing Health Care Leadership (associate) representing the consortium of Harvard-affiliated nursing services. She has published AIDS-related articles in respected journals and has been an invited speaker on the DNP topic at both the state and national levels, where she maintains an active presence.

**Linda C. Andrist, PhD, RN, WHNP-BC,** is a professor and assistant dean of graduate programs at the MGH Institute of Health Professions School of Nursing, Boston. She has directed the DNP program since 2007 and has been instrumental in curriculum development. She teaches courses relevant to the capstone experience, such as Knowledge and Inquiry, Doctoral Practicum, Capstone Development, and Residency. She is active in the DNP movement at the national level. Dr. Andrist previously coordinated the women's health nurse practitioner program at the institute and was one of the authors of the *NONPF Nurse Practitioner Primary Care Competencies in Specialty Areas: Adult, Family, Gerontological, Pediatrics, and Women's Health* (2002). Dr. Andrist has many years of practice as a WHNP in reproductive health care and has been teaching at the graduate level for more than 30 years. She is a CCNE accreditation site visitor, and a consultant to the Ohio Board of Regents for accreditation of new DNP programs. She was a 2010–2011 Fellow in the AACN Leadership for Academic Nursing Programs. Dr. Andrist has over 30 publications in peer-reviewed and invited book chapters. She is the first author of *A History of Nursing Ideas.*

**Sheila M. Davis, DNP, ANP-BC, FAAN,** is assistant clinical professor in nursing at the MGH Institute of Health Professions, and is the director of Global Nursing at Partners In Health, an international nongovernmental organization working in 12 countries providing comprehensive health care and services for the poor. Dr. Davis has had a clinical practice as an APN (DNP) in the Infectious Diseases clinic at MGH, Boston, since 1997. Since 1992, Dr. Davis has been on faculty or a guest lecturer at a number of schools of nursing, including Howard University, Simmons College, Northeastern University, University of Natal (Durban, South Africa), and Boston College. She is the recipient of numerous awards and has served in a variety of organizations, including Physicians for Human Rights (nurse member/HIV-AIDS, Healthy Women Summit), Clinton Foundation (nurse member, 12-person team to develop comprehensive HIV/AIDS National Treatment Plan for South Africa), APHA (member, Expert Panel on Adherence), and currently is on the editorial board of the *International Journal of Health and Human Rights*. She cofounded a nurse-run nongovernmental organization in South Africa and a rural nurse-run clinic and orphan-feeding program in an urban township. Her publications include 17 papers, 9 abstracts, and 2 book chapters. Dr. Davis is deeply involved with the Association of Nurses in AIDS/HIV Care (ANAC), was the founding/elected president of the Washington, DC chapter, and has been a locally, nationally, and internationally invited speaker on AIDS/HIV for ANAC since the mid-1980s. She has presented on a number of topics in global health and infectious diseases, nationally and internationally.

**Valerie J. Fuller, DNP, ACNP-BC, FNP-BC, GNP-BC,** is a nurse practitioner in the Department of Surgery, Maine Medical Center, Portland, ME, and assistant professor of surgery at Tufts University School of Medicine, Boston, MA. In addition, Dr. Fuller holds certifications as a wound ostomy nurse, foot care nurse, and RN first assistant. She has worked in a variety of positions in medicine and surgery in both Maine and Oregon. She is the past president of the Maine Nurse Practitioner Association, having served on its executive board for 5 years. She is the APRN representative to the Maine State Board of Nursing and advanced practice registered nurse representative to the National Council of State Boards of Nursing. The focus of her doctoral work was delirium education, and she continues to lecture extensively on the topic.

# DNP Education, Practice, and Policy

## Redesigning Advanced Practice Roles for the 21st Century

Stephanie W. Ahmed, DNP, FNP-BC, DPNAP

Linda C. Andrist, PhD, RN, WHNP-BC

Sheila M. Davis, DNP, ANP-BC, FAAN

Valerie J. Fuller, DNP, ACNP-BC, FNP-BC, GNP-BC

*Editors*

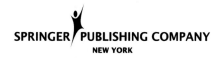

SPRINGER PUBLISHING COMPANY
NEW YORK

Springer Publishing Company, LLC
11 West 42nd Street
New York, NY 10036
www.springerpub.com

*Acquisitions Editor:* Margaret Zuccarini
*Composition:* Newgen Imaging

ISBN: 978-0-8261-0815-9
E-book ISBN: 978-0-8261-0816-6

12 13 14/ 5 4 3 2

The author and the publisher of this Work have made every effort to use sources believed to be reliable to provide information that is accurate and compatible with the standards generally accepted at the time of publication. Because medical science is continually advancing, our knowledge base continues to expand. Therefore, as new information becomes available, changes in procedures become necessary. We recommend that the reader always consult current research and specific institutional policies before performing any clinical procedure. The author and publisher shall not be liable for any special, consequential, or exemplary damages resulting, in whole or in part, from the readers' use of, or reliance on, the information contained in this book. The publisher has no responsibility for the persistence or accuracy of URLs for external or third-party Internet Web sites referred to in this publication and does not guarantee that any content on such websites is, or will remain, accurate or appropriate.

**Library of Congress Cataloging-in-Publication Data**

DNP education, practice, and policy : redesigning advanced practice roles for the 21st century / editors, Stephanie Ahmed ... [et al.].
    p. ; cm.
  Includes bibliographical references and index.
  ISBN 978-0-8261-0815-9—ISBN 978-0-8261-0816-6 (e-book)
  I. Ahmed, Stephanie.
  [DNLM: 1. Advanced Practice Nursing. 2. Education, Nursing, Graduate. 3. Evidence-Based Nursing.
  4. Leadership. 5. Nurse Practitioners. 6. Nurse's Role. WY 128]

  610.7306'92—dc23
                                                                                        2012012459

Printed in the United States of America by Gasch Printing.

*For my mother Dorothy, the nurse who provided my earliest instruction in carative theory, and for my patients, who serve as an endless source of inspiration.*
—Stephanie W. Ahmed

*To all of my students—past and present—with whom I proudly share our excitement about shaping the future of nursing.*
—Linda C. Andrist

*To my mom who has been my biggest supporter, to my dad who showed me the way, to Martin and Karen who are courageous every day, and, lastly, to my daughter Eva, who is going to change the world.*
—Sheila M. Davis

*In memory of my father Alfred R. Fuller, who proved that the difference between the possible and the impossible lies in a person's determination.*
—Valerie J. Fuller

# Contents

# Contributors

**Margaret Ackerman, DNP, GNP-BC, ANP-BC, ADM-BC**
Director of Education & Research, Commonwealth Care Alliance Clinical Group
Assistant Professor of Nursing
Graduate School of Nursing
University of Massachusetts
Worcester, MA

**Jeffrey M. Adams, PhD, RN**
Yvonne L. Munn Center for Nursing Research
Massachusetts General Hospital
Boston, MA

**Richard Ahern, DNP, ANP**
Adult Nurse Practitioner Infectious Diseases
Massachusetts General Hospital
Lecturer, MGH Institute of Health Professions, School of Nursing
Boston, MA

**Stephanie W. Ahmed, DNP, FNP-BC, DPNAP**
Nursing Director, Ambulatory
Brigham and Women's Hospital
Boston, MA
Assistant Professor of Nursing
University of Massachusetts
Graduate School of Nursing
Worcester, MA

**Linda C. Andrist, PhD, RN, WHNP-BC**
Professor and Assistant Dean of Graduate Programs
MGH Institute of Health Professions School of Nursing
Boston, MA

**Elaine Bridge, DNP, MBA, RN**
Senior Vice President Patient Care Services and Chief Nursing Officer
Newton-Wellesley Hospital
Newton, MA
Lecturer, MGH Institute of Health Professions, School of Nursing
Boston, MA

**Dawn Carpenter, DNP, ACNP-BC**
Assistant Professor and Coordinator ACNP Track
Graduate School of Nursing
University of Massachusetts
Worcester, MA

**Ann H. Cary, PhD, MPH, RN**
Robert Wood Johnson Foundation Executive Nurse Fellow 2008–2011
Director, School of Nursing
Loyola University
New Orleans, LA

**Lisa Colombo, DNP, MHA, RN**
Corporate Vice President and Chief Nursing Officer
UMASS HealthAlliance Hospitals, Inc.
Leominster, MA
Assistant Professor
Graduate School of Nursing
University of Massachusetts
Worcester, MA

**Inge Corless, RN, PhD, FAAN**
Professor, MGH Institute of Health Professions, School of Nursing
Boston, MA

**Katherine Crabtree, DNSc., FAAN, APRN, BC**
Professor, Associate Dean for Graduate Studies
University of Portland
School of Nursing, Portland, OR

**Sheila M. Davis, DNP, ANP-BC, FAAN**
Assistant Clinical Professor in Nursing
MGH Institute of Health Professions, School of Nursing
Boston, MA
Director of Global Nursing at Partners In Health

**Marianne Ditomassi, DNP, MBA, RN**
Executive Director, Patient Care Services
Operations and Magnet Program Director
Massachusetts General Hospital
Boston, MA

**Jeanette Ives Erickson, DNP, RN, FAAN**
Chief Nurse and Senior Vice President, Patient Care
Massachusetts General Hospital
Boston, MA

**Valerie J. Fuller, DNP, ACNP-BC, FNP-BC, GNP-BC**
Nurse Practitioner
Department of Surgery
Maine Medical Center
Portland, ME
Assistant Professor of Surgery
Tufts University School of Medicine, Boston, MA

**Daisy Goodman, DNP, WHNP-BC, CNM**
Certified Nurse Midwife
Women's Health Nurse Practitioner
Franklin Women's Health Care
Farmington, ME

**Kristiina Hyrkäs, PhD, LicNSc, MNSc, RN**
Director, Center for Nursing Research & Quality Outcomes
Adjunct Professor, University of Southern Maine
Associate Editor, *Journal of Nursing Management*
Maine Medical Center
Portland, ME

**Lisa J. Hogan, CRNA, DNP**
Assistant Program Director
Assistant Clinical Professor
University of New England
School of Nurse Anesthesia
Portland, ME

**Susan Jacoby, DNP, CNM**
Certified Nurse Midwife
Central Maine Ob/Gyn & Midwifery
Lewiston, ME

**Amanda D. Jojola, DNP, FNP**
Nursing Director
Adams State College
Alamosa, CO

**Nancy Ann Kelly, GNP-BC, DNP**
Nurse Practitioner, Patient Care Services
Medical Nursing
Massachusetts General Hospital
Boston, MA

**Debra Kramlich, MSN, RN, CCRN**
Assistant Professor of Nursing
Saint Joseph's College of Maine
Standish, ME
Co-owner, Zebra Consulting, LLC
Child Care Health Consultant
Chapter Consultant, Tourette Syndrome Association of Maine/NH

**Jeffrey Kwong, DNP, MPH, ANP-BC, ACRN**
Clinical Assistant Professor
Rutgers College, College of Nursing
The State University of New Jersey
Newark, NJ

**Patricia Lussier-Duynstee, PhD, RN**
Assistant Professor and Assistant Dean, Academic Affairs
MGH Institute of Health Professions
School of Nursing, Boston, MA

**Leah McKinnon-Howe, MS, ANP-BC**
Health Service Coordinator
HCA College Health Program
BIDMC New England Conservatory of Music
Boston, MA

**Thomas J. McQuaid, DNP, FNP**
Medical Liaison
Norwalk, CT

**Kathleen H. Miller, EdD, ANCP-BC, GNP-BC, FAANP**
Professor of Nursing and Medicine
Associate Dean for Clinical Scholarship, Diversity, and Evaluation
Professor and Associate Dean for Advanced Practice Programs
University of Massachusetts
Graduate School of Nursing
Worcester, MA

**Patrice Nicholas, DNSc, DHL (Hon.), MPH, RN, ANP, FAAN**
Professor
MGH Institute of Health Professions, School of Nursing
Director of Global Health and Academic Partnerships
Division of Global Health Equity
Center for Nursing Excellence
Brigham and Women's Hospital
Boston, MA

**David G. O'Dell, DNP, ARNP, FNP-BC**
Co-Founder and Administrator
Doctor of Nursing Practice, LLC
Graduate Nursing Program Director
Assistant Professor
South University
Royal Palm Beach, FL

**Nancy C. O'Rourke, MSN, ACNP, ANP, RnC, FAANP**
Manager, Critical Care Affiliate Practitioner Program
University of Massachusetts Medical Center
Worcester, MA
PhD Candidate
University of Massachusetts Graduate School of Nursing
Worcester, MA

**Debra Palmer, RN, MS**
Data Coordinator
Maine Medical Center
Portland, ME
Co-owner, Zebra Consulting, LLC

**Teresa Kuta Reske, MSN, MPA, RN**
Practice Manager Bay State Children's Hospital Ambulatory Services
    and DYS Community Services
Graduate School of Nursing Faculty
American International College
Springfield, MA

**Lena Sorensen, RN, PhD**
Associate Professor
School of Nursing and Center for Interprofessional Studies and Innovation
MGH Institute of Health Professions
Boston, MA

**Maureen Sroczynski, DNP, RN**
President and CEO
Farley Associates, Inc.
Norton, MA

**Lynda A. Tyer-Viola, RNC, PhD**
Associate Professor
MGH Institute of Health Professions, School of Nursing
Senior Advisor
Division of Global Health & Human Rights
Massachusetts General Hospital
Boston, MA

**Judith L. Webb, DNP, ANP-BC**
Palliative Care NP-BC
Clinical Assistant Professor
School of Nursing
MGH Institute of Health Professions
Boston, MA

**Marjorie Splaine Wiggins, DNP, MBA, RN, NEA-BC**
Chief Nurse Executive of Maine Medical Center
Chief Nurse Executive of the Maine Health System
Portland, ME

**Joyce P. Williams, DNP, RN, AFN**
Clinical Instructor
Johns Hopkins University School of Nursing
Doctors of Nursing Practice, LLC
Forensic Nurse Consultant
Baltimore, MD

**Karen Anne Wolf, PhD, ANP-BC, DPNAP**
Professor and Faculty Development Coordinator
School of Nursing
Samuel Merritt University
Oakland, CA

# Preface

With the passage of the Affordable Care Act and the Institute of Medicine (IOM) report on the future of nursing, the discipline of nursing is situated to make a strong impact on the U.S. health care system. We need nursing leaders to step up and pave the way for the work that lies ahead in the 21st century. Doctors of nursing practice (DNP) will be the change agents, and as Cary asks in Chapter 2, "Could the DNP be the future in the Future of Nursing report?" We think so.

We offer this text as food for thought, to serve as a guide for students and DNPs engaged in advance practice in the following specialty areas; leadership, policy, and information technology. Presented in a framework that addresses DNP education, practice, and policy, the text seeks to challenge the reader, and is at times provocative. We hope the content will stimulate discussion at many levels.

Ahmed and Wolf retrace the rich history of advanced nursing practice in Part I, offering the reader a sense of how societal forces have long contributed to the shaping of advanced nursing practice. Transporting the reader to the present, this section further addresses the evolution of the DNP in the context of contemporary health care challenges and culminates in a discussion of how the DNP can influence the essential changes identified in the Future of Nursing report.

Part II takes the reader through the process of clinical scholarship, beginning with Crabtree's definition of clinical scholarship and the evolution of students into scholars. She discusses how the role of the DNP is to generate nursing knowledge from practice. Miller and Andrist continue with the process of carrying out the culminating piece of scholarship in DNP education programs, which is here referred to as the capstone project. Nurse executives and administrators contributed examples of the capstone projects in which they were involved, while advanced practice DNPs share their experience of the challenges and opportunities presented during the capstone experience. It is hearing the student voice that makes this section particularly strong.

Part III explores the DNP degree and role, and the continual evolution of the nursing profession. Tyer-Viola and Davis discuss the benefits of a practice doctorate in nursing and further illustrate how the "Essentials" for doctoral education for advanced practice may be articulated into practice. Recommendations are made on the importance of role definition and integration, as well as the key role that DNPs will play in health care reform. Seven DNP graduates who work in different practice settings discuss their real-life experiences in integrating their learnings from their education, and further outline opportunities and challenges they have experienced since graduation. The DNP will be a leader in health care, and Kwong gives concrete guidance on how to gain valuable leadership experience in the clinical setting. lves Erickson, Ditomassi, and Adams take leadership to the next level in their chapter, discussing the unique skill set needed for an executive nurse leader.

Part IV highlights three important essentials of the DNP curriculum: evidence-based practice (EBP), information technology, and outcomes measurement. In Chapters 11 and 12, EBP is viewed from the perspective of the practicing clinician as well as the nurse executive, whose responsibility it is to promote the use of EBP within organizations and systems. In Chapter 11, Fuller, Kramlich, and Palmer provide an overview of EBP and share a new nursing framework to assist practitioners in moving evidence into practice. In Chapter 12, Wiggins and Hyrkäs discuss the organizational barriers and facilitators of implementing EBP and the theories and methods that can be used to promote change. In Chapter 13, Sorenson reviews the essential role that information technology plays in transforming health care. In the final chapter in this section, Colombo discusses outcomes measurement and its importance in driving processes of care that will result in better outcomes for patients and health care organizations. An understanding of these essentials prepares the DNP graduate to lead at the highest level in both the clinical and organizational environment.

The final section of this text addresses policy, politics, and the DNP. With the advent of the DNP degree, national organizations and nursing leaders were engaged in discussion to define the objectives for the practice doctorate. With the relative newness of the degree, a person with a DNP clearly was absent from the exchange, and therefore unable to participate in the shaping of the degree or its influence upon the DNP role. It is in this context that O'Dell discusses the importance of developing a community for DNPs as a place to connect within the discipline. He outlines how a DNP-led organization called DNP, LLC employed social networking techniques that linked DNPs, students, and faculty across the nation. Jointly, Ahmed and O'Dell describe early initiatives to engage national nursing organizations in the development of an agenda that was inclusive of the new DNP. Together they chronicle initiatives that encouraged DNPs to move beyond external definitions, to find their own voices and develop their own agendas for DNP education, practice, and policy. Health care economics and health reform unquestioningly represent both obstacles and opportunities for nurses engaged in advanced practice. O'Rourke, Ackerman, and McKinnon-Howe lead a high-level discussion around the national issues that are most pressing in our current health care setting. The text culminates in a discussion by Davis, Corless, and Nicholas around the need for global nursing leadership and the DNP.

It is our hope that upon reading this text you will have achieved a greater understanding of DNP education, practice, and policy.

*Stephanie W. Ahmed, DNP, FNP-BC, DPNAP*
*Linda C. Andrist, PhD, RN, WHNP-BC*
*Sheila M. Davis, DNP, ANP-BC, FAAN*
*Valerie J. Fuller, DNP, ACNP-BC, FNP-BC, GNP-BC*

# Acknowledgments

The editors wish to acknowledge the many committed people who have served to both inspire us and support us as we have embarked on this literary journey.

We are indebted to

- The Institute for Nursing Healthcare Leadership, Inc., and more specifically the late Joyce Clifford, RN, PhD, FAAN, who offered three new DNP graduates the support and political clout needed to attract an audience and conduct a small focus group in Burlington, MA, which explored DNP education and the impact upon role.
  Dr. Clifford's influence and this event helped to develop the framework upon which this text, exploring the DNP in the context of *education, practice, and policy*, was developed.
- The MGH Institute of Health Professions leadership and faculty who had faith in the first three graduates. President Janis P. Bellack, PhD, RN, FAAN, for her inspiration; former Dean Margery Chisholm, EdD, RN, CS, ABPP, who early on envisioned the role of the DNP; Dean Laurie Lauzon Clabo, PhD, RN, who continues to provide leadership and support; Linda C. Andrist, PhD, RN, WHNP-BC, who championed the program.
- All DNP students, past, present, and future, who share in our excitement of shaping the future of nursing.
- Inge Corless, RN, PhD, FAAN, and Patrice Nicholas, DNSc, DHL (Hon.), MPH, RN, ANP-C, FAAN, for their ongoing mentorship and support, and Lynda Tyer-Viola, PhD, RN, for her reliability and vision.
- Jackie Somerville, RN, PhD, CNO, and Joanne Hogan, MS, RN, associate chief nurse for ambulatory and care coordination and the Department of Nursing at Brigham and Women's Hospital, Boston, MA.
- Mairead Hickey, PhD, RN, FAHA, Brigham and Women's COO, and Mary Lou Etheredge, RN, MS, PMHCNS-BC, executive director, Nursing Practice Development, for creating opportunity and inspiration.
- The nursing, medical, and support staff of the Infectious Diseases Clinic at Massachusetts General Hospital.
- The nurses and medical assistants at the Brigham and Women's/Mass General Health Care Center in Foxborough and the nurses working across the larger Brigham and Women's Hospital ambulatory enterprise.

- The nurses, surgeons, and support staff in the Department of Surgery and Richards 3, Maine Medical Center, Portland, ME.
- Sally Rankin and Kathy Crabtree, who never fail to inspire and support.
- Paulette Seymour Rout, PhD, RN, MS, Kathleen Miller, EdD, RN, APRN-BC, and the students and faculty at the Graduate School of Nursing at the University of Massachusetts in Worcester, MA.
- Elof Eriksson, MD, and the faculty, nurses, residents, and clinical support staff from the Division of Plastic Surgery at Brigham and Women's Hospital in Boston, MA.
- Donna Barry, RN, NP, MPH, Meredith Eves, Dr. Joia Mukherjee, Kathryn Oas, and Sarah Roberto from Partners In Health.
- The Massachusetts Coalition of Nurse Practitioners and the Maine Nurse Practitioner Association.
- Tammy Robitsek, ANP, APRN-BC, and Jennifer Russell, ACNP-BC, who kindly offered their services to chronicle the rich discussion of the Burlington focus groups.

Finally, much gratitude is due to our families, spouses, and friends, who offered endless love and support, thereby making this process possible.

*Stephanie W. Ahmed*
*Linda C. Andrist*
*Sheila M. Davis*
*Valerie F. Fuller*

# PART I

# Through the Looking Glass: The Growth and Development of Doctor of Nursing Practice Role

*Whoever wishes to foresee the future must consult the past; for human events ever resemble those of preceding times.*

—Niccolo Machiavelli

Contemporary health care challenges include escalating costs, poor access to care coupled with a rise in number of older Americans, and the birth of a quality movement that has created a demand for improved outcomes and transparency. From Nightingale in the Crimea to the new DNP graduate of today, nursing history provides testimony to the strong impact such societal forces have historically exerted in the shaping of nursing education, practice, and policy.

Seeking to mitigate the impact of current U.S. health care challenges, Congress proposed the much debated Affordable Care Act. Subsequently, the Institute of Medicine (IOM, 2011) released a landmark report entitled *The Future of Nursing: Leading Change, Advancing Health* (IOM report). With an acknowledgment that nurses are the most prevalent of health care providers and therefore best positioned to make a strong impact on the ailing U.S. health care system, the IOM issued a national call for the removal of barriers that prohibit nurses from optimally responding to the evolving health care needs of the nation and further recommended that, at all levels, nursing must practice to the full extent of both their education and training. Additionally, the IOM (2011) stated that nurses must be positioned to lead and advance health.

With leadership reflected in the curriculum, the DNP nurse is prepared to lead such initiatives. However, in order to best understand how we arrived at this present juncture, it is helpful to reflect back upon our history and take notice of how through the years nurses have challenged the constraints of their scope of practice, expanding skill sets in an effort to best meet the needs of society.

In this part, the reader is offered a thoughtful explanation of the history of advanced practice, while jointly engaging the IOM Report as compass, propelling the DNP closer to the intended future of nursing.

## ■ REFERENCE

Institute of Medicine (IOM). (2011). *The future of nursing: Leading change, advancing health.* Washington, DC: U.S. Government Printing Office.

# CHAPTER 1

# Evolution to Revolution: Positioning Advanced Practice to Influence Contemporary Health Care Arenas

Stephanie W. Ahmed and Karen Anne Wolf

The evolution of the doctorate of nursing practice (DNP) degree occurred rapidly in the United States. Forged by a coalition of nursing organizations, the DNP degree emerged in the midst to calls for greater accountability in the health care system. The DNP curricula are reflective of this concern and the belief that leadership by advanced practice nurses can make a substantial contribution to improve health care system costs, quality, and access. While educational parity of advanced nursing practice with other health professions is justified, the most compelling rationale and sustaining drive for the DNP is the need for transparency and change in the health care system. Advanced practice nurses, historically subordinated to medicine as "mid-level providers," now lay claim to greater practice liberty. Emboldened by support from groups such as the Institute of Medicine (IOM) and the Robert Wood Johnson Foundation, advanced practice nurses are seeking to take a central role in the evolving health care reform. As policy changes in health reform move forward, it is evident that advanced practice nurses cannot afford to be passive. Advanced practice nurses are challenged to break from the patterns of the past and assert their claims to practice leadership.

The history of advanced practice nursing demonstrates our commitment to meeting societal and health care systems needs. But, over the past 20 years, growing concern about "how" needs are met has reframed our professional accountability. As health care costs escalated and the perceived quality of care declined, health care quality, long measured by process and structural characteristics, shifted toward practice outcomes. By 1990, health research began to focus on the outcome measures (Epstein, 1990). Many of our physician colleagues went "back to school" to study health financing and economics, outcome research, and epidemiology. The measurement of clinical practice is now a central component of health care. Amidst the stresses of system changes and demand for greater accountability, innovation in the advanced practice education has flourished.

## ■ REFLECTIONS FROM OUR PAST

The evolution of advanced nursing practice is both chaotic and continuous. Looking back over the past century, the development of roles in advanced nursing practice is marked by different chronologies and practice patterns. A diversity of advanced nursing practice roles emerged out of the complexity of the nursing educational and practice environments. Despite the apparent differences, there are common themes that have shaped their trajectory, including the following: (1) the adaptation of nursing practice to meet the needs of society, (2) the transfer of knowledge and skills and role negotiation between nursing and medicine, and (3) the influence of a dialectical culture of managerialism and professionalism in shaping nursing roles. Both sides are evident in the unique history of advanced practice roles.

The development of advanced practice roles has reshaped nursing, forging new opportunities for autonomy in practice. At the same time, the changes in nursing roles have brought to light the political and economic constraints faced when pursuing such practice. Nursing has been defined and redefined in modern history in relation to hospitals and medicine. This initial set of conditions provides the basis for the constraints and barriers that advanced practice roles have faced. For most of modern history, advanced practice nurses have repeatedly stretched the acceptable boundaries of nursing to meet societal needs and institutional demands, only to be asked to recoil when economic and political pressures mounted. Advanced practice roles such as midwifery, nurse anesthesia, clinical specialists, and nurse practitioners (NPs) found the path to legitimacy twisted and strewn with obstacles often placed by forces external to the discipline and at times from within. Some nurse leaders resisted the development of advanced practice roles, arguing that this eroded the professional identity, while others embraced the opportunity and new identities. Repeat efforts by groups such as the American Medical Association (AMA) have attempted to block the advanced practice nurses legislation; yet, many advanced practice nursing roles were shaped by close educational and practice partnerships with physicians.

Advanced nursing practice, reflective of nursing, shares a history that is also marked by distinctly gendered roles, as well as class and racial differentiation of roles (Hines, 1994). The feminization of nursing in America was both a source of strength and constraint. While nurses forged their way to engage in caring work, they were also restrained from engaging in self-advocacy for much of their first century.

## ■ NURSING, SOCIAL JUSTICE, AND THE DRIVE TO MEET SOCIETAL NEEDS

Nursing has been characterized as having a strong ethic of service. The profession grew in tandem with social reformism. Nurses attribute this to the foundation laid by Florence Nightingale. Best known for her work in addressing the care of hospitalized soldiers in the Crimean War, her efforts extended beyond hospital reformism to address the health of the poor in the British Empire (Rafferty & Wall, 2010). Nightingale's concern for vulnerable populations and their environment (Beck, 2006; Dossey, Selanders, Beck, & Atwell, 2005) is the foundation for advance nursing practice. The ethic of service was also a legacy of the religious and military culture of early hospitals. The advancement of professional nursing in the United States perpetuated this legacy through the system of hospital schools of nursing, which created a contradiction, as nurses were "ordered to care" (Reverby, 1987).

While much of nursing was rooted in hospitals, the majority of nurses educated in the early part of the twentieth century worked in the community doing private duty nursing or in public health nursing. The surge of immigration and industrialization was well underway.

Public health and nursing practice in settings such as the Henry Street Settlement House and the Frontier Nursing Service provided outreach to populations at risk, and embraced efforts toward social justice and advocacy (Drevdahl, 2002; Jenkins, 2006). The work of nurses in outreach to underserved urban and rural settings created a foundation for the evolution of advanced practice roles.

## ■ KNOWLEDGE AND SKILL TRANSFER

The growth in knowledge and technology has reshaped nurses' roles over the past 150 years. From thermography to genetic testing, there has been a consistent transfer of knowledge between nursing and medicine. For much of nursing history, the transfer of technology has expanded the scope of nursing responsibility and the work of patient care. While physicians may have initially controlled diagnostics and therapeutic interventions, as Sandelowski (2000) notes, more often than not, it was nurses who operationalized them. Nurses were expected to contribute their skill in assessing patients' status without making judgment. However, it became clear to many nurses and physicians that the boundaries of practice were much more fluid, and once knowledge and skills have crossed the boundary, they do not recede (Allen, 1997). The continuous flow of technology in health care has reshaped nursing work with greater demand for information management. But along with information comes the question of how it is to be used. As nurses gained competence in knowledge and skills, they were challenged to reject a passive stance and actively use their expertise in patient care. For the nurse anesthetist, it was through the administration and regulation of anesthesia, midwives in the care of mothers through the prenatal to the postnatal period, and NPs and clinical nurse specialists (CNSs) as they engaged in the management of patients with acute and chronic health challenges.

## ■ DIALECTICAL CULTURES OF MANAGERIALISM AND PROFESSIONAL NURSING

From the well-known work of Nightingale to the more recent emergence of professional models of nursing practice, nursing identity was fused to hospitals. By the mid-twentieth century, hospitals became the centerpiece of U.S. health care and nursing education was viewed as a means to supply hospitals with a ready supply of nursing workers. Despite efforts to advance nursing education through raising standards and accreditation, the education of nurses in diploma schools of nursing subordinated education to hospital interests until the 1960s. Hospital and medical paternalism subordinated nursing, and a good nurse followed orders within the hospital hierarchy (Ashley, 1976). Efforts to move nursing education into colleges and universities were directed at preparing nursing superintendents to manage hospitals and teach in schools of nursing. The oversight of the day-to-day management of hospitals gave nurses the power to protect and further structure their expertise, and to set the basis for nursing definition and professionalism efforts (Abbott, 1988). By claiming hospital nursing as the primary basis for professionalization, nursing further intertwined with medicine, and further thwarted efforts to achieve autonomy in practice. Over time, as hospital bureaucracy grew and became highly corporatized, nursing knowledge and skills were subjugated to organizational rationality (Wolf, 2006). For the first half of the twentieth century, the slow march to professional practice took nurses into management and away from direct patient care.

By mid-century, nurses began to work more consistently as staff nurses (Reverby, 1987). Collegiate nursing education grew along with efforts to advance nursing knowledge and skills. The dialectic of managerialism and professionalism converged in the role of the institutionally based CNS. By the late 1960s, nurses, empowered by organized interests of nursing and feminism, began to organize and reclaim professionalism. Educational programs were developed to support clinician expertise, with formalized movement to universities supported through federal legislation and monies. By the end of the 1970s, the expanded scope of nurses' practice was slowly codified by state laws, professional certification developed, and advanced practice nurses organized to advance to their professional interests.

## ■ NURSE-MIDWIFERY

Before professional nursing and allopathic medicine, midwifery was a major source of health care in the United States. Midwives, historically trained through apprenticeships, lost ground to physician "male midwives." With medicalization, childbearing was viewed as a problem to be controlled (Wertz & Wertz, 1977). As medicine and professional nursing grew in status and power, efforts mounted to abolish midwives. The ideological battle to professionalize and control childbearing practices served both the interests of nursing and medicine. While medicine viewed the "granny midwife" as competition, the nursing community viewed midwifery as a threat to professionalization. Nursing joined forces with physicians in a campaign to eliminate the midwife in the name of social reformism (Dawley, 2001). Midwives were made scapegoats for the rise in maternal mortality. The mortality was in fact due to the increased physician use of unclean equipment such as forceps (Varney, Kriebs, & Gegor, 2004). Nurses joined with physicians to stop the practice of midwives. Nursing leaders began a movement to claim midwifery services as within the scope of nursing practice. Nurses began to train as midwives under the umbrella of public health nursing. The scope of nurse-midwifery expanded to become maternity care, financially supported by the Children's Bureau and the Sheppard-Towner Act. Nurse-midwifery took off slowly, providing care to immigrant and poor women in urban areas such as New York City and Philadelphia and rural areas such as Appalachia. Lay-midwifery practice was largely eliminated and or forced underground. Physicians, freed from the threat of lay-midwifery, achieved legitimacy with wealthier patients. Nurse-midwives, in such settings, became subordinated to physicians by law and practice, serving as the physicians' eyes (Varney et al., 2004).

Nurse-midwives attempted to follow the path to professionalism. Training schools were opened in major cities; standards were set first in the 1930s and again in the 1960s. The first unifying organization, the American College of Nurse Midwives (ACNM), was formed in the 1940s. As the nurse-midwives began to pursue legitimacy in education and practice in the 1950s, the number of programs in midwifery remained small, and it was overshadowed by the "scientific" approach of medicine. By the 1960s, legal recognition of nurse-midwives was limited to only Kentucky, New Mexico, and New York. By the 1970s, nurse-midwives were rediscovered as the women's movement reframed pregnancy and childbearing as natural life experiences rather than pathological states. The public demand for nurse-midwives increased, further fueled by the growth of federally qualified health centers and a shortage of obstetrician–gynecologists. A 1971 joint statement between the ACNM and the American College of Obstetrician–Gynecologists voiced support for nurse-midwives as members of the obstetrical team but also reinforced physician supervision over the team. The 1980s ushered in a new era of regulation with legal recognition for nurse-midwives in all states by the end of the decade (Rooks, 1997).

The quest to obtain prescriptive authority and third party reimbursement moved nurse-midwives to align more closely with other advanced practice nurses. The nurse-midwives achieved the latter, first through the federal Campus program for military dependents and then Medicaid payments in many states. The 1990s led to a gain in prescriptive authority, which was authorized state by state for the Certified Nurse Midwives (CNMs) alongside other advanced practice registered nurse (APRNs) (Hamric, Spross, & Hanson, 2005).

Over the past few decades, nurse-midwives not only gained legitimacy but also scope for practice. Nurse-midwives took on technology in hospital centers, managing increasingly high-risk patients in collaborative relations with physicians. The infusion of technology into midwifery shifted the "natural-birthing" stance of midwifery. As a result of the changing practice patterns, there was an increase in cost of the malpractice insurance. The high costs of malpractice insurance further constrained the availability of sites for practice, as well as the education of nurse-midwives. The move to managed care in the 1990s has brought midwifery practices under new scrutiny. Constraints on choices continue to marginalize midwifery services (Brodsky, 2008). The demands on health care systems to reduce cost and improve quality and safety through evidence-based practice has further challenged nurse-midwifery practice (Sinclair, 2010). A disturbing trend is the increasing medicalization of childbirth, with cesarean births once again on the rise. Midwives, hindered in many states from homebirths, now practice predominantly in hospital settings (Rooks, Ernst, Norsigian, & Guran, 2008). Once again thrust into a managerial role, many midwives provide leadership for ensuring nursing and medical care. The 2010 health reform legislation renewed the call for nurse-midwives to provide care to underserved populations. The nurse-midwife, similar to other advanced practice roles, is challenged to meet the demands for improved access, quality, and contained costs.

## ■ NURSE ANESTHESIA

The role of the nurse anesthetist is acknowledged as the first advanced practice role to emerge with formal recognition in the United States. The nursing role in the administration of anesthetics arose during 1861–1865, during the Civil War, when Catherine S. Lawrence and other nurses provided anesthesia for surgeons operating on the wounded (AANA, n.d.).

This wartime experience would be repeated throughout history, as nurses provided anesthesia to meet the needs of injured soldier-patients and expanded both the knowledge base and skills of the nurse. Nurse anesthetists have been a consistent presence working in the United States and abroad to train and care for military troops. In the late 1870s, Sister Mary Bernard, a catholic nursing sister at St. Vincent's hospital in the industrial and shipping center of Erie, Pennsylvania, became the first nurse known to specialize in anesthesia. The practice of anesthesia continued as nurses were schooled on the job in hospitals from Philadelphia to Chicago. The need for professional anesthetists was discussed across the country, as surgery outcomes were compromised at the "hands of skilled anesthetizers" (Galloway cited in Harris & Hunzikar-Dean, 2001). Nurses and the wives of physician-surgeons frequently provided the anesthesia, as few physicians were willing to accept the limited fee provided from the surgeon for services (Harris & Hunzikar-Dean, 2001). Formal nurse anesthesia education developed as discovery of new agents and techniques made surgery and the demand for anesthesia "administrators" more common in hospitals. Industrialization and the tandem growth of hospitals would expand the role across the United States. In 1893, Alice Magaw began her practice in nurse anesthesia at the Mayo Clinic, and was later proclaimed the "Mother of Anesthesia" by Dr. Charles H. Mayo. Miss Magaw, a leader in the nurse anesthesia, published the first major paper (McGaw, 1900) by a nurse on anesthesia practices in medical journals in 1900. The

Lakeside Hospital in Cleveland, Ohio, became the site of the school of anesthesia in 1915, under the direction of Agatha Hodgins. The Lakeside alumni association evolved to become the Organization of Nurse Anesthesia. Typical of professionalization efforts, the subsequent organization, the Association of Nurse Anesthetists, began an official publication. In 1952, the association was granted the authority to serve as the accrediting agency for schools of anesthesia. In the post–World War II and Korean conflict, the growing complexity and economics of surgery made anesthesia more viable and attractive (AANA, n.d.; Hamric et al., 2005).

During the 1950s medical practitioners began to enter into anesthesia in greater numbers, setting the stage for future challenges to the nurse authority and creating the image of anesthesia as a main field of practice. The development of all-male nurse anesthesia programs followed in the late 1950s, leading to the nurse anesthesia becoming the area of nursing most inclusive for men (Hamric et al., 2005). Nurse anesthesia, similar to other advanced practice roles, established practice ahead of regulation. The passage of regulation was difficult, as the field of anesthesia, once ignored by medicine as a specialty, grew of interest. As the government, through programs such as Medicare and Medicaid, joined the realm of payers for surgical services, regulation and challenges to nurse anesthesia practice grew. The nurse anesthetists responded by raising the educational association standards to a master's degree. This elevation in requirements occurred during a period of program closure and growing physician opposition. For over 40 years, the American Association of Nurse Anesthetists (AANA) met in conjunction with the American Hospital Association meetings, evidence of the central role that surgery and anesthesia played in hospital growth and prosperity (Hamric et al., 2005). This relationship changed in 1976, in tandem with mounting physician attempts to take control over anesthesia practice. These unsuccessful efforts were reflected at both the state and national levels. From the start, nurse anesthesia practice reflected both an area of shared knowledge and skill and, further, a concern by nurses for the safety and quality of anesthesia practice. But nurse anesthesia, by occupying this negotiated space, faced ambivalence from nurses and repeated resistance from physicians.

## ■ CLINICAL SPECIALISTS

The emergence of CNS marked an expansion of specialty practice in nursing. Nurses have typically evolved their practice along specialty lines, seeking out individual opportunities to develop competence in specialty practice. In the early decades of the twentieth century, specialty practice was in areas such as public health, maternity care, and pediatrics. In the post-WWII period, primed by the development of new knowledge and technologies, interest in the formal process and recognition of specialization was generated (Christman, 1968). Hildegard Peplau (1965), viewed as the mother of the psychiatric CNS role, states that the role originated in 1938. The concept of an expert clinician was proposed by Frances Reiter in 1943 as a generic title for a nurse with clinical competence demonstrated in function, depth of understanding, and breadth of service. The nurse clinician and nurse clinical specialist have been used synonymously through the years and reflect a common focus on specialized knowledge and function (Reiter, 1966; Reihl & McVay, 1973).

As the role of CNS evolved, more and more of the CNS practice was institutionally bound to hospitals. By mid-century, the CNS role began to parallel medical specialization to medicine in areas such as medical–surgical, pediatric, or psychiatric nursing. Clinical specialists were hired into roles based on their education, knowledge, and skills. Certification was not yet developed or required (Hudspeth, 2011). During the 1970s, despite the lack of consensus over the CNS role, the number increased dramatically along with graduate education funding. By the mid-1970s, the American Nurses Association (ANA) advocated for the master's degree as a requirement for the CNS (ANA Congress on Nursing Practice, 1974). Despite the growing number of nurses educated in CNS roles, confusion over the role persisted. Some CNSs were working in direct care or in physician-led teams in specialty practice and were reshaped by the transfer of specialized knowledge skills. The direct care of clinical specialist appealed to many CNSs as a means to expand access and address the needs of patients in crisis. The psychiatric CNSs exemplified this trend with practices that, more often than not, provided care to underserved populations. A larger number of CNSs were expert consultants to nursing staff, bridging clinical expertise with managerialism at the unit or nursing service level. The CNS working in areas such as gerontology, psychiatry, and cardiovascular nursing has supported the development of implementation of guidelines and rational systems of care. The inability to show direct cost saving through the integration of the CNS in nursing services remained a problem.

CNSs organized and sought legitimacy through certification. Certification slowly evolved beginning in the late 1970s but was not the panacea; with the exception of the psychiatric CNS, it was rarely required by employers. By the 1980s, psychiatric CNS aligned with nurse-midwives and NPs in the pursuit of legislative goals for reimbursement and prescriptive authority (Lyon, 2000). This move supported the successful campaign for legislative and regulatory changes in many states.

As changes in hospital reimbursement constrained budgets, the CNS became an easy target, as their role did not generate income for the hospitals systems. In many institutions, the CNS positions were eliminated or combined into administrative or teaching positions such as unit-based clinical teaching, nurse managers, and/or case managers. By 1990, CNSs found themselves at an economic disadvantage to NPs, who were beginning to secure positions in specialty practices with their clinical skills and eligibility for billing. Thousands of clinical specialists returned to school to seek NP certification. Within the advanced practice community, there was an increasing talk about the blended role of CNS–NP (Hamric et al., 2005).

The medical outcomes era was well underway by the time the first major wave of CNS completed their NP education. The release of the 2001 IOM report, *Crossing the Quality Chasm* (IOM, 2001), generated close attention on system improvements for quality and safety. A decade after, there was fear that the CNS might become extinct; there was renewed focus on the CNS as nursing change agent.

The 2004 National Association of Clinical Nurse Specialists (NACNS) statement on CNS practice and education reaffirmed the importance of preparing the CNS with skills in leadership, collaboration, and consultation; professionalism; ethical practice; and professional citizenship. The NACNS further elaborated these in 2010 as it outlined new core competencies such as (1) direct care; (2) consultation; (3) systems leadership; (4) collaboration; (5) coaching; (6) research including interpretation, use, translation, evaluation, and conduct; and (7) ethical decision making, moral agency, and advocacy. These were presumed to occur with leadership, collaboration, and consultation; professionalism; ethical practice; and professional citizenship (NACNS, 2010b).

The CNS role continued to be broadly focused on specialty knowledge for populations, nursing staff education, consultation, and organizational change (Sparacino, 2005).

The 2010 passage of the Patient Protection and Affordable Health Care Act raised questions once again on the economic viability of the CNS role. As many CNSs were working in direct care roles in areas such as gerontology, oncology, palliative care, and maternal child health, NACNS (2010a) reaffirmed the position that CNSs are valuable members of primary care teams. Brenda Lyon, former chairperson of the American Association of CNS legislative/regulatory committee, noted the following: "although several barriers to CNS practice were identified in the analysis, the two most prevalent were (1) not recognizing CNS practice at all or requiring a CNS to meet requirements to practice as an NP and (2) requiring a CNS to be certified in specialty areas even in the absence of availability of CNS certification in the specialty." The development of the 2011 consensus report on advanced nursing practice did not resolve the regulatory issues for the CNS. Many CNSs practice in states that do not recognize or require certification.

Despite gains in professional legitimacy, the role of the CNS continues to be at risk. The future of CNS practice, constrained by fiscal trends, requires a political savvy to maneuver the straits of health care reforms, such as the Patient Protection and the Affordable Care Act. The CNS has the potential to help reshape health systems to guide chronic care and patients' transitions inside and out of hospitals.

## ■ NURSE PRACTITIONERS

The NP was the last of the direct practice advance nursing roles to develop in the twentieth century. The history of NPs is commonly dated back to 1965 with the opening of the pediatric NP program by Loretta Ford and Henry Silver, MD, in Colorado. In reality, the NP role evolved after decades of expanding nursing practice in community settings such as public health and outpatient centers (Norris, 1977). The formal creation of the role was observed by Loretta Ford to legitimize the reality of nurses practice (Fairman, 2008). In the 1960s, the great society movement led to a dual concern for easing social tensions with major policy reforms. These included the development of new forms of health care payment under Medicare and Medicaid, as well as the development of new settings of care such as community health centers. As Medicare and Medicaid policies created an unprecedented demand for health care services, interest in a new expanded role grew. Primary care physicians were few and far between, as the culture of medicine placed greater value on specialization and, as a result, diverted physicians into more lucrative areas of surgery and medical specialties. The growing shortage of general practitioners and the limited availability of pediatricians created an opportunity for the first programs for pediatric NPs (Andrews, Yankauer, & Connelly, 1970).

Many nurses had already demonstrated the ability and a willingness to take on the assessment and management of patients with common acute and chronic health care needs. NP education began with support from medicine, causing many leaders in nursing to cast a jaundiced eye on NPs. The NP movement took off, just as the nursing profession and feminist ideology converged, offering a critical view and fear of further subjugation. As the numbers of NPs grew and gained positive reviews from patients and collaborating physicians, efforts to sustain the movement took shape through policy-making. With the support of federal funding, the nursing profession began to acknowledge NPs, opening the doors in the 1970s to offer training, first as certificate programs and a few years later, as graduate programs. Nursing organizations such as the ANA and their state constituent organizations, despite ambivalence, facilitated NP practice groups' efforts. Legal recognition of NP practice was slowly achieved on a state-by-state basis. This also helped to advance efforts to establish standards and certification. At the national level, NPs organized as the American Academy of Nurse Practitioners in 1985 as a "unified way to network and advocate for NP issues." This was the first national organization created to advocate politically for NPs of all specialties. This step in organizing NPs helped to advance legislation and set standards of practice. Regulatory efforts at the state level were initially sought to recognize and control the scope of practice and later to prescriptive practices and reimbursement (Keeling, 2007). The varieties of state policy outcomes vary widely, as evidence of the strength of physician attempts to assert control and nursing power to resist this. NP autonomy of practice became a goal but elusive to NPs in most states. Barbara Safriet, in a (1992) Yale Law Journal, argued for the greater consistency and criteria for NP education and practice. As NPs demonstrated the ability to provide cost-effective quality care, the public and private insurance markets began to open up to NP practice. The 2011 Patient Protection and Affordable Heath Care Act renewed debate about the future of NPs and other advanced practice nurses despite language that recognized advanced practice nurses as providers; the supportive regulatory agencies such as Center for Medicare and Medicaid Services (CMS) offered contradictory language in proposed regulations.

## ■ BEYOND DIRECT CARE: ENGAGING IN ADVANCED PRACTICE

Advanced practice nursing (APN), as defined by the National Council of State Boards of Nursing (2011) in the Campaign for APRN Consensus, includes the previously introduced direct care roles of the certified registered nurse anesthetist (CRNA), CNM, CNS, and the certified nurse practitioner (CNP). However, there is an acknowledgment that new and emerging nursing roles will continue to evolve and perhaps, in some instances, even migrate away from direct patient care, which has long been the hallmark of advanced practice. Nurses engaged in administration, policy work, or the emerging role of the informatics nurse specialist provide us with such example. The inclusion of nondirect care roles under the umbrella of engaging in advance practice is an acknowledgment of the broad sphere of influence and specialized nature of the work undertaken by nurses practicing in these areas.

### Nursing Administration

The ANA developed *Nursing Administration: Scope and Standards of Practice* (2009), which serves to outline competencies and provide a framework for the administrative practice of nurses today. Nurse administrators are registered nurses responsible for communicating the shared vision of an organization, and they further orchestrate and influence the work of others toward the achievement of important organizational outcomes (ANA, 2009).

With her appointment to the position of superintendent of the Upper Harley Street Hospital, Florence Nightingale is often credited with developing the management role in nursing. Like much of nursing, history suggests that it is unlikely that this role would have developed outside of the influence of the social and political forces of the time (Wildman, 2009). Historically, female superintendents held responsibility for the oversight of nursing practice, as was chronicled by Nightingale. However, the literature suggests that similar structures of nursing workforce oversight existed among nineteenth-century religious sisterhoods, alluding to the idea that some early form of nursing management may have predated Nightingale. Despite this ambiguity, what remains significant today is that this structure of clinical oversight establishes a foundation for the nurse management role and precedence that nurses are responsible for the management of other nurses (Wildman, 2009).

From Nightingale to Clifford, who served as the senior vice president and nurse-in-chief of the Beth Israel Deaconess Hospital in Boston, Massachusetts, and who is credited with the development of a professional nursing model that is considered the benchmark for professionalism in nursing, history is rich with examples of nurses engaged in administration and leadership.

Early nursing leaders often lacked formalized management training; however, the 1899 development of a "Hospital Economy" certificate program at Teacher's College at Columbia University in New York represented an important step toward formalizing the education of the nurse administrator (Alexander, 1997). Designed to train nurses for administrative positions in hospitals, the Columbia program is credited with establishing the foundation for early baccalaureate and master's degree programs (Alexander, 1997).

Over the years, the migration of nurses from the bedside to the boardroom has been both tenuous and tentative. In the early 1900s, the American Medical Association (AMA) reported that more than 1,500 charitable or church-affiliated institutions were being managed by nurses (Alexander, 1997). However, secondary to an evolving perception that nurses lacked the acumen necessary to lead, the presence of women in hospital leadership began a trajectory of decline, often substituted by men who possessed proficiency in business and medicine (Alexander, 1997).

The march for nurse administrators to evolve their roles and maintain organizational footing was slow and required significant help from private funders, including The Kellogg Foundation and, later, the Commonwealth Fund (Alexander, 1997). During the 1950s, graduate programs for nursing administration became more prevalent. However, as greater value was placed on growing the body of nursing knowledge and developing the clinical practice, these academic opportunities for nursing administration again began a decline. It was not until the 1970s and 1980s that interdisciplinary master's programs in nursing administration were developed within university schools of business, public health, and health care administration. Eventually, with recognition that management within the nursing services required improvement, dual degree programs such as the MSN/MBA were initiated. The aforementioned degree programs provided a long-overdue opportunity for the nurse administrator role to flourish as this degree soon became the preparation of choice for the nurse executive; producing a master's prepared nurse with a master's in business administration (Alexander, 1997).

The contemporary role of the nurse administrator has evolved from the "head nurse" with a defined unit-based responsibility to include executive-level roles with broad organizational influence and responsibility such as the vice president of Patient Care Services, chief nursing officer (CNO), chief executive officer (CEO), chief operating officer (COO), or dean (ANA, 2009). Certification for nursing administration has been offered through the American Nurse Credentialing Center (ANCC) since 1979. However, in 2008, the organization announced that the certification title would be changed to the Nurse Executive Certification with basic and advanced competencies. With broad applicability across diverse administrative roles, this move was designed to both align and contemporize the nurse administrator title with current health care culture and remains standard today (ANCC, 2008). Despite such changes in titles and a high public trust rating, a recent Gallup poll suggests that the nurses remain largely absent at the highest decision-making levels and lack a meaningful presence in the boardroom when compared to physician colleagues (Khoury, Blizzard, Wright Moore & Hassmiller, 2011). Clearly, there is much work to be done to move advanced practice nurses out of the margins of health care leadership.

## ■ EMERGING ROLES FOR ADVANCED PRACTICE

Over the past two decades, the restructuring of health care systems toward consolidation and integration of services has led to new roles such as case managers and informatics nurse specialists. The support for such roles has risen amidst expanding governmental regulations to address quality and safety. Both roles represent a significant solution toward addressing the health care system dysfunctions that contribute to injuries and high costs of rehospitalization.

Case management, acknowledged as an advanced practice role function, is in transition to become a distinct role for advanced practice nurses. Graduate-level education programs for case management are emerging throughout the United States and efforts are underway to provide master's-level case management certification by the ANCC. The recent passage of health reforms has strengthened the impetus of case management. As health care institutions tackle new mandates in chronic disease management and care transitions, nurse management has an opportunity to demonstrate greater expertise and control over health care decision making.

Nursing informatics has slowly become integrated into nursing education and practice. The first documented computer technology course was offered in New York for undergraduate nursing students in 1976 (Guenther, 2006). Over time, nurses have assumed increasingly larger roles in the management of health-related data, but the phrase "nursing informatics" reportedly did not appear in the literature until 1985. A decade later, the ANA defined nursing informatics as a specialty and published the *Scope of Practice in Nursing Informatics* and *Nursing Informatics Standards of Practice* (Guenther, 2006).

The evolution toward a nursing informatics specialty necessitated that the nursing informatics roles evolve from the already well-established medical and health care informatics specialties (Guenther, 2006). As core content and competencies for nursing informatics have become better developed, there has been an emergence of coursework to support the growing specialty. Offering the first certifying exam in November of 1995, the ANCC remains the official certifying organization for informatics nurse specialists (Tietze, 2008). While certification was offered, it is important to note that it was not until 2001 that the ANA *Scope of Practice in Nursing Informatics* and *Nursing Informatics Standards of Practice* were integrated and the *Scope and Standards of Nursing Informatics* was published (Guenther, 2006). Accordingly, it is with this process that the ANA set the stage to truly legitimize the specialty and define nursing informatics; the integration of nursing, computer, and information sciences to manage and communicate data, knowledge, and nursing practice (Guenther, 2006). An additional necessity is the integration of such data to support decision making across all health care roles and settings (Tietze, 2008).

Reinforced by the tendency for chief information officers (CIOs) to value technology, the early roles for the information nurse specialists were largely related to the insertion of technology into practice settings (Staggers, 2002). Today, there are numerous programs across the country preparing nurses to engage in the advanced practice of nursing informatics and their graduates have prominent roles in staff education, quality, and safety, as well as the protection of the privacy and confidentiality of patients (Tietze, 2008). Informatics nurse specialists are integral to ensuring the delivery of safe patient care and may serve as systems analysts, consultants, programmers, researchers, or decision support/outcomes managers (Tietze, 2008). Indeed, the roles are likely to continue to evolve as the infusion of technology and the need to effectively manage data continue to exert an impact upon the dynamic health care environments in which nurses are engaged in practice. The leveraging of technology to manage aggregates of patients or perhaps for predictive modeling purposes will be as routine as the blood pressure cuff in the exam room.

### ■ DNP: PREPARING THE APRN FOR THE FUTURE—OR IS THE FUTURE NOW?

The move to a practice doctorate for advanced nursing practice is again a response by nursing to societal demands and anticipated challenges. There is no question that the master's-prepared nurses have demonstrated well-documented outcomes that include safe, cost-effective care and high patient satisfaction rates (Mundinger, 2008; Newhouse et al., 2011). The American Association of Colleges of Nursing (AACN, 2004) makes the case for reshaping the education for advanced practice nursing, citing demographic imperatives, and population health trends. In 2006, as the AACN was considering the transformative shift of specialty education to the doctoral level, the U.S. Census Bureau reported that the number of Americans with employer-based access to health insurance had markedly declined, and an estimated 47 million Americans were living without health insurance (Johnson, 2007). In 2010, the U.S. Census Bureau (2011) reports the number of uninsured had increased to 49.9 million and in the current state, the health care system is no better positioned to meet the access needs of the people.

Further complicating, the United States is potentially facing a geriatric crisis, as unprecedented growth in the number of older adults is anticipated (CDC, 2007). As societal and health care advances in prevention have reduced the threat of infectious diseases, a demographic shift toward longevity and chronic disease has emerged. The number of Americans aged 65 or older is predicted to double, and by 2030, this population could reach a staggering 71 million older adults with documented health care costs exceeding that of a younger demographic (CDC, 2007).

An examination of health care outcomes for Medicare beneficiaries suggests that there is a strong case for cost-containment and coordinated care if we are to meet the health care needs of an aging population (Jencks, Williams, and Coleman, 2009). A recent analysis of Medicare claims data revealed that one fifth of discharged Medicare beneficiaries were readmitted within 30 days. Those readmitted had a longer than average length of stay and many had not had post-discharge follow-up—a clear case for improved access and coordination of care. The estimated cost of unplanned hospital readmissions in 2004 alone was a staggering $17.4 billion (Jencks et al., 2009). In the backdrop is an IOM report (Kohn, Corrigan, & Donaldson, 2000) that estimates as many as 98,000 Americans may die annually as a result of errors in care. Primary care is virtually nonexistent as medical students continue to gravitate toward lucrative specialty training and, by 2020, a deficit of 200,000 generalist physicians has been projected (Schwartz, Basco, Grey, Elmore, & Rubenstein, 2005). Should this deleterious trend continue, the fragmented health care system will likely be ill-positioned to meet the complex medical needs of an aging U.S. population (Schwartz et al., 2005). The increased complexities of the health care environment, coupled with a rising population of older Americans and decreased access to care, can be cited as major drivers in the health care crisis, the direction of health reforms, and the need to move specialty education in nursing to the doctoral level.

Citing concern related to the quality and safety of patient care delivery, as well as the increasing complexity of the current health care system, the AACN published the *Essentials of Doctoral Education for Advanced Nursing Practice* (2006) and issued a call for transformational change in the educational preparedness for nurses practicing at the most advanced level in nursing. With a recommended implementation date of 2015, the AACN boldly asserted that nurses effectively engaged in practice at advanced levels would require doctoral-level preparedness. At that time, identified benefits of repositioning specialty education to the doctoral level further included closing the gap on evolving advance nursing competencies for practice, leadership, and faculty shortages (AACN, 2006).

Having born witness to the rise and fall of the ND and DNSc degrees, a practice-oriented doctorate was not novel for nursing. However, of significance, the AACN-proposed DNP would impact broadly the scope of advanced nursing practice, and the AACN Position Statement on the Practice Doctorate in Nursing (AACN, 2004) was foundational in defining it as:

> nursing interventions that influence health care outcomes for individuals or populations, including the direct care of individual patients, management of care for individuals and populations, administration of nursing and health care organizations, and the development and implementation of health policy. Preparation at the practice doctorate level includes advanced preparation in nursing, based on nursing science, and is at the highest level of nursing practice.

Given the divergence from direct clinical care in scope, framing the DNP as a "clinical doctorate" is a misnomer. Reflecting upon this broad definition, the DNP-prepared nurse is either an APN with specialization in direct patient care, or a nurse with a specialized focus in administration, health care policy, informatics, or population-based care who is engaged in practice at an aggregate, systems, or organizational level (AACN, 2006). This move by the AACN to ensure the inclusion and doctoral preparation of nurses engaged in "nondirect care" roles under the rubric of advanced nursing practice thoughtfully ensures the migration of these roles toward a formalized plan of education. The aforementioned strategizes to develop the transformational leaders needed to respond to an evolving health care crisis, assuming greater responsibility for patient and organizational outcomes. Such a move is not merely good for patients but further positions the larger body of nursing professionals toward better representation with respect to ongoing national health care–related discussions and, further, to be responsive to evolving health care needs. With consideration of the diverse roles that nurses engaged in advanced practice assume, DNP curricula are designed to meet both foundational competencies considered core to engaging in advanced nursing practice, as well as specialty content (AACN, 2006).

While nursing continues to ruminate around the very basics, including standardizing education requirements for entry-level practice, the IOM (2011), recognizing the complexity of the current health care environment, issued a report entitled *The Future of Nursing: Leading Change, Advancing Health*. This landmark piece of work, funded by the Robert Wood Johnson Foundation, offers strong recommendations with implications for nursing practice at all levels. Significant attention has been paid to the need to reconceptualize existing nursing roles, innovate, attract and retain new nurses, and increase the numbers of nursing faculty. Recognizing a need to strategize to develop and retain nursing faculty, the IOM (2011) issued a call to double the number of nurses with a doctoral degree by 2020. Alarmingly, this call to action was issued at a time when the AACN (2011) has acknowledged that in 2010, more than 1,200 qualified doctoral applicants were denied entry into programs. The aforementioned was largely attributed to the faculty shortage. If nursing is to succeed in preparing greater numbers of nurses at the doctoral level, there is no question that preparing DNPs will be essential to the successful attainment of such a goal.

■ SUMMARY

The DNP-prepared nurse is a nurse of the future, positioned to deliver evidence-based direct care, manage systems and lead quality initiatives, integrate technology into care delivery systems and models, and further impact organizations and policy at the highest levels—all critical to transforming our broken health care system and ensuring the health of the nation. Such a demand for advanced education is likely to contribute to the evolution of nursing roles as it challenges both the master's degree as the cornerstone of nursing specialty education and the traditional outcomes of doctoral education, where clinical research has historically been the hallmark.

The second decade of the twenty-first century shepherded in a new era of health care policy and debate. The passage of the Patient Protection and Affordable Health Act catapults nurses, particularly advanced practice nurses, into a new prominence in health care. As advanced practice nurses seek to expand practice into a variety of settings and secure reimbursement for their services, they must be prepared to demonstrate effective outcomes of care (Newhouse et al., 2011). The DNP, with the emphasis on practice-based research, supports the attainment of a higher level of accountability in health care (Florczak, 2010). The future of advanced nursing practice rests on a rich and complex history of nursing practice. The DNP presents an opportunity to renegotiate and legitimize the APRN role in the evolving health care system. With this opportunity comes the challenge to hold onto our values and to transcend the age of intra- and interprofessional politics to participate fully in the health care system change.

## ■ REFERENCES

AANA. (n.d). *Timeline of AANA history, pre AANA.* Retrieved March 29, 2012, from http://www. aana.com/resources2/archives-library/Pages/Timeline-of-AANA-History,-Pre-AANA.aspx

Abbott, A. (1988). *A system of professions, An essay on the division of expert labor.* Chicago, IL: University of Chicago Press.

Alexander, C. C. (1997). The nurse executive in the 21st century: How do we prepare? *Nursing Administration Quarterly, 22,* 76–82.

Allen, D. (1997). The nursing–medical boundary: A negotiated order. *Sociology of Health and Illness, 19,* 498–520.

American Association of Colleges of Nursing (AACN) (October 2004). *AACN position statement on the practice doctorate in nursing.* Retrieved July 10, 2011, from http://www.aacn.nche.edu/ dnp/pdf/DNP.pdf

American Association of Colleges of Nursing (AACN). (October 2006). *The essentials of doctoral education for advanced nursing practice.* Retrieved July 10, 2011, from http://www.aacn.nche. edu/dnp/pdf/essentials.pdf

American Association of Colleges of Nursing (AACN). (2011). 2011 Annual report: *Shaping the future of nursing education.* Retrieved April 11, 2012, from http://www.aacn.nche.edu/aacn-publications/annual-reports/AR2011.pdf

American Nurses Association (ANA) Congress for Nursing Practice. (1974). *Definition: Nurse practitioner, nurse clinician and clinical nurse specialist.* Kansas City, MO: American Nurses Association Practice.

American Nurse Credentialing Center (ANCC) (April 24, 2008). *ANCC updates nursing administration certifications and credentials.* Retrieved August 12, 2011, from http://nursecredentialing. org/Documents/Certification/Articles/NurseExecAnnouncement.aspx

American Nurses Association (ANA). (2009). *Nursing administration: Scope and standards of practice.* Silver Spring, MD: Nursesbooks.org.

Andrews, P., Yankauer, A., & Connelly, Y. (1970). Changing the patterns of ambulatory pediatric caretaking: An action-oriented training program for nurses. *American Journal of Public Health, 60,* 870–879.

Andrist, L., Nicholas, P., & Wolf, K. A. (2006). *A history of nursing ideas.* Sudbury, MA: Jones & Bartlett.

Ashley, J. A. (1976). *Hospital, paternalism and the role of the nurse.* New York, NY: Teachers College Press.

Beck, D. M. (2006). Nightingale's passion for advocacy: Local to global. In L. Andrist, P. Nicholas, & K. Wolf (Eds.), *A history of nursing ideas* (pp. 473–487). Sudbury, MA: Jones & Bartlett.

Bekemeier, B. & Butterfield, P. (2005). Unreconciled inconsistencies: A critical review of the concept of social justice in 3 national nursing documents. *Advances in Nursing Science, 28,* 152–162.

Brodsky, P. (2008). Where have all the midwives gone? *Journal of Perinatal Education, 17,* 48–51.

Centers for Disease Control (CDC) and Prevention & the Merck Company Foundation (2007). *The state of aging and health in America.* Retrieved August 28, 2011, from http://www.cdc. gov/Aging/pdf/saha_2007.pdf

Christman, L. (1968). The nurse clinical specialist. *Hospital Progress, 49,* 14–16.

Dawley, K. (2001). Ideology and self-interest, nursing, medicine and the elimination of the nurse-midwife. *Nursing History Review, 9,* 99–126.

Dossey, B. M., Selanders, L., Beck, D. M., & Atwell, A. (2005). *Florence Nightingale today: Healing leadership and global action.* Silver Spring, MD: Nursebooks.org.

Drevdahl, D. (2002). Social justice or market justice? The paradoxes of public health partnerships with managed care. *Public Health Nursing, 19,* 161–169.

Epstein, L. (1990). The outcomes movement- will it get us where we want to go? *New England Journal of Medicine, 323*(4): 266–270.

Fairman, J. (2008). *Making room in the clinic, nurse practitioners and the evolution of modern health care.* Piscataway, NJ: Rutgers University Press.

Florczak, K. (2010). Research and the doctor of nursing practice: A cause for consternation. *Nursing Science Quarterly, 23,* 13–17.

Galloway, D. H. (May 29, 1899). The anesthetizer as a specialist. *The Philadelphia Medical Journal,* 1173.

Guenther, J. T. (2006). Mapping the literature of nursing informatics. *Journal of the Medical Library Association, 94,* E-92–E-98.

Harris, N. & Hunzikar-Dean, J. (2001). The art of open-drop ether. *Nursing History Review, 9,* 159–184.

Hamric, A., Spross, J., & Hanson, C. (2005). *Advanced practice nursing* (3rd ed.). Philadelphia, PA: Elsevier/Saunders.

Hines, D. C. (1994). The intersection of race, class and gender in the nursing profession. In *Critical issues in American nursing profession in the twentieth century: Perspective and case studies.* New York, NY: Foundation of the New York State Nurses Association, Inc.

Hudspeth, R. (2011). Changes for the valuable clinical nurse specialist: A regulatory conundrum. *Nursing Administration Quarterly, 35,* 282–284.

Institute of Medicine (IOM). (2001). *Crossing the quality chasm.* Washington, DC: National Academies Press.

Institute of Medicine (IOM). (2011). *The future of nursing: Leading change, advancing health.* Washington, DC: U.S. Government Printing Office.

Jenkins, M. (2006). Nursing centers and the autonomy of nursing work. In L. Andrist, P. Nicholas, & K. Wolf, *A history of nursing ideas* (pp. 319–332). Sudbury, MA: Jones & Bartlett.

Jencks, S. F., Williams, M. V., & Coleman, E. A. (2009). Rehospitalizations among patients in the Medicare fee-for-service program. *The New England Journal of Medicine, 360,* 1418–1428.

Johnson, T. D. (2007). *Census bureau: Number of U.S. uninsured rises to 47 million Americans are uninsured: Almost 5 percent increase since 2005.* Retrieved August 12, 2011, from http://www.medscape.com/viewarticle/567737

Keeling, A. (2007). *Nursing and the privilege of prescription 1893–2000.* Columbus, OH: Ohio State University Press.

Khoury, C., Blizzard, R., Wright Moore, L., Hassmiller, S. (2011). Nursing leadership from bedside to boardroom: A Gallup National Survey of Opinion Leaders. *Journal of Nursing Administration, 41* (7/8), 299–305.

Kohn, L. T., Corrigan, J. J., & Donaldson, M. S. (Eds.). (2000). *To err is human: Building a safer health system.* Washington, DC: National Academy of Sciences.

Lyon, B. (2000). Enhancing the public's access to CNS services: Model statutory and regulatory language for CNS practice. *Clinical Nurse Specialist, 14,* 156–157.

Magaw, A. (1900). Observations on 1092 cases of anesthesia from January 1, 1989 to January 1, 1900. *St. Paul Medical Journal, 2,* 306–311.

Mundinger, M. (2008, May). *Growing role of nurse practitioners.* Retrieved August 12, 2011, from http://www.lifeupenn.org/Growing%20role%20of%20nurse%20practitioners.pdf

National Association of Clinical Nurse Specialists (NACNS). (2010a). Clinical nurse specialists–practitioner contributing to primary care: A briefing paper. *Clinical Nurse Specialist, 24,* 271–272.

National Association of Clinical Nurse Specialists (NACNS). (2010b). *Organizing framework and core competencies.* Retrieved from http://nacns.org/LinkClick.aspx?fileticket=22R8AaNmrU I%3d&tabid=139

National Association of Clinical Nurse Specialists. (2004). *Statement on clinical nurse specialist practice and education* (2nd ed.). Harrisburg, PA: National Association of Clinical Nurse Specialists.

National Council of the State Boards of Nursing (NCSBN). (2011). *Campaign for APRN Consensus.* Retrieved August 21, 2011, from https://www.ncsbn.org/aprn.htm#definition

National Council of the State Boards of Nursing Consensus Model for APRN Regulation. (2008). Retrieved August 11, 2011, from https://www.ncsbn.org/Consensus_Model_for_APRN_Regulation_July_2008.pdf

Norris, D. M. (1977). One perspective on the nurse practitioner movement. In A. Jacox & D. Norris (Eds.), *Organizing for independent nursing practice* (pp. 21–33). New York, NY: Appleton-Century-Crofts.

Newhouse, R., Stanik-Jutt, J., White, K., Johantgen, M., Bass, E., Zangaro, G., et al. (2011). Advanced practice nurse outcomes 1990–2008: A systematic review. *Nursing Economics, 29,* 1–21.

Peplau, H. E. (1965). Specialization in professional nursing. *Nursing Science, 3,* 268–287.

Rafferty, A. M., & Wall, R. (2010). An icon for today and iconoclast for today. In S. Nelson & A. M. Rafferty, *Notes on Nightingale, the influence and legacy of a nursing icon* (pp. 130–143). Ithaca, NY: Cornell University Press.

Reiter, F. (1966). The nurse-clinician. *American Journal of Nursing, 66*(2), 274–280.

Reverby, S. (1987). *Ordered to care: The dilemma of American nursing, 1850–1985.* New York, NY: Cambridge University Press.

Reihl, J., & McVay, J. (1973). *The clinical nurse specialist: Interpretations.* Appleton, WI: Century Crofts.

Rooks, J. (1997). *Midwifery and childbirth in America.* Philadelphia, PA: Temple University Press.

Rooks, J., Ernst, E., Norsigian, J., & Guran, L. (2008). Marginalization of midwives in the United States: New responses to an old story. *Birth Issues in Perinatal Care, 35,* 158–161.

Safreit, B. J. (1992). Health care dollars and regulatory sense: The role of advance practice nursing. *Yale Journal of Regulation, 9,* 417–477.

Sandelowski, M. (2000). The physician's eyes: American nursing and the diagnostic revolution in medicine. *Nursing History Review, 8,* 2–38.

Schwartz, M. D., Basco, W. T., Grey, M. R., Elmore, J. G., & Rubenstein, A. (2005). Rekindling student interest in generalist careers. *Annals of Internal Medicine, 142,* 715–724.

Sinclair, M. (2010). Moving midwifery research forward in the revolutionary information and high-tech era. *Evidence Based Midwifery, 8,* 111.

Sparacino, P. (2005). The clinical nurse specialist. In A. Hamric, J. Spross, & C. Hanson, *Advanced practice nursing: An integrative approach* (pp. 414–446). Philadelphia, PA: Saunders.

Staggers, N. (2002). The evolution of definitions for nursing informatics: A critical analysis and revised definition. *Journal of the American Medical Informatics Association, 9,* 255–261.

Tietze, M. (August 2008). *Nursing informatics: What's it all about?* Retrieved August 12, 2011, from http://www.uta.edu/ced/static/onlinecne/CEAugust08.pdf

U.S. Census Bureau. (2011). *Highlights: 2010.* Retrieved April 11, 2011, from http://www.census.gov/hhes/www/hlthins/data/incpovhlth/2010/highlights.html

Varney, H., Kriebs, J. M., & Gegor, J. M. (2004). *Varney's midwifery* (4th ed.). Sudbury, MA: Jones & Bartlett.

Wertz, R. & Wertz, D. (1977). *Lying in: A history of childbirth in America.* New York, NY: Free Press.

Wolf, K. (2006). The slow march to professional practice. In L. Andrist, P. Nicolas, & K. Wolf (Eds.), *A history of nursing ideas* (pp. 305–318). Boston, MA: Jones & Bartlett.

Wildman, S., & Hewiston, A. (2009). Rediscovering a history of nursing management: From Nightingale to the modern matron. *International Journal of Nursing Studies, 46*(12), 1650–1661.

# CHAPTER 2

# Could the DNP Be the "Future" in the Future of Nursing (2011) Report?

Ann H. Cary

Imagination blended with opportunity leads to highly effective innovations in society. No one can dispute that there are ample opportunities for the profession of nursing to lead innovation in health care during this second decade of the twenty-first century. Nurses must be willing strategists, committed to harnessing their intellectual and political capital toward the creation of the next-generation delivery systems. The largest discipline in health care, over 3 million U.S. nurses are capable of harnessing their political advocacy, leadership, and human capital efforts toward an efficacious and just delivery system. Nurses provide an essential and strategic force for change. The U.S. health care system continues to demonstrate a voracious appetite for amassing an increasing share of the gross domestic product, entitlement of government programs, and personal budgets. It is oxymoronic that while consuming greater costs, U.S. health care rankings globally are only moderate, access to care is not politically funded as a "individual right," quality remains uneven and slow to be adopted, and sustainability is doubtful.

The perfect storm for serious change in U.S. health care and the mandate for nurses to create innovative systems, financing, and practice models have been placed at the foot of the profession by the Institute for Medicine (IOM) and the Robert Wood Johnson Foundation (RWJF) in The Future of Nursing: Leading Change, Advancing Health (2011), http://www.IOM.edu/reports/2010/The-Future-of-Nursing-Leading-Change-Advancing-Health.aspx. The IOM was founded to convene experts and use science to discuss, debate, and examine possible solutions to real issues in health care (Fineberg, 2011). In addition, RWJF is investing $20 million with the American Association of Retired Persons (AARP) to establish the Center to Champion Nursing in America by stimulating real change for and by the nursing profession, which can maximize the impact of the IOM report. This chapter will describe the overall recommendations from the IOM and assert that nurses prepared with the doctor of nursing practice (DNP) degree have a critical mandate to create, translate, evaluate, and advocate for innovations in the new health care system.

Knowing is not enough; we must apply. Willing is not enough, we must do

Goethe (IOM, 2011)

## ■ MANDATE FOR CHANGE: PRELUDE TO REDESIGNING HEALTH CARE IMPACT

Four key messages frame the eight recommendations in the Future of Nursing (2011) to the public:

- Nurses should practice to the full extent of their education and training.
- Nurses should achieve higher levels of education and training through improved educational systems that promote seamless academic progression.
- Nurses should be full partners with other health professionals in redesigning health care in the United States.
- Effective workforce planning and policy require better data collection and an improved information infrastructure. (IOM, 2010, 2011, p. 4)

An intriguing dimension of these key messages is that while addressing nursing specifically there is explicit recognition of the interdependent, adjuvant, and systemic changes among all providers and policymakers to assure any successful health care transformation. The DNP provider and the national guidelines (AACN, 2006) for DNP programs are critical in assuring that DNPs and their impact on systems reflect knowledge of the science and practice of systems thinking and application in real-world venues. Strategy, leadership, teamwork, policy competencies, and informatics knowledge and translation, implementation, and evaluation science are minimal requisites for the DNP provider to successfully innovate all of the components of a redesigned health care system. Education, practice, workforce data modeling and surveillance, policy, and effective, intentional interprofessional teamwork preparation and practice are domains of action embedded in these messages. Described below are some of the issues that undergird the key messages by the IOM (2011).

### Full Practice to the Limits of Credentials, Training, and Education

State-specific regulatory models for advanced practice registered nurse (APRN) practice have created a barrier to the ability of DNPs to practice to the full extent of preparation. Disciplinary "guilds" assure that economic redistribution of income potential among interprofessional providers is prevented to maintain adequate levels of expected disciplinary standards of living. Organizations, payers, and insurers maintain policies that may prevent the DNP provider from being credentialed or privileged as well as set reimbursement rules for direct or "incident to" reimbursement. In the majority of cases, the entity that pays the provider decides how they will value the DNP provider, even though the DNP may have outcomes that are equal to or better than another provider. In fact, Newhouse and her coworkers published a systematic review of the literature on whether nurse practitioners and certified midwives who worked collaboratively with physicians had patient outcomes similar to physicians working without advanced practice nurses (APNs). Their review encompassed 18 years of literature and they found that outcomes were similar and sometimes better, depending on the patient population and setting (Newhouse et al., 2011).

Institutional policies limit nurses at both the bedside and in the boardroom. However, barriers to full practice are not limited to nurse providers (DNPs or PhDs) with the highest credentials. All members of the health care team who are credentialed also work in organizations that place boundaries around their unique and overlapping practice abilities. This is achieved through institutional policies that guide actual "institutional" scopes of practice and memberships on key policy boards such as medical privileging committees and boards of directors. Few organizations have evaluated frameworks in which the work of providers at the lowest-paid level are matched to their competency to perform work based on training and education, from community worker and health coach to bedside nurse, DNP, and physician.

## Seamless Academic Progression to Assure Higher Educational Preparation Within the Discipline

The fault line within nursing between levels of preparation for entry into practice at one end and the debate about the PhD versus DNP as an appropriate academic and practice scholar at the other end fractures the ability of nurses to speak with one voice in their role as a full partner in the future of health care. In an RWJF 2010 Gallup poll, opinion leaders ranked doctors and nurses first and second in providing trusted information, but noted that nurses who had relatively weak influence on increasing access to care were not perceived as important decision players or revenue assets and did not speak with one voice on national issues. However, these same opinion leaders suggested that nurses should demonstrate more leadership and higher expectations (RWJF, 2010). The same registered nurse (RN) licensure is provided for multiple routes of entry whereby eligibility relies on at least three degree/diploma pathways or only a graduate degree. In addition, nurses earn multiple "professional initials" as testimony to advanced practice or specialty designations and academic credentials. These are clearly not understood or differentiated by the public and, in many cases, within the profession.

While the Consensus Model for APRNs (2008) has been supported by all 50 states, implementation is slow as it winds through the state regulatory review processes. The majority of nurses (80%) who are educated for licensure at the associate-degree level do not seek higher educational preparation even if they eventually earn a BSN (Aiken, Cheung, & Olds, 2009) and, thus, are not eligible to provide higher levels of care to patients or amass the knowledge to generate or translate research/science on nursing or health care. Similarly, these nurses are not eligible to assume faculty positions to educate the next generation of nurses, nor are they able to sit equitably with highly educated peers to influence next-generation practices and policies. Various levels of nursing degree programs easily maintain themselves as silos in which the ability of the nurse to transition between levels is fraught with redundancy requirements and lengthy curriculums to satisfy perceived higher education requirements. It is likely that a nurse who earns an associate degree (AD) and then seeks a Bachelor of Science in Nursing (BSN) degree will spend much longer total time to achieve the BSN post–high school than to earn the BSN degree initially.

Our current nursing licensure/certification renewal process is often based on continuing education courses that do not demonstrate any evidence of additional learning or behavioral competency. Some states have no requirements for continuing education. Thus much of the skill development of nurses who decline to seek higher educational preparation is just-in-time or on-the-job training, which can vary tremendously by region and institution in terms of quality practice expectations. Lifelong learning, while providing lip service, is not a consistent expectation for high-value practice.

Access to progress in degree attainment is enhanced by the availability of distance and online educational programs. These provide convenient access from distance sites and flexibility in schedules to accommodate multiple commitments of the nurse and assure a more user-friendly path for educational advancement. The need to redesign educational pathways, articulation requirements, dual enrollment options, and entry to terminal degree pathways efficiently walks hand-in-hand with health care systems redesign.

The rate of knowledge explosion in health care and nursing demands that curriculum content reflect immediate advancements. Nursing education is constantly challenged to anticipate and teach the latest in science, practice, and technology to assure that students and graduates access knowledge rapidly for translation to patients and systems (Benner, Sutphen, Leonard, & Day, 2009). The DNP graduate has acquired such capabilities as a hallmark of his or her educational competencies and thus is an optimal clinical and theoretical teacher for all levels of students as they learn the process for rapid acquisition of specific knowledge, skills, and behaviors for improved competence.

## Full Partnership in Systems Redesign

Full partnerships necessarily imply equitable accountability for assuring the process and outcomes for systems design. All partners must come to the table with an exquisite capacity to negotiate and leverage their professional assets, communicate a vision, contribute resources, create and maintain energy, and provide influence, power, and stamina to achieve the desired redesign impact. The ability to work in collaborative and interprofessional groups will be critical to a successful effort.

Earlier reference was made to the Opinion Leaders survey results (RWJF, 2010), questioning the effectiveness of nurses to successfully influence change in our systems. However, interprofessional preparation and practice is fraught with uneven science outcomes across systems, as well as a disciplinary climate of "silo mentality," and in some cases, "imagined" boundaries of unique competencies and delayed care delivery due to team processes. Interprofessional teams as a fulcrum in the educational and provider culture appear to suffer from a lack of implementation leadership within systems of care for populations. Catalysts for selecting the power brokers in systems redesign have typically been achieved through the alignment of organizational consultants, health care administrators, chief financial officers, and medical committees. Recent evidence of the effectiveness of nursing leadership in redesign has been revealed in TCAB (transforming care at the bedside) projects, a national program that incentivizes nurses to lead process improvement for health and fiscal outcomes through small tests of change, rapid adoption, and improvement (Bolton & Aronow, 2009). Evaluations of systems that efficiently create, manage, and assure outcomes of interprofessional team structures, processes, and outcomes are emerging (e.g., the Department of Veterans Affairs [VA] system of organizing primary care providers into health teams and linking integrated information technology to teams and services; http://www1.va.gov/health/; Barr, 2002; Barr, Koppel, Reeves, Hammick, & Freeth, 2005; Reeves et al., 2008).

Systems redesign by nature requires the assessment of information flow, efficiency, and the ability of digitalization and health information technology (HIT) to improve quality of work, care, and system effectiveness. Health care is in the midst of a commitment to digital interoperability and digital workflow schemata to test and improve the impact. Nurse leaders must be engaged in the design and knowledgeable in the technologies and opportunities of application to support these HIT efforts if early success is to be achieved. Technology–digital workflow impacts how nurses and team members document, deliver, and review clinical care. Redesigned systems will incorporate computerized knowledge management and decision support that releases providers to address complex care and high-touch needs of patients not addressed by the technology. It also promotes the ability to provide many types of care without regard to location of the provider or the patient. Today, patient and population care is radically influenced by information technology and digitalization.

Research shows how it influences the increase or decrease in documentation requirements (Thompson, Johnston, & Spurr, 2009) and quality indicators (DesRoches, Donelan, Buerhaus, & Zhonghe, 2008; Waneka & Spetz, 2009), and it is improved by the participation of nurses in the design. The Patient Protection and Affordable Care Act (ACA) and Health Care and Education Affordability Reconciliation Act (2010) contains incentives to assure the "meaningful use" of HIT by providers to improve patient care and to add to the aggregate picture of quality clinical care nationally. The DNP, having been educated in systems, informatics, and leadership, is well-positioned to advance the concept of digital redesign within the redesign team.

In 2011, the Interprofessional Education Collaborative (IPEC) Expert Panel published a vision and explicated competencies of interprofessional collaborative practice as essential to safe, high quality, accessible, patient-centered care. Building on the concept of interprofessionality as a process to develop practice, the panel adopted the definition of D'Amour and Oandasan to describe it:

> the process by which professionals reflect on and develop ways of practicing that provide an integrated and cohesive answer to the needs of clients/family/population … involves continuous interaction and knowledge sharing between professionals, organized to solve or explore a variety of education and care issues, all while seeking to optimize the patient's participation … Interprofessional practice has unique characteristics in terms of values, codes of conduct, and ways of working.
>
> (D'Amour & Oandasan, 2005, p. 9)

Key challenges exist, however, to successfully operationalize full partnerships through interprofessional practices (IP) in a redesigned system (IPEC, 2011). These include the following:

- The support of top leadership to dismantle barriers to design, education, and practice within an interprofessional concept.
- Limited professional schools within an institution; the need for outreach agreements to embrace interinstitutional collaboratives to achieve interprofessional training.
- Scheduling issues for conflicting classes/clinicals among the professional schools.
- Faculty development training and practice to articulate and integrate new behaviors and attitudes about processes of engagement in interprofessional culture.
- Early stage development of assessment instruments and metrics to capture processes and outcomes of IP.
- Regulatory expectations of "learning together to work together" need to be developed to affirm the concept and commit to transformational changes in accreditation and certification of institutions and providers.

These issues can be solved through intentional solutions by all parties who value effective execution of health care delivery.

Exemplars of redesign efforts are amply described here from the IOM report (2011). Nurses are reminded that the ACA also provides additional opportunities to advance "disruptive innovation" strategies in an effort to change health care delivery and practice through the creation and funding of the new Center for Medicare and Medicaid Innovation (CMMI) within the Department of Health and Human Services (DHHS). Four current initiatives that are receiving expanded funding support include accountable care organizations (ACOs), the medical/health homes (MHHs), community health centers (CHCs), and nurse-managed health clinics (NMHCs). Each of these strategies needs to incorporate highly functioning interprofessional teams in which nurses are used as full partners in the design and operate to the full extent of their education and training. Interprofessional research teams are critical to assure that the production will incorporate nurse-sensitive indicators as well as collaborative indicators.

ACOs are structured around the coordination of primary care providers (including APRNs), hospitals, and some specialists. Payment models may include shared savings or capitated payments, and move well beyond the traditional fee for service, which encourages more service, redundancy, and costs. The goals of the ACO are to improve quality, contain growth and costs, and improve coordination of care (IOM, 2011; Exhibit 2.1).

MHHs are not a new concept, originally created by pediatricians in the 1960s. The ACA indicates that the interprofessional teams that include physicians, nurses, and other health professionals should support these structures. This particular type of primary care coordinates and provides comprehensive services, strengthens the relationship between provider and patient/family, and measures and monitors quality. As the IOM notes, the language in the ACA uses the terms medical/health sometimes interchangeably, allowing the interpretation by funders to exclude APRNs at will. The VA system uses this concept (primary care medical home) and has expanded it to include staff nurses who function as care managers and coordinators, provide health risk appraisals, as well as promotion and disease prevention. Other terms for this model include patient-centered medical or health home (IOM, 2011; Exhibit 2.2).

CHCs have a proven record of providing high value primary and preventive care for the underserved and have been allocated additional funds (in the billions) through ACA (IOM, 2011). CHCs offer comprehensive services for dental, mental, and behavioral health as well as access to pharmacies. Nurses have traditionally played a central role on the team, as APRN primary care providers and in outreach and home care services. Outcome indicators show that CHC patients have fewer unmet needs, underutilize emergency department services, avoid hospitalizations, and have lower medical costs (NACHC, the Robert Graham Center and Capital Link, 2007; Exhibit 2.3).

NMHCs have existed since the 1960s to serve Medicare and Medicaid recipients, the uninsured, and children in communities across the nation. Although run by nurses with APRNs providing primary care, NMHCs employ an array of health care providers including physicians, health educators, social workers, and outreach workers using a collaborative team model. Services may include primary care, family planning, mental/behavioral health, prenatal care, health promotion, and disease prevention (IOM, 2011). A major challenge for NMHCs is financial sustainability from patient revenues so that fiscal models employed in any redesign of a transformational health care system will dramatically impact the sustainability of a center. The ACA authorized $50 million to NMHCs funding in 2010 and additional sums as possible (NNCC, 2011).

---

### EXHIBIT 2.1
#### DNP Leadership in Accountable Care Organizations

---

With a sufficient number of DNP providers in each ACO, can you envision the articulation of practices, data and systems requirements, technology, regulatory reform, and teamwork required to be successful in this environment?

---

**EXHIBIT 2.2**

**DNP Leadership in Medical/Health Homes**

- With a sufficient number of DNP providers in each MHH, can you envision your role, function, and effectiveness in planning the model, measuring the processes and outcomes, adjusting the system components for improvement, and disseminating the results for replication?

- Can you imagine the information technology needs, the training for interprofessional high-level functioning, and the cost and quality metrics that can inform replication and dissemination?

- How will your participation provide the value-added component to this model in terms of substitution and expansion of provider roles?

- What will it take for DNPs to demonstrate leadership and a successful outcome for sustainable regulatory reform?

---

**EXHIBIT 2.3**

**DNP Leadership in Community Health Centers**

- With a sufficient number of DNP providers in each CHC, can you envision an expanded role for DNPs?

- What new skills do DNPs add to CHCs due to the education and training received in the DNP program?

- What disruptive innovations do you imagine could be provided to make the impact of CHCs on the community's health even more dramatic?

- What are the expanded metrics required to capture the impact of CHC care on the populations they serve?

---

The national nursing centers consortium (NNCC, 2011) explicates the reasons nurse-managed centers are successful in patient care as follows:

- As a neighborhood initiative, they understand patient and community needs and earn their trust.
- NMHCs strive to identify and coordinate the social services that are essential to maintain all avenues of health support.
- By bringing care to the "people," NMHCs build community capacity in areas such as safety and violence abatement, after-school programs, and community advocacy.

Outcomes for improved patient care at lower costs in NMHCs give this model another dimension of credibility to funders. Regulatory and other disciplinary support will be needed to advance this model. Clearly, national incentives through grants, demonstration projects, and other mechanisms will be key to assure innovative projects by nurses, in interprofessional teams, and through strategic and thoughtful leadership (Exhibit 2.4).

---

**EXHIBIT 2.4**

**DNP Leadership in Nurse-Managed Health Centers**

---

- With a sufficient number of DNP providers in each NMHC, can you envision an expanded role for DNPs?

- What new skills do DNPs add to NMHCs due to the education and training received in the DNP program?

- What disruptive innovations do you imagine could be provided to make the impact of NMHCs on the community's health even more dramatic?

- What are the expanded metrics needed to capture the impact of NMHC care on the populations they serve?

### Better Workforce Policy Influence Through Improved Information Infrastructure

Health professions workforce data are critical to forecasting, planning, and resourcing the right mix, distribution, and competencies needed by a transformed health care system. Systematic and timely collection of data and new models of provider mix to supply efficacious and cost-effective care to more patients in the new era of health care are essential to its success. For example, national data indicate that 50 million people were uninsured in 2009, an increase of 4.3 million people (Kaiser Family Foundation, 2010). Workforce data provide the early warning mechanism for this "tsunami" of patients likely to overwhelm current achievements in quality, not to mention improvements that are at risk for failing in an overwhelmed system. While past efforts in workforce surveillance have yielded various modeling approaches, the science is far from precise. Often, adjustments in assumptions are later discovered to mediate the implications of the data for programming and workforce policy decisions. While the need for primary care providers is forecasted, political will of self-interests among disciplines, new educational programs (DNP), and politicians mediate the ability of workforce models to redesign sufficient incentives to meet the needs of populations needing primary care. The evidence that primary care can be provided by nonphysician APRN providers with equal or better outcomes for patients appear to get lost in the modeling assumptions. The impact by the DNP workforce on care and systems redesign is not yet evident since these providers are a relatively new entry to the health care system, although anecdotal examples exist. The disconnect between what is, what should be, and what will be is often traced to political "spin" on data as well as too many data variations and analysis options.

A balance of providers to impact the vision of the redesigned health care system must be achieved with careful attention to improved modeling for supply. The critical elements in such a system are included in Exhibit 2.5.

Demand can be created to match the supply, which can either harm or help the redesign impact.

The three key areas explicated for workforce data across the health professions in the IOM (2011, p. 261) report include the following:

*(1)* Core data sets on health care workforce supply and demand
*(2)* Surveillance of workforce market conditions
*(3)* Health care workforce effectiveness research

---

**EXHIBIT 2.5**

**Critical Elements in a Redesigned Health Care System**

The necessary shift to ambulatory care

Telehealth

Information technology

Prioritization of health care resource consumption among an increasingly diverse patient population

Global market competition

Newly prepared evidence-based providers and teams

"Medicalization" of events in the life of a patient

---

Some of these areas are addressed in the ACA. Specifically, the law creates a National Health Workforce Commission (NHWC) to "develop and evaluate training activities to determine whether demand is being met, identify barriers to improved coordination at federal, state and local levels and recommend solutions" (p. 256). It also supports the National Center for Workforce Analysis (NWC) as well as state and regional centers for improved data collection and analysis.

Finally, it is pertinent to recognize that a severe shortage of faculty, forecasted between 5,000 and 5,500 instructional faculty during the next 15 years, looms on the horizon as the demand for educating health professions and nursing providers is realized (Kovner, Fairchild, & Jacobson, 2006). Educational systems must ready their resources today to be able to meet the production cycle of preparing new faculty for tomorrow. Creative models of faculty sharing, rapid preparation, and partnerships with the business community in strategic planning and execution will all be "on the table" as partial solutions.

Regulatory issues emerge when attempting to innovate in any of the key areas or to implement any of the recommendations noted below. Disruptive innovation is just that; it questions and repositions all assumptions that maintain the current system. Transformational health care will require regulatory experimentation and timely responses. For each of the four key areas, successful solutions are at the mercy of regulatory and policy reforms. DNP graduates must always be thoughtful and action-oriented toward the policy and regulatory dimensions necessary to assure any redesign change is executed. By committing to be thoughtful strategists, the likelihood of success is greatly improved.

■ **EIGHT RECOMMENDATIONS FOR TRANSFORMATION OF THE FUTURE OF NURSING (IOM, 2011, PP. 9–15)**

The eight recommendations published by the IOM are repeated below, practically verbatim, to preserve the consensus of the IOM committee for the reader.

### 1. Remove scope of practice barriers

APRNs should be able to practice to the full extent of education and training. This will be possible with federal recognition by the Centers for Medicare & Medicaid Services, Office of Policy and Management; federal reimbursement models for APRN parity; institutional participation, which assures APRNs are eligible for credentialing and privileging; and state scopes of practice, which conform to National Council of State Boards Model act. The Federal Trade Commission and the Antitrust Division of the Department of Justice should review existing and proposed state regulations for needless anticompetitive effects.

### 2. Expand opportunities for nurses to lead and diffuse collaborative improvement efforts

Private and public funders, health care organizations (HCOs), nursing education programs, and nursing associations should expand opportunities for nurses to lead and manage collaborative efforts with interprofessional health care team members to conduct research and redesign and improve practice environments and health systems. Nurses must diffuse successful practices and identify administrative waste and redundancies to improve efficiencies. Nurses should be part of medical device and HIT design and evaluation teams. Nurses are capable of using their experiences to design entrepreneurial care systems.

### 3. Implement nurse residency programs

State boards of nursing, accrediting bodies, the federal government, and HCOs should take actions that support nurses' completion of a transition-to-practice nurse residency program after they have completed a prelicensure or APRN degree program or when they transition to a new clinical practice area. Policymakers should redirect the Graduate Medical Education funding from diploma programs to support BSN and nurse residency programs.

### 4. Increase the proportion of nurses with baccalaureate degrees to 80% by 2020

Academic nurse leaders should work together to increase the proportion of nurses with baccalaureate degrees from 50% to 80%. Higher education should partner with accrediting bodies, private and public funders, and employers to ensure funding, monitor progress, and increase diversity of students. The workforce must be prepared to meet the demands of diverse populations across the lifespan. Education and training with interprofessional students and teams should be done early in the educational process to affirm the culture of team practice.

### 5. Double the number of nurses with doctorates by 2020

Schools of nursing, with support from private and public funders, academic administrators, university trustees, and accrediting bodies should double the number of nurses with a doctorate to add to the cadre of nurse faculty, practitioners, and researchers. Attention should be directed to increasing diversity. Policymakers should monitor the progression of entry nurses through masters and doctoral programs and incentivize rapid and efficient matriculation. Higher education must create compensation packages to reward recruitment and retention of highly educated nurse faculty who are responsible to create and deliver the next generation of educational innovations in nursing.

### 6. Ensure that nurses engage in lifelong learning

Accrediting bodies, schools of nursing, HCOs, and continuing competency educators from multiple health professions should collaborate to ensure that nurses, nursing students, and faculty continue their education to engage in lifelong learning. Competencies need to be refined to provide care for diverse populations across the life span. Special attention to the inclusion of interprofessional competency development in integrated disciplinary learning teams within delivery systems is key to ensuring sustainable performance and improved quality improvements.

**7. Prepare and enable nurses to lead change to advance health**

Nurses, nursing education programs, and nursing associations should prepare nurses for leadership at all levels in health care. Private and governmental health care decision makers should ensure that leadership positions are available and filled by nurses. Nurses should receive priority for inclusion on boards, executive teams, and other key leadership areas commensurate with their competencies. Leadership development must recognize the power of interprofessional development with others in the business and health care enterprise.

**8. Build an infrastructure for the collection and analysis of interprofessional health care workforce data**

The National Health Care Workforce Commission, with oversight from the Government Accountability Office and the Health Resources and Services Administration (HRSA) should lead a collaborative effort to improve research and collection and analysis of data on health care workforce requirements. The Workforce Commission and HRSA should collaborate with state licensing boards, state nursing workforce centers, and the Department of Labor in this effort to ensure that the data are timely and publicly accessible.

It is worthwhile to read the details in the IOM Future of Nursing report in its entirety as it is composed of rich and solid research from which these timely recommendations emerge. The report challenges the responsibility and the accountability of the nursing profession to unify its position on policy, education, practice, leadership, and research to build logical propositions and articulate solid leverage points for transformational change in health care today. It seeks allies and collaborators outside of nursing who commit to create the larger pie of health care access, quality, and value rather than continue the downward spiral by positioning for the size of the piece for each provider. Patients and population health lose ground in the current politics of fragmented financing, education, and delivery systems.

## ■ COULD THE DNP BE THE FUTURE OF NURSING AND HEALTH CARE?

For many reasons, the answer is YES!

- The AACN (2006) eight essentials document referenced to prepare nurses with the DNP clearly articulates the areas of competence expected by DNP graduates. In doing so, it unifies and standardizes expectations for systems and advanced practice knowledge so that DNPs will translate science rapidly to improve health care delivery, policy, and leadership impact. Curriculum should be producing "big picture" change agents who are capable of testing disruptive innovations in systems and with populations, understanding replication implications, and rapidly disseminating these to other researchers, policymakers, and interested parties.
- The DNP has a vital "stake in the game" for regulatory reform within advanced practice, among other disciplinary regulations that impinge on full scope of practice, and within institutions and systems in which they practice. Leading the way in all of these areas in a coordinated manner will be critical to open the window of policy reform necessary to execute transformational systems for health care.
- DNPs should be facile with information and knowledge to advance translation and implementation science as they redesign practice and systems. Traditional practices cannot be used as leverage against evidence-based practices if the DNP is to adhere to the ethical mandate of beneficence. All patients deserve a right to high-value

health care and systems deserve the right to expect high-performing providers. The DNP provider is mandated to bring expertise equitably to the patient, the institution, the system, policymakers, and team members.

- Key evidence gaps are identified below by the IOM (2011, pp. 274–277) to transform practice, education, and leadership—for which the DNP can make substantive contributions to study and execute:

1. Studying personal and professional characteristics, knowledge, and skills most important to leaders of redesigned organizations and quality initiatives, including ACOs, MHHs, CHCs, NMHCs, and other innovative delivery systems.
2. Identifying spheres of influence used by nurses in health care decision making and on boards and health care committees at a variety of levels.
3. Identifying mentoring and coaching characteristics most successful in recruiting, retaining, and promoting optimal performance in interprofessional teams, individual providers, and within an array of institutions.
4. Examining how alternative faculty/student ratios affect the acquisition of competence and student retention as well as the impact of distance technologies and simulation to expand capacity for educating a more highly competent nurse at every level and setting.
5. Identifying faculty, staff, environmental, and organizational characteristics that best support a diverse nurse population to successfully pursue and complete BSN, graduate, and doctoral degrees.
6. Testing new models of nursing education and residency options incorporating Benner et al.'s (2009) characteristics, interprofessional paradigms, continuing competence for lifelong learning, technology efficiencies, and benefit structures for attracting highly qualified nurses to faculty roles.
7. Comparing programs, providers, provider teams, and health exchange models on costs, quality, access, and impact of current and innovative delivery models.
8. Identifying and evaluating decision support technologies on care delivery, high-value performance, quality, provider satisfaction, and rapid dissemination of science to the bedside and articulating measures of "meaningful use" of HIT to nurses and the team.
9. Examining trends and the impact of innovations and incubators of redesign in which "concept to execution processes" are tested for efficacy, policy impact, human capital requirements, and community sustainability.
10. Testing the characteristics of translation research that improve uptake and sustainability for diverse communities, organizations, providers, financiers, and policymakers.

- DNP and PhD providers can demonstrate the power of collaboration from the scientist and the executer "team" approach as they iteratively discover, test, refine, and evaluate bench and applied evidence in current and emergent care systems. Program planning and evaluation capabilities are strengthened with systematic approaches that yield both qualitative and quantitative outcomes.

The "future" of nursing is a future of possibilities, imagination, leadership, radical incentives, and new paradigms. It cannot be created by using the same patterns of thinking and expectations that maintain the currently fragmented and fractured health delivery system. Patients deserve a system that promotes health and access to high value care options. High value care options can only be borne by limitations on self interests, a willingness to risk new ventures, highly educated provider teams composed of diverse and flexibly skilled personnel, and a market that tolerates social capital as part of the market advantage. To truly change our expectations that the U.S. health care system is "good enough," passionate providers, politicians, markets, and communities must demand better and be willing to leverage a spirit of adventure combined with applied science. DNP leaders must demonstrate courage, innovation, and adaptability to complexity while avoiding the noise of detractors who stand to lose when the status quo is dismantled. Developing this next chapter in the U.S. health care system is not for the faint of heart—indeed it will be made whole through the appropriate utilization of the DNP professional.

Aim high, aim for something that will make a difference.

(Drucker & Maciariello, 2006, p. 111)

## ■  ACKNOWLEDGMENTS

Partial support for creation of this chapter by the author was provided by funds from the Division of Nursing (DN), Bureau of Health Professions (BHPr), Health Resources and Services Administration (HRSA), Department of Health and Human Services (DHHS) to Loyola University New Orleans, School of Nursing under grant number D09HP18996–01-00, for the Post-Masters Doctor of Nursing Practice: Access to Comprehensive Care Systems for $1,213,924 for 2010 to 2013. The information or content and conclusions are those of the author and should not be construed as the official position or policy of, nor should any official endorsement be inferred by, the DN, BHPr, HRSA, DHHS, or the U.S. government.

## ■  REFERENCES

Aiken, L. H., Cheung, R. B., & Olds, D. M. (2009). Education policy initiatives to address the nurse shortage in the United States. *Health Affairs, 28,* w646–w656.

American Association of Colleges of Nursing (AACN). (2006). *Essentials of doctoral education for advanced practice nursing.* Washington, DC: AACN.

APRN Consensus Model. Retrieved August 1, 2011, from https://www.ncsbn.org/consensus_model_forAPRN_Regulation_July_2008.pdf

Barr, H. (2002). *Interprofessional education today, yesterday and tomorrow: A review.* London, England: LTSN Hs&P.

Barr, H., Koppel, I., Reeves, S., Hammick, M., & Freeth, D. (2005). *Effective interprofessional education: Argument, assumption and evidence.* Oxford, England: Blackwell Publishing.

Benner, P., Sutphen, M., Leonard, V., & Day, L. (2009). *Educating nurses: A call for radical transformation.* San Francisco, CA: Jossey-Bass.

Bolton, L., & Aronow, H. (2009). The business case for TCAB: Estimates of cost savings with sustained improvement. *American Journal of Nursing, 109,* 77–80.

D'Amour, D., & Oandasan, I. (2005). Interprofessionality as the field of interprofessional practice and interprofessional education: An emerging concept. *Journal of Interprofessional Care, 19,* 8–20.

DesRoches, C., Donelan, K., Buerhaus, P., & Zhonghe, L. (2008). Registered nurses' use of electronic health records: Findings from a national survey. *Medscape Journal of Medicine, 10,* 164.

Drucker, P. F., & Maciariello, J. A. (2006). *The effective executive in action: A journal for getting the right things done.* New York, NY: Harper Collins.

Fineberg, H. V. (2011). Foreword. In *Institute of Medicine, The future of nursing: Leading change, advancing health.* Washington, DC: The National Academies Press.

Institute of Medicine (IOM). (2011). *The future of nursing: Leading change, advancing health.* Washington, DC: The National Academies Press.

Institute of Medicine (IOM). (2010). *Report brief.* Washington, DC: The National Academies Press.

Interprofessional Education Collaborative Expert (IPEC) Panel. (2011). *Core competencies for interprofessional collaborative practice: Report of an expert panel.* Washington, DC: Interprofessional Education Collaborative.

Kaiser Family Foundation. (2010). *The uninsured: A primer.* Retrieved August 5, 2011, from http://www.kff.org/uninsured/upload/7451-06.pdf

Kovner, C. T., Fairchild, S., & Jacobson, L. (2006). *Nurse educators 2006: A report of the faculty census survey of RN and graduate programs.* Washington, DC: NLN.

NACHC, The Robert Graham Center and Capital Link. (2007). *Access granted: The primary care payoff.* Washington, DC: The Robert Graham Center, Capital Link.

National Nursing Centers Consortium (NNCC). (2011). *Who we are.* Retrieved August 1, 2011, from http://www.nncc.us/site/index.php/about-nurse-managed-care

Newhouse, R. P., Stanik-Hutt, J., White, K. M., Johantgen, M., Bass, E. B., Zangaro, G., et al. (2011). Advanced practice nurse outcomes 1990–2008: A systematic review. *Nursing Economics, 29*(5), 230–250.

Patient Protection and Affordable Care Act (ACA) (PL 111–148) and Health Care and Education Affordability Reconciliation Act (PL 111–52). (2010).

Reeves, S., Zwarenstein, M., Goldman, J., Barr, H., Freeth, D., Hammick, M., & Koppel, I. (2008). *Interprofessional education: Effects on professional practice and health care outcomes.* Cochrane Database of Systematic Reviews, (1), CD002213.

Robert Wood Johnson Foundation (RWJF). (2010). *Nursing leadership from bedside to boardroom: Opinion leaders' perceptions.* Retrieved August 1, 2011, from http://www.rwjf.org/pr/product

Thompson, D., Johnston, P., & Spurr, C. (2009). The impact of electronic medical records on nursing efficiency. *Journal of Nursing Administration, 39,* 444–451.

Waneka, R., & Spetz, J. (2009). *2007–2008 annual school report: Data summary and historical trend analysis.* Sacramento, CA: California Board of Registered Nurses.

# PART II

# *Scholarship and the DNP*

Doctors of nursing practice (DNP) degree programs prepare nurse leaders who will be instrumental in transforming the profession to meet the challenges of the burgeoning health care system of our nation. Clinical scholarship is at the heart of doctoral education and practice. Part II takes the reader through the process of clinical scholarship, beginning with Crabtree's definition of clinical scholarship and the evolution of students into scholars. She discusses how the role of the DNP is to generate nursing knowledge from practice.

Miller and Andrist continue this part with the process of carrying out the culminating piece of scholarship in DNP education programs—here referred to as the capstone project. They begin with the research or burning question from clinical practice and then guide the reader through the development, implementation, evaluation, and dissemination of the project.

The authors in Chapter 5, all nurse executives or administrators, write about some of the kinds of projects that DNPs carry out, including systematic reviews, organizational analysis, practice change initiative, and quality improvement projects. These are all examples of nurse executive scholarship that contribute to changing nursing practice.

Chapter 6 is written by former students and contains their stories in their own voices of the scholarship/capstone experience. They share how they came to develop their burning question into a project and some of the challenges and opportunities they encountered along the path. As a testament to DNP scholarship and disseminating capstone projects, four of the five papers have been published or are in press and the fifth is in process.

CHAPTER 3

# The Formation of Clinical Scholars: The Generation of Nursing Knowledge From Practice

Katherine Crabtree

The focus of Doctor of Nursing Practice degree programs is to prepare nurse leaders who can transform nursing to meet the burgeoning health care challenges of our nation. The curriculum leading to the DNP degree emphasizes a clear vision of nursing's future during this era of health care reform. Transforming nursing practice requires the preparation of leaders who can articulate nursing science and integrate knowledge and practice. A DNP-prepared nurse is expected to create new models of care, change practice, and improve health outcomes. The premise of this chapter is that clinical nurse scholars prepared in DNP programs acquire an inquiry approach to their practice that enables them to generate knowledge from practice. Expert clinicians are prepared to give voice to the need for change, and design and evaluate practice improvements through collaboration. Working with patients, families, and communities to implement population health goals and reduce disparities requires collaborating with other professionals and it requires policy change. The DNP program offers a curriculum that engages nurses in these activities to ensure that graduates are capable of envisioning the exciting possibilities for the profession and actualizing them.

■ CONVERGENCE OF NEED AND OPPORTUNITIES FOR THE DEVELOPMENT
   OF THE DNP DEGREE PROGRAMS

The health care crisis fueled by rising costs, poor outcomes, and increasing health disparities has launched an era of health care reform that is long overdue. The work of reforming the fragmented U.S. health care system is underway with three major work groups providing direction for parallel reform of nursing education, practice, and regulation. These reforms are paramount to ensure nursing's leadership role in health care delivery as nurses develop scientific evidence for practice and translate that evidence into practice to achieve optimal health outcomes. The American Association of Colleges of Nursing (AACN, 2004) recommended educational reform and development of the DNP degree. These recommendations are congruent with the Institute of Medicine's (2010) report on the future of nursing and with the Advanced Practice Registered Nurse (APRN) Consensus Work Group's (2008) development of a consensus model for licensure, accreditation, certification, and education of advanced practice nurses.

The AACN's (2006) eight curricular essentials for DNP programs describe new areas of emphasis in preparing nurse leaders to meet the challenges arising from an explosion in scientific knowledge that requires use of technology to manage that knowledge; new skill sets that enable nurses to contribute to practice knowledge development; and advanced preparation to transform practice through the application of that new knowledge.

The full recommendations of The Institute of Medicine (2010) report on the future of nursing have been published online at www.nap.edu. The IOM report advocates for increased educational preparation of nurses. The goal is to ensure that 80% of nurses earn baccalaureate degrees by 2020. Another recommendation relevant here is a 100% increase in the number of nurses with doctoral preparation. Doctoral preparation helps nurses develop and evaluate scientific evidence, create and evaluate innovative care models, evaluate policy outcomes, and collaboratively change health policies that are essential to realizing the future of nursing.

In addition to the AACN Essentials and the IOM report recommendations, the landmark work of the APRN Consensus Group must be noted here for its impact on the future of advanced practice nursing. The work of this Group was devoted to the removal of barriers arising from the lack of consistency in APRN licensure, accreditation, certification, and education across the United States. The work entailed designing a national model encompassing four components: education of APRNs, accreditation of APRN educational programs, licensing, and certification of APRNs. The consensus model addresses four roles (nurse practitioner, nurse anesthetist, clinical nurse specialist, and nurse midwife) as the basis for licensure as an advanced practice nurse. The educational preparation for each role and population focus must match the accreditation and certification criteria set forth by national bodies. The model (Figure 3.1) has been endorsed by over 70 organizations and allows for greater consistency and favors APRN mobility. These standards are expected to raise the level of practice for states whose practice acts have not kept abreast of changes in practice and educational preparation of advanced practice nurses (APRN Consensus Group, 2008).

In addition to these three landmark reports, Benner and colleagues called for a "radical transformation" in nursing education (Benner, Sutphen, Leonard, & Day, 2010). Doctors of nursing practice find themselves well positioned to meet the challenges of the twenty-first century. One of the contributions of the DNP is to produce knowledge from practice—this is clinical scholarship.

### ■ NURSING SCHOLARSHIP

As the profession strove to legitimize its science, we neglected the scholarship of practice and the knowledge that can be acquired through practice. Fawcett (1999) called for all nurses to become nurse scholars to save the professional discipline from extinction by merging research and practice and closing the research–practice gap. She advocated for the post-baccalaureate nurse doctorate (ND), the early precursor of the DNP, as an entry to nursing practice. Although the ND did not survive, the concept of doctoral preparation of nurses who can bridge the gap between research and practice to achieve better outcomes for patients is alive and well, as demonstrated by the growing number of schools offering the DNP.

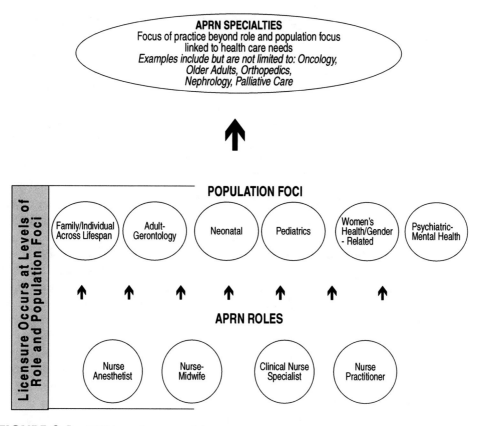

**FIGURE 3.1**  APRN regulatory model.

## Scholarship Traditions

The focus on the discovery of new knowledge via accepted quantitative research has garnered respect for the discipline and enhanced its standing in the scientific community as evidenced by the development and funding of the National Institute of Nursing Research. Furthermore, nurse theorists have developed broad theories addressing person, environment, health, and nursing to define the scope and substance of the discipline. While these theories and nursing philosophies have been used to guide research and advance the profession, we have lagged in valuing knowledge generated from practice. The grand theories of pioneering nurse philosophers such as Martha Rogers gave way to theories narrower in scope. These mid-range theories provided frameworks for investigating clinical phenomena such as pain and uncertainty. Mid-range theories linked concepts more closely to practice phenomena (Fawcett & Alligood, 2005; Peterson & Bredow, 2009) and better outcomes of care. Because these mid-range theories were more closely tied to practice phenomena, they also fostered the development of quantitative measures to capture human responses to health and illness states for further research. Social science theories such as role theory, self-efficacy, resilience, and hardiness were imported into nursing to further study and explain phenomena of interest to nurses. Nurse researchers, using quantitative research methods, adapted or devised new tools to study these concepts.

The development of postmodern philosophies of science and the use of qualitative methods has also shaped our view of nursing science. Research methods such as ethnography, phenomenology, grounded theory, critical social theory, and feminist theory were adopted by nurse researchers to better understand the patient's experience of health and illness through more holistic approaches (Rew & Barrow, 2007). These researchers expanded the use of qualitative methods to explore phenomena and processes that describe and explain the lived experience of patients and families adapting to life-changing experiences that impact health outcomes.

Nurses are drawn to qualitative approaches to research in part because of the connection they feel to patients and families as they seek to understand how best to provide support for health, healing, recovery, and resilience. Nurses encounter patients during times of transition, when there are rich opportunities for teaching, coaching, and for changing patients' perspectives and health behaviors. Qualitative research methods bring together the researcher and patient informant in a type of relationship that is not sought or possible with quantitative research. Narrative methods enhance story telling arising from interaction with patients. Fawcett and Rawnsley described these research methods as approaches that "...disclose a universal meaning of a lived experience that can be universally understood" (2002, p. 43). Knowledge arising from practice may be used to create interventions and new models of care. However, Rawnsley cautioned against direct application of knowledge generated from practice before it has been tested. Partnering with nurse researchers for testing and evaluation of these interventions and models may lead to generalizable knowledge that can be shared and applied elsewhere.

The accelerating popularity of naturalistic research and mixed-method studies blending quantitative and qualitative methods stems from the desire for a more comprehensive understanding of the human experience of health and illness. Recognizing that a combination of quantitative and qualitative methods provides a more complete picture, nurse researchers are using mixed methods to ensure greater understanding of clinical phenomena. Often, this comprehensive approach to discovery would be best served through partnerships between researchers and clinical nurse scholars as they uncover practice knowledge. Using an inquiry approach to practice, nurse scholars conceptualize clinical phenomena needing further investigation, thus providing a fruitful basis for partnering with nurse researchers that enriches the discipline.

## Definitions of Clinical Scholarship and Development of Practice Knowledge

As Donna Diers (1983), a previous editor of *Image,* once described, defining clinical scholarship "is like trying to nail Jello to the wall" (p. 35). Yet recognition of the need for clinical scholarship is evident throughout the literature. Clinical scholarship contributes to the knowledge of the discipline through conceptualization, investigation, evaluation, and dissemination of knowledge to inform practice, education, policy, and research. Although clinical scholarship includes research and theory development, it is not limited to these two forms of scholarship. The advancement of nursing science requires nurses to contribute through research, theory, and *practice.* Accordingly, Diers (1995) placed clinical scholarship within a context of discovery which involves "observation of patients or practice including one's own participation or reaction to patients or situations" (p. 24).

Woods and colleagues defined clinical scholarship (Figure 3.2) as comprised of three entities: practice-based theory, clinical research, and practice inquiry (Woods, 2009).

The University of Washington School of Nursing coined the title *practice inquiry* in 2004 to capture the investigative focus of the DNP: Practice inquiry is an ongoing,

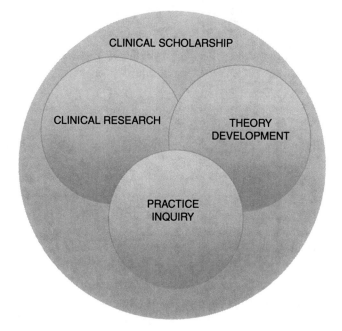

**FIGURE 3.2** Clinical scholarship.

*Source:* From Woods (2009).

systematic investigation of questions about nursing therapeutics and clinical phenomena with the intent to appraise and translate all forms of "best evidence" to practice, and to evaluate the translational impact on the quality of health care and health outcomes. Through the process of translating science to practice, APRNs observe, describe, understand, and appraise clinical phenomena and their interface with empirically and theoretically based knowledge. The investigative focus integrates scientific curiosity and inquiry with the realities of everyday practice (Magyary, Whitney, & Brown, 2006, p. 143). We could now propose that the DNP is a clinical scholar who does practice inquiry to produce practice knowledge.

The definition of practice knowledge proposed by this author is "the knowledge gained through examination of experience and study that leads to mastery of (or expertise in) a defined area of practice that is shared with others for evaluation, validation, and application." In this manner, practice knowledge improves the health of patients, families, and communities, and contributes to knowledge within the profession.

Practice-derived knowledge leads to clinical scholarship when it is exposed to further evaluation, validation, and eventually to dissemination. Schon's (1983) reflective practitioner is an example of a clinical scholar who is able to use practice encounters to reflect on and to conceptualize practice experiences that guide future encounters. However, the knowledge acquired by the nurse remains private knowledge until it is vetted through peer review, then disseminated and evaluated by the profession. Once articulated and validated, this knowledge can be developed into systematic approaches to care delivery and used to promote the development of professional standards and guidelines (Exhibit 3.1).

---

**EXHIBIT 3.1**

**An Iterative Process for Development and Dissemination
of Practice Knowledge Using an Inquiry Perspective**

---

1. Advanced practice knowledge and skills (competencies) within a population focus
   a. Clinical literature
   b. Research literature
2. Passion for caring, excellence, and learning
3. Reflection on practice experiences (e.g., micro: health processes, healing behaviors, illness trajectories, interventions that promote recovery and resilience; macro: collaborations and continuity across boundaries, systems, care processes)
4. Dialogue with peers and colleagues to evaluate, validate, and refine
   a. Conceptualization and recognition of clinical problems
   b. Data on patterns, variations, outcomes of care
   c. Development of interventions that address clinical problems, improve processes, reduce cost
5. Pilot testing (care models, creative approaches, etc.)
6. Evaluation of results with practice application
7. Dissemination of outcomes

## The Inquiry Continuum: Research and Other Forms of Inquiry

The inquiry projects conducted by DNP-prepared nurses span a broad continuum. At one end, inquiry overlaps with research. The continuum also includes translation of research into practice, quality improvement and program evaluation, and practice improvement projects. The purpose, scope, methods, and resources used to mount inquiry projects also vary considerably. As quality improvement standards become more rigorous, the data generated may have use beyond local application.

Dreher (2011) has asked important questions about the type of knowledge produced in a DNP program and inquiry processes used to produce it. Action research is appropriate for students engaged in inquiry projects within their work environment as it is designed to simultaneously study and make changes in practice. He also describes another approach to clinical inquiry that is conducted within a "context of application," that emphasizes generation of knowledge from clinical interactions taking place outside of traditional controlled research. Originally proposed by Gibbons (1994) as distinct from traditional research, this alternate mode of inquiry produces knowledge that crosses disciplinary boundaries with multiple participants contributing to the generation, appraisal, and diffusion of the knowledge and evidence acquired. Dreher considers the forms of inquiry in a DNP program as still evolving and varying across the research–inquiry continuum with potential transdiciplinary application. He advocates for keeping a full range of options open as dialogue about clinical knowledge generation continues.

If a school has both a PhD and a DNP program, there may be separation of clinical inquiry from pure research based on the faculty's philosophies, research skills, and resources.

In other universities, graduate studies require all doctoral degree programs to meet certain standards of research and designate the type of product acceptable for awarding a doctoral degree. It is hoped that the future of clinical inquiry will involve partnerships between clinical experts and researchers who bring their expertise in methods to bear on the study of the problem. In the past, dissertations from PhD programs often generated knowledge that had little or no impact as they were shelved and forgotten after the degree was awarded. To avoid this outcome, both PhD and DNP programs are requiring different types of formats for products of inquiry. If the goal is for clinically based inquiry projects to impact care delivery, policy, future research, and nursing education, the requirement may be to submit a document in a format suitable for publication in a peer-reviewed journal. Just as practice continues to change and evolve over time, it is incumbent upon faculty and educational institutions to adopt strategies that communicate this knowledge widely. Dissemination is also a way to examine outcomes, for example, products of the scholarly endeavor, potential impact, and productivity of DNP program scholars.

Rolfe and Davies (2008) point out that Gibbons is challenging our traditional assumptions about how knowledge is generated and how its value is judged. The answers to the questions that were raised offer a vision of future transdisciplinary doctoral programs where contextualized knowledge is generated and applied immediately. The conceptualization of knowledge generation from practice and application in practice has implications for transforming doctoral education. Transdiciplinary practice doctoral programs might produce rich dividends for nursing and society to augment the contribution to knowledge from traditional research doctorates. Recognition of the contribution of nurses with practice doctorates to knowledge generation and practice improvement is needed, rather than insisting that only traditional research doctorates are rigorous enough to produce knowledge.

There is not yet an infusion of DNP-prepared faculty teaching in DNP programs. The majority of DNP program faculty who are teaching methods of inquiry to DNP students are PhD-prepared. Teaching research is familiar to PhD faculty whereas practice inquiry may be foreign to them. Consequently, the DNP projects may be research oriented rather than a translation of research findings into practice. Practicing doctoral faculty may help balance the emphasis on research with other forms of inquiry more adapted to study of clinical phenomena in rapidly paced practice settings. Valuing both research and translation of research into practice enhances partnerships among faculty with research-focused and practice-focused doctoral preparation.

## ■ DEVELOPING CLINICAL SCHOLARS

Walker and his colleagues (Walker, Golde, Jones, Buesche, & Hutchins, 2008) reported the results of a 5-year Carnegie Foundation study of doctoral education in over 100 programs spanning six disciplines in *The Formation of Scholars*. Personal identity as a scholar who is committed to professional integrity and accountability for the future of the discipline is internalized during doctoral study. Similarly, the DNP curriculum shapes the identity of the clinical scholar by nurturing curiosity, passion for learning, commitment to excellence, and ethics in order to make a meaningful difference in the health of patients.

Expert nurses illustrate the development of practice knowledge. Riley, Beal, and Lancaster (2007) studied 36 nurse clinicians from four acute-care magnet hospitals. Peers within their practice environments recognized these nurses as expert nurses. When asked about scholarly nursing practice, these experienced nurses described themselves as "active learners, out-of-the-box thinkers, passionate about nursing, available and confident"

(p. 429). They described a tolerance for ambiguity and uncertainty in practice settings that were often chaotic. They were flexible adapters and innovators "committed to the highest professional standards" who at times were also "rule bender(s)" and "risk taker(s)" who "buck the system" (pp. 427–431). They accepted challenges and took responsibility as leaders to achieve excellence in care. Their self-descriptions of their nursing identity as they engaged in practice represented the values of the profession. They were eager to share their practice knowledge and instill a passion for practice in others. They described their nursing practice not as a list of skills they had mastered or tasks to be performed. They described themselves as "being leaders, caring, sharing knowledge with others, evolving and reflecting on practice" (Riley et al., p. 425). These are the characteristics of clinical scholars.

Nursing's social contract with society obligates clinical scholars to develop unfolding practice knowledge fully, to validate it, and to use it to benefit society. To accomplish this, the DNP program provides transformative experiences via immersion in practice. Through personal and vicarious encounters, DNP students learn to identify practice knowledge and its potential for application.

## Scholarly Role Models

Faculty in DNP programs who are actively engaged in practice-knowledge generation and dissemination provide role models for emerging clinical scholars. Clinical experts who are immersed in the practice area can serve as mentors to promote professional development of clinical nurse scholars as well. These experts may be nurses or colleagues outside of nursing (physicians, epidemiologists, behavioral or nonbehavioral scientists, methodologists, policy makers, etc.). Mentors open doors to professional networks, and provide access to patient populations for scholarly projects. As mentors engage DNP nurses in dialogue about substantive issues in the area of practice, those nurses learn to appraise the clinical and research literature. The mentoring relationship also helps students cope with anxieties as they take on greater responsibility for decision making in complex situations and as they act as agents for change in practice or policy. Mentors help students acquire the competencies, experience, and assurance needed to be a leader.

Delivery of quality care requires interprofessional communication and collaboration. Team approaches are needed to integrate contributions from multiple disciplines. However, we have not determined when, where, and how collaboration with other disciplines is best learned. Clearly this too often takes place on the "firing line," which is too late to attain the quality of cooperative care needed. Clinical nurse scholars who become involved in interprofessional journal clubs learn to share their perspectives and expertise as they evaluate the literature for practice application. Their colleagues learn what DNP nurses can contribute to the dialogue and what perspective they bring to understanding health problems and health services. When DNP-prepared nurses provide grand rounds on cases that demonstrate complex decision making, they showcase their clinical expertise. As they conduct practice improvement projects to improve quality of care, evaluate clinical programs, and translate research into practice, they demonstrate the value they bring to the table in clinical arenas, whether that influence affects practice, research, policy, or nursing education.

As clinical nurse scholars describe the expanding boundaries of the discipline, they also promote understanding of areas where these boundaries overlap with other disciplines. Diers (1995) acknowledged that nurse scholars, through education and practice experiences, are prepared to make a "creative leap" to move the discipline forward. Thus, they enlarge the discipline by pushing its borders and collaborating with colleagues from other disciplines to redefine knowledge in their specialty. Integration of knowledge derived from the field of genetics is an example of how nurses are working collaboratively to advance the application of new knowledge in advanced practice nursing. Joint educational opportunities that provide learning together are needed to enable the highest level of interprofessional collaboration. Quality practice does not occur in isolation from other disciplines. Mentors of DNP students can facilitate interprofessional collaboration through peer review, quality improvement projects, and serving together on standards, ethics, or policy committees. The communication of knowledge to a variety of audiences promotes and reinforces successful interprofessional collaboration. Opportunities for joint inquiry and publication abound.

Accountability is key to leadership roles. To paraphrase Melanie Dreher (1999), clinical scholars are leaders prepared to own the outcomes of their actions. The clinical scholar holds himself or herself accountable for learning and growth and is open to feedback. Doctoral programs that encourage peer review processes, constructive collegial exchange, and scholarly feedback provide opportunities for professional development. Engaging faculty and students in open dialogue models a community of scholars to appraise practice knowledge and examine implications for practice application.

The challenge before us as nursing faculty and mentors is how to prepare nurse scholars who value practice knowledge and recognize and regularly reflect on it. Clinical nurse scholars give voice to this knowledge and share with others the outcomes achieved. Clinical nurse scholars are setting new benchmarks for practice as they evaluate care against the national standards and devise new clinical guidelines to improve practice.

## ■ CLINICAL SCHOLARS AS LEADERS IN HEALTH CARE DELIVERY

Health care reform is drastically changing the landscape of health care delivery. The fragmented health care system has created formidable barriers to quality and safety. Competing priorities, rapid change, and professional shortages are accelerating the implosion of the entire system. Health disparities have escalated with the economic recession. Despite growing recognition of health disparities, reallocation of resources to abolish these inequities remains inadequate. Equal access to affordable quality health care services is a verbalized goal that continues to remain out of reach in the United States. While reform is expected to provide health coverage to 32 million more individuals, another 10 million will remain uninsured. The commitment of clinical nurse scholars to improving health and access to quality care includes devising strategies that bridge this gap through health promotion programs, education, and screening. Providing care for populations who have been left out of the mainstream requires leadership, commitment, planning, and new models of care involving community outreach efforts. The move from master's preparation to DNP preparation of the advanced practice nurse emphasizes the move to a population perspective for delivery of care, and partnering with communities to make services available to more individuals and their families. Nurses have a strong sense of social justice. As nurses advocate for health equity with access to affordable quality health care, DNP-prepared nurse scholars are providing leadership in forming interprofessional coalitions to advance the agenda of equitable, cost-effective health care.

Another leadership strategy for improving quality of care encompassed in DNP education is the integration of evidence-based practice (Frewin, 2009). The DNP-prepared nurse learns to access information, evaluate it, and integrate that knowledge in practice. Preparation of clinical scholars who take an inquiry approach to practice requires learning new skills and using knowledge management technologies to improve health outcomes. Knowledge management technologies are transforming the clinical environment. Using best practices, the DNP-prepared nurse maximizes implementation of those strategies known to be effective. As research grows, scholarly systematic reviews and other strategies are needed for synthesis of research results. Working in collaboration with other health care providers, the clinical nurse scholar can introduce evidence-based practices through innovative models of care to improve care quality. As clinical scholars learn to use sophisticated search strategies and new technologies for knowledge management, they become better puzzle solvers. They discover patterns in practice problems and develop possible solutions. Skills in using the latest evidence to solve clinical problems require efficient retrieval of relevant information and its appraisal. Clinical nurse scholars with doctoral preparation and expertise in the health of populations will be at the table with other decision makers because they will know how to appraise research findings and can contribute to the development, implementation, and evaluation of evidence-based practice guidelines.

Drawing on practice expertise, the clinical nurse scholar integrates practice knowledge with the formal knowledge derived from research and the clinical literature to develop new approaches to care. As leaders of change, scholars also use these technologies to monitor rapidly expanding knowledge bases from which to retrieve relevant research and practice information for quality improvement and translation of research into practice. Technology can alert them to the publication of new guidelines or research in specified areas of practice, allowing them to remain updated. Ongoing review of practice and the latest evidence continually offers potential improvements to be evaluated. As clinical scholars analyze and interpret new knowledge for its practice implications, they integrate and adapt knowledge from expanding scientific fields such as genomics, ethics, and the humanities.

Technology is also changing the patient/provider interface. Patients can retrieve information on the Internet and query their care provider about it or supply regular updates on physiological data and their response to treatments. Learning how to fully use this technology to communicate with patients allows the clinical scholar multiple opportunities to expand electronic feedback to patients and to elicit further information when symptoms recur. Tele-health is making care possible across geographical distances that would otherwise limit or even deny access to care. Sharing of data and consultation with specialists electronically allows improved access to care and more patients to be served. Clinical nurse scholars need to examine and describe how technology and tele-health influence the knowledge arising from practice.

The electronic health record is also changing the way clinical information is stored, retrieved, and made accessible to multiple care providers in multiple sites. Involvement of clinical nurse scholars in the development of these systems ensures that the data captured can be used for generating nursing practice knowledge. Previously, the technology was organized for business purposes rather than for use by clinicians to evaluate and change practice. In harnessing the power of these technologies for practice, clinical scholars are able to identify patterns, track trends, monitor their population, notify themselves and patients of the need for periodic screening, follow up interventions, evaluate outcomes against national benchmarks, and appraise the quality of practice. DNP-prepared nurses and their practice partners can evaluate the sustainability of evidence-based changes made in practice. Furthermore, clinical inquiry is facilitated as databases describing practice allow retrieval, analysis, and evaluation of care and its outcomes.

As astute observers, clinical nurse scholars discern knowledge from practice encounters, whether from databases or through reflection on a sentinel patient encounter. Through examination of unanticipated outcomes of care processes, the clinical nurse scholar may gain insights for validation and pursue additional data gleaned from the database for the larger patient population. These technologies allow the clinical nurse scholar to explore whether variations are health-promoting or health-limiting. Using technology to retrieve data, clinical scholars can examine processes and evaluate responses to various types of interventions. Observing patterns of care outcomes over time will allow clinical scholars to advance practice more quickly and to share their practice-based data as evidence that care is meeting national standards.

The clinical scholar conveys practice knowledge and clinical wisdom to others through clinical case reports, explicates lessons learned when launching innovative care models, and discontinues practices that are ineffective. As these scholars merge practice knowledge formed through experience and expertise with scientific knowledge to inform decision making, they are advancing practice to its highest level.

Nurse researchers, nurse theorists, and nurse clinicians all value nursing knowledge, but they approach discovery of knowledge in different ways. The discipline of nursing will benefit most through recognition of each of their unique contributions. Their talents and skills enrich the profession and ultimately benefit the recipients of our care and teaching.

## ■ ACKNOWLEDGMENT

The author wishes to acknowledge Donna G. Nativio, PhD, CRNP, FAAN, University of Pittsburgh, for her thoughtful review of this chapter.

## ■ REFERENCES

Advanced Practice Registered Nurse (APRN) Consensus Work Group. (2008). *Consensus model for APRN regulation: Licensure, accreditation, certification & education.* Retrieved from www.nonpf.org

American Association of Colleges of Nursing. (2004). *Position statement on practice doctorate. Approved October 2004.* Retrieved from http://www.aacn.nche.edu

American Association of Colleges of Nursing. (2006). Essentials *of doctoral education for advanced nursing practice.* Retrieved from http://www.aacn.nche.edu

Benner, P., Sutphen, M., Leonard, V., & Day, L. (2009). *Educating nurses: A call for radical transformation of nursing education.* New York, NY: John Wiley & Sons.

Diers, D. (1983). Clinical scholarship II. *Image: The Journal of Nursing Scholarship, 15*(2), 35.

Diers, D. (1995). Clinical scholarship. *Journal of Professional Nursing, 11*(1), 24–30.

Dreher, M. (1999). Clinical scholarship: Nursing practice as an intellectual endeavor. In Clinical Scholarship Task Force Resource Paper. *Sigma Theta Tau International,* 26–33.

Dreher, H. M. (2011). Next steps toward practice knowledge development: An emerging epistemology in nursing. In M. Dahnke & H. M. Dreher (Eds.). *Philosophy of science for nursing practice: Concepts and application* (pp. 301–331). New York, NY: Springer Publishing Company.

Fawcett, J. (1999). The state of nursing science: Hallmarks of the 20th and 21st centuries. *Nursing Science Quarterly, 12* (4), 311–315.

Fawcett, J., & Alligood, M. (2005). Influences on the advancement of nursing knowledge. *Nursing Science Quarterly, 18*(3), 227–232.

Fawcett, J., & Rawnsley, M. (2002). On science and human science: A conversation with M. Rawnsley. *Nursing Science Quarterly, 15*(10), 41–45.

Frewin, D. (2009). Elements of evidence-based health care. *International Journal of Evidence Based Healthcare, 7,* 1–2.

Gibbons, M. (1994). Preface. In M. Gibbons, C. Lomoges, H. Nowotny, S. Schwartzman, P. Scott, & M. Trow (Eds.), *The new production of knowledge* (pp vii–ix). London, UK: Sage.

Institute of Medicine. (2010). *The future of nursing: Leading change, advancing health.* Washington, DC: The National Academies.

Magyary, D., Whitney, J. D., & Brown, D.M. (2006). Advancing practice inquiry: Research foundations of the practice doctorate in nursing. *Nursing Outlook, 54,* 139–151.

Peterson, S. J., & Bredow, T. S. (2009). *Middle range theories: Application to nursing research* (2nd ed.). New York, NY: Lippincott Williams & Wilkins.

Rew, L. R., & Barrow, E. M. (2007). State of the science: Intuition in nursing, a generation of studying the phenomenon. *Advances in Nursing Science, 30*(1), E15–E25.

Riley, J., Beal, J. A., & Lancaster, D. (2007). Scholarly nursing practice from the perspectives of experienced nurses. *Journal of Advanced Nursing, 61*(4), 425–435.

Rolfe, G., & Davies, R. (2009). Second generation professional doctorates in nursing. *International Journal of Nursing Studies, 46*(9), 1265–1273.

Schon, D. (1983). *The reflective practitioner: How professionals think in action.* London, UK: Basic Books.

Walker, G. E., Golde, C. M., Jones, L., Bueschel, A., & Hutchins, P. (2008). *The formation of scholars: Rethinking doctoral education for the twenty-first century.* Stanford, CA: Carnegie Foundation for the Advancement of Teaching.

Woods, N. F. (2009). *Clinical practice and scholarship inquiry: Contributions of DNP and PhD-prepared nurses to evidence-informed practice.* Retrieved August 1, 2011, from http//www. nursing.columbia.edu/research/pdf/Woods_Presentation.pdf

# CHAPTER 4

# Capstone Project: Development, Implementation, Evaluation, and Dissemination

Kathleen H. Miller and Linda C. Andrist

## ■ CAPSTONE PROJECT DEVELOPMENT: THE PROPOSAL

The capstone project is a scholarly work that is often a requirement of Doctor of Nursing Practice programs. There are other terminologies used for this work, including scholarly project or practice inquiry. The expectations for the capstone project vary across institutions depending upon the focus. Some schools of nursing may require more in-depth assignments such as a thesis or practice dissertation. The general premise is that the student will complete scholarly work that translates evidence into practice.

There has been a debate in the literature as to whether the capstone project should be a quality improvement initiative or research (Gardenier, Stanik-Hutt, & Selway, 2010). Arguments on research capstone projects are that the DNP-prepared graduate will contribute to nursing knowledge by focusing on research grounded in practice. Those against research for capstone projects state that the curricula of DNP programs do not prepare the students for this competency. Additionally, the focus on research may distract from the attainment of the DNP competencies developed by AACN (2006). However, in the year 2011, at least four new texts were published with the growing opinion that DNP clinical scholars acquire an inquiry approach to their practice in order to generate knowledge from practice (see Chapter 3, The Formation of Clinical Scholars). Knowledge generated from practice involves research.

The capstone project is focused on an advanced nursing practice specialty or interprofessional intervention that may benefit a group, population, or community (NONPF, 2007). This work is usually based on clinical practice and involves partnerships with other entities such as health care organizations, schools, community agencies, or groups. The capstone project can take different forms, including practice change initiatives, evidence-based protocols, clinical guidelines, and health policy. Other capstone projects may focus on the development, implementation, and evaluation of interprofessional strategies to improve health care. The completion of the capstone project also demonstrates the attainment of the DNP competencies by the student.

The development of this scholarly work is a step-by-step process that includes a systematic approach and translation of evidence into practice. These processes include (1) description of the innovation or clinical inquiry, (2) application of the best evidence from the literature, (3) collection of data using methods or tools that are standard and acceptable, and (4) definition of outcomes to be measured. Additionally, the projected should be conducted according to ethical principles and the dissemination methods peer reviewed, whether public and/or professional (NONPF, 2007).

The Institute of Medicine has set as a goal that by 2020, approximately 90% of clinical decisions be grounded in the best evidence (Olsen, Aisner, & McGinnis, 2007). Although there is not a universally accepted hierarchy of evidence, a frequently cited document for biomedical research states systematic reviews are at the highest level. This evidence is followed by randomized controlled clinical trials. It is important to be aware that not all research or capstone questions can be investigated using this design because some inquiries may be more amenable to a qualitative approach. The bottom of the hierarchy includes approaches such as cased controlled studies. The focus is finding the best evidence to support practice changes. The components of this hierarchy developed by Greenhalgh (1997) are depicted in Table 4.1.

Nursing has adapted this model and has recommended changes to address the issue of translation of evidence to practice. This approach may be facilitated by the outcomes of well-designed capstone projects grounded in the best evidence. The first step in this process is the identification of a question from clinical practice.

## Project Development

### The "Burning Question" From Practice

Sister Callista Roy wrote that "practice…is the unifying factor for all of knowledge development. For example, nurses often enter doctoral education with burning questions from advanced practice" (Roy & Jones, 2007, p. 4). This is the premise that underlies project development; it is grounded in practice and designed to add to practice knowledge. The burning question may arise from a practice situation in which the student wonders if an observation is evidence based or coincidental, or from reading the research literature and thinking about replicating a study with a different population (Terry, 2012).

## TABLE 4.1   Hierarchy of Evidence

| Level of Evidence | Type of Evidence |
|---|---|
| 1. | Systematic reviews and meta-analyses |
| 2. | Randomized controlled trials with definitive results (confidence intervals that do not overlap the threshold clinically significant effect) |
| 3. | Randomized controlled trials with nondefinitive results (a point estimate that suggests a clinically significant effect but with confidence intervals overlapping the threshold for this effect) |
| 4. | Cohort studies |
| 5. | Case-control studies |
| 6. | Cross-sectional surveys |
| 7. | Case reports |

*Source:* Adapted from Greenhalgh (1997).

Students should plan to develop their question in each doctoral course, concentrating on building their literature to fine tune the question. For example, in an outcomes measurement course, a student might examine patient dissatisfaction in the emergency department due to compassion fatigue on the part of staff. In an epidemiology/population health course this student then could look at aggregate populations regarding the same subject.

Several cautionary words are needed regarding the capstone project question. Students should consider the following:

(1) Will they have sufficient time to carry out the project within the scope of the DNP program? (Terry, 2012)

(2) Is the project within the scope of the DNP?

(3) Do they have sufficient resources—such as financial resources (Terry, 2012) and available faculty expertise in the area?

A faculty advisor should be involved in each step of the process to ensure that the student is on target and is proceeding in a reasonable fashion. In one of the author's knowledge and inquiry courses, faculty have students discuss their "burning" questions, critique each other, and search the literature for theoretical models to apply to their question. In the research analysis and critique course, they search for the best evidence, analyze and critique the literature, and begin a review of the literature. These two courses form the foundation for the proposal.

### Formulating a PICO(T) Question

After the identification of a topic from clinical practice, the student uses the literature to guide the development of the initial question or practice inquiry to develop the PICO(T) question. PICO(T) is a framework that can be used to develop clinical questions in a systematic manner (Nollan, Fineout-Overholt, & Stephenson, 2005). The use of the PICO(T) framework facilitates the development of questions with the scientific underpinnings of evidence-based practice to diagnosis, treat, and facilitate patient understanding of their prognosis (Melnyk & Fineout-Overholt, 2011). This framework is useful for developing clinical questions to examine the best evidence to answer these questions and is associated with improved quality reporting from randomized controlled clinical trials (RCTs) (Rios, Ye, & Thabane, 2010). It is important that these randomized controlled clinical trials are well designed so that the evidence is generalizable. For a DNP student, the PICO(T) question can be used in an evidence-based practice search or for a systematic review of the literature. With a more focused PICO(T) question, the search will yield appropriate studies targeted to the practice inquiry.

The acronym PICO(T) stands for *P*, the population of interest; *I*, intervention or issue of interest; *C*, comparison of interest or intervention/issue; *O*, the outcome of interest or what will be improved for the population of interest; and *T*, for time, which is optional for the PICO(T) question (Stillwell, Fineout-Overholt, Melnyck, & Williamson, 2010). These are explained below.

*P* is the specific population of interest. What is the population of interest that is the focus of the practice inquiry? There should be specific detail to identification of the population including age, ethnicity, gender, or diagnosis. This information can be used to focus the scope of the practice inquiry while not excluding other relevant groups from the question. The population can also be a specific position category such as nurse practitioners, registered nurses, nurse executives, informaticists, and the like. These can further be delineated by population foci for advanced practice nurses, for example, as identified in the *Consensus Model for APRN Regulation: Licensure, Accreditation, Certification, and Education* (APRN

Consensus Work Group & National Council of State Boards of Nursing APN Advisory Committee, 2008).

*I* is focused on the intervention or issue of interest or what the investigator will do for the patient or population of interest. It is important to depict a clear and concise statement of the intervention or issue of interest. This strategy will focus the question so that the project or study may be evaluating a new clinical practice guideline, model, protocol, or therapy.

*C* stands for the comparison of interest or intervention/issue. What are the alternatives to the identified intervention? This section is relevant for those populations of interest that may have treatment alternatives or different interventions that may influence the outcomes.

*O* is focused on the outcome of interest or what will be improved for the population of interest. Capstone projects are frequently initiated to improve the quality of patient care or to enhance organizational processes. The project or study will evaluate the effect of the intervention on the outcomes of the population to determine if they were improved, had no effect, or resulted in adverse or negative results.

*T* is for time and is optional for the PICO(T) question. Time is referenced in relation to the scholarly project. This approach is particularly helpful for work that is either time limited or if there is data collection at specific periods that are examining changes over time. The use of time is also helpful for determining the starting and ending points of the intervention. An explanation of PICO(T) and recommended items for each component of the framework are identified in Table 4.2.

Using a standardized format such as the PICO(T) will guide the inquiry to develop questions that are searchable using the best evidence. The data to answer the question may vary depending upon the question and the information in the literature. Some questions are best answered by systematic reviews or meta-analyses while others may be developed so that qualitative studies are the source of the evidence. The question will then guide the design of the project or study. Examples of PICO(T) are in Table 4.3.

### Exploring Theoretical Frameworks

Theory-based nursing is central to advanced nursing practice and defines the DNP. Nursing theory distinguishes the DNP from the medical model because, rather than working with decontextualized pieces of data, nursing practice occurs in the exchanges between patient and nurse. The advanced practice nurse has a relationship with the patient and their unique values and goals, not with the disease (Eldridge, 2011). Nursing theories help guide practice by providing a foundation to understand patients, their problems, and to formulate interventions to help them. Eldridge noted:

> Nursing theory improves our care by giving it structure and unity, by providing more efficient continuity of care, by achieving congruence between process and product, by defining the boundaries and goals of nursing actions, and by giving us a framework in which to examine the effectiveness of our interventions. (p. 13)

We recognize that DNP students are also nurse administrators, health policy experts, informaticists, and educators. There are many social science, organizational, and educational theories and models to bring to the capstone project.

Theory-based nursing practice applies theories, principles, and models from a variety of sources to practice. Conceptual models and grand theories are broad in scope and focused on the large nursing arena, while middle range theories are more specific, focused, and narrow. They concentrate on specific health experiences, health or illness problems, or a particular patient population (Reed, 2011).

McEwen and Wills, in their second edition of *Theoretical Basis for Nursing* (2007), commented that nursing theory books have failed to keep up with trends in theory, specifically

**TABLE 4.2  Components of a PICO(T) Question**

| PICO(T) | Question | Examples |
|---|---|---|
| Population | What is the population of interest that is the focus of the practice inquiry? | Age<br>Ethnicity<br>Gender<br>Health status<br>Diagnoses |
| Intervention | What will the investigator do for the patient or population of interest? | Clinical practice guideline<br>Model<br>Protocol<br>Therapy |
| Comparison | What are the alternatives to the identified intervention? | Alternative intervention<br>No intervention<br>Placebo<br>No diagnosis<br>No risk factor |
| Outcome | What will be improved for the population of interest? | Improvement based on intervention<br>Intervention results in more positive outcomes than no intervention<br>Placebo has no effect on outcome<br>Intervention results in decreased diagnoses<br>Intervention results in decreased risk factors |
| Time | What is the time to demonstrate the outcome? | Time for the intervention to achieve an outcome<br>Time for subjects observed for the outcome |

**TABLE 4.3  Examples of PICO(T) Questions**

| PICO(T) | Question 1 | Question 2 |
|---|---|---|
| Population | In opiate dependence users completing a detoxification program who are risk for relapse, | In elders being transferred to a long-term care facility after hospitalization for pneumonia who are at risk for medication errors, |
| Intervention | how does receiving intensive outpatient therapy ... | how does a new medication reconciliation form ... |
| Comparison | compared to the standard of care (weekly support groups) ... | compared to the hospital's standard discharge form ... |
| Outcome | affect their relapse rate ... | affect the number of medication errors on admission ... |
| Time | three months after treatment? | two weeks after discharge? |

with middle range theories, application to practice, and evidence-based practice. In the last few years, more attention has been placed on this trend and there is now an extensive selection of texts and resources for students to use. Theory experts believe that middle range theory is the preferred direction for knowledge development (Peterson, 2009).

Middle range theory is defined as a "set of related ideas that are focused on a limited dimension of the reality of nursing" (Smith & Liehr, 2008, p. xvii). They grow and develop at the intersection of research and practice and provide guidelines for nursing practice (Smith & Liehr, 2008). Examples of middle range theories are in Table 4.4.

**TABLE 4.4   Examples of Middle Range Theories**

| Middle Range Theory | Reference |
| --- | --- |
| Uncertainty in illness (uncertainty during diagnosis and treatment of illness) | Mishel, M. H. (1988). Uncertainty in illness. *Image: Journal of Nursing Scholarship, 20,* 225–231 |
| Comfort (needs for ease, relief, and transcendence) | Kolcaba, K. (1994). A theory of holistic comfort for nursing. *Journal of Advanced Nursing, 19,* 1178–1184 |
| Community empowerment (improving health in communities) | Hildebrandt, E. (1996). Building community participation in health care: A model and example from South Africa. *Image: Journal of Nursing Scholarship, 28,* 155–159 |
| Story theory (story as the context for a nurse-person health-promoting process) | Smith, M. J., & Liehr, P. (1999). Attentively embracing story: A middle range theory with practice and research implications. *Scholarly Inquiry for Nursing Practice: An International Journal, 13,* 187–204 |
| The synergy model (critical care) | Hardin, S. R. (2005). Introduction to the AACN Synergy Model for patient care. In S. R. Hardin & R. Kaplow (Eds.), *Synergy for clinical excellence: The AACN Synergy Model for Patient Care.* Sudbury, MA: Jones and Bartlett |
| Unpleasant symptoms (symptom management) | Lenz, E. R., Pugh, L. C., Milligan, R. A., Gift, A., & Suppe, F. (1997). The middle range theory of unpleasant symptoms: An update. *Advances in Nursing Science, 19*(3), 14–27 |
| The tidal model of mental health recovery (psychiatric mental health nursing) | Barker, P. J. (2001). The Tidal Model: Developing an empowering, person-centered approach to recovery within psychiatric and mental health nursing. *Journal of Psychiatric and Mental Health Nursing, 8,* 233–240 |
| Postpartum depression theory (psychiatric mental health nursing, obstetrical nursing, women's health care) | Beck, C. T. (1993). Teetering on the edge: A substantive theory of postpartum depression. *Nursing Research, 42,* 42–48 |

Throughout their course of study, DNP students are exposed to a variety of frameworks, both in nursing and other disciplines. Before examing which would guide your capstone, consider Kenney's guide to selecting a theory in Table 4.5.

### TABLE 4.5  Guidelines for Selecting Models and Theories for Nursing Practice

| Afaf Meleis (1997) | Hugh McKenna (1997) | Kenney (2006) |
| --- | --- | --- |
| Personal—the nurse's comfort with the theory and congruency with the nurse's own philosophical views of life | Personal values and beliefs—the theory must be congruent with the nurse's own views about humans, health, and nursing | Consider your personal values and beliefs about nursing, clients, health, and environment |
|  |  | Identify several models that are congruent with your own values and beliefs about nursing, clients, and health |
| Mentor—the model or theory learned from a nurse mentor or educator | Health care setting—the type of clinical setting and nursing practice are contextual factors that affect selection of theories |  |
| Theorist—their reputation in the discipline and degree of recognition | Origins of the theory—the credibility, prior use, and testing of the theory should also be considered | Examine the underlying assumptions, values, and beliefs of various nursing models and how the major concepts are defined |
| Literature—support the amount of literature available about the theory and the theory's significance for one's specialty | Type of client—the client's needs should direct the choice because the theory provides guidelines to achieve the client's goals | Identify the similarities and differences in client focus, nursing actions, and client outcomes of these models |
| Sociopolitical congruency—the model or theory's acceptability within the nurse's workplace and whether major structural or practice changes are required | Paradigms as a basis for choice—nurses must decide between the totality or simultaneity paradigm, as each provides a different view of clients and nursing actions |  |
| Utility—the ease in which nurses can understand and apply the model or theory in practice settings | Parsimony/simplicity—simple and realistic theories are more likely to be understood and applied in practice | Practice applying the models and theories to clients with different health concerns to determine which ones best "fit" specific situations and guide nursing actions that will achieve desired client outcomes |
|  | Understandability—nurses must understand a theory if they are expected to use it |  |

*Source:* Kenney, J. W. (2006). Theory-based advanced nursing practice. In W. K. Cody (Ed.), *Philosophical and theoretical perspectives for advanced nursing practice* (4th ed.) (pp. 295–310). Sudbury, MA: Jones and Bartlett.

## Synthesis of the Literature

A thorough review of the literature provides the best evidence to support the development, implementation, and evaluation of the capstone project. Each component of the PICO(T) question can be used to guide the process of gathering evidence from the literature. There are several rating systems for the hierarchy of evidence for addressing the PICO(T) question, some that are specifically tailored to biomedical research, nursing, or health care.

After the development of the PICO(T) question, there are many databases that can be used to determine the best evidence. The rating system for hierarchy of evidence ranges from systematic reviews to reports of expert committees (Melnyk & Fineout-Overholt, 2011). A systematic review is a literature review of published studies focused on a research question that identifies, analyzes, and synthesizes evidence from randomized controlled trials or RCTs, while meta-analyses are systematic reviews that use quantitative methodologies to summarize the results of these findings. Both of these are considered Level I that yield the best evidence for practice. This model of hierarchy for evidence is more inclusive of the different types of research, including qualitative and descriptive studies. Levels I through VII are depicted in Table 4.6.

There are many databases that can be used to gather evidence to answer the PICO(T) question. An initial inquiry may be with resources such as CINAHL®, MEDLINE®, and/or PsycINFO® depending upon the type of question. These information resources often have a large repository of articles on a variety of topics. The use of one or more of these databases will be dependent upon the focus of the PICO(T) question. Clearly, the aim of gathering this information for quantitative studies is to identify Level I evidence and then move to other sources in the hierarchy that provide the best evidence on the topic. The databases available to search for studies are identified in Table 4.7.

A systematic review is an investigation of the scientific literature on an identified topic whereby the participants of the articles are being evaluated (Cook, Mulrow, & Haynes, 1997). Thus, before the student implements a systematic review, a protocol must be developed that includes (1) a targeted study question; (2) identified databases to be searched including inclusion and exclusion criteria for the participants; (3) types of data to be collected including interventions that are clearly described and risks and benefits clearly identified; and (4) plan for synthesizing the data with key elements identified so critical appraisal and replication can be done (West et al., 2002). Key elements to grade the strength of the evidence include the quality ratings for individual studies, quantity, effect size of the studies or sample size, and consistency or the number of similar or different studies with the same outcomes (West et al., 2002).

## TABLE 4.6  Rating System for the Hierarchy of Evidence

| Levels | Evidence |
|--------|----------|
| I | Systematic review or meta-analysis of RCTs |
| II | Well-designed RCTs |
| III | Well-designed controlled trials without randomization |
| IV | Well-designed case control and cohort studies |
| V | Systematic reviews of descriptive and qualitative studies |
| VI | Single descriptive or qualitative studies |
| VII | Authority opinions or expert committees |

*Source:* Melnyk & Fineout-Overholt, 2011. Adapted from Guyatt & Rennie, 2002.

**TABLE 4.7  Sources of Best Evidence**

| Name | Database |
| --- | --- |
| Cochrane Database of Systematic Review | Systematic reviews and protocols |
| DynaMed | Evidence-based clinical review summaries |
| Database of Abstracts of Reviews of Effects (DARE) | Abstracts of systematic reviews |
| American College of Physicians (ACP) Journal Club | Abstracts with strong evidence in the primary literature |
| United States Preventive Services Task Force | Evidence-based recommendations in prevention and screen |
| PubMed Clinical Queries | Articles supported by evidence |
| National Guideline Clearinghouse | Guidelines from the Agency for Healthcare Research and Quality (AHRQ) and professional medical organizations |
| TRIP Database | Search engine for multiple evidence-based sites |

The translation of evidence to practice should be based on research rather than on clinical experience or opinions. The systematic review compiles scientific evidence from research using a rigorous approach to answer health care questions. In this way, the best evidence from research is used to improve the practice of health care professionals. This information is important for students to use as they develop, implement, and evaluate their capstone project.

### Building the Committee

The development of the committee is an important process of the capstone project. The committee should have representation of doctorally prepared advanced practice nurses and/or interprofessional providers, depending upon the scope of the capstone project. The number of committee members is usually set by the program or the complexity of the PICO(T) question that may require additional content experts. Many schools have at least one faculty and one clinical site member. There should be a content expert on the committee who is knowledgeable about the evidence-based topic and/or clinical expert. Some schools may also require a committee member knowledgeable about the project methods or statistical procedures.

Typically, the proposal may be developed, implemented, and evaluated in the DNP capstone courses. The committee should be identified prior to writing the proposal as the PICO(T) question is being developed. The committee will oversee all aspects of the capstone project, including the approval by the Institutional Review Board, if indicated. There are often formal signatures during this process, including the agreement to serve on the DNP capstone project committee along with the final approval of the completed work.

The student and the committee will work together for at least two to three semesters until completion of the project. The expectations for this relationship need to be established prior to the formulation of the DNP capstone project committee. The relationship between committee members and the student needs to be collaborative as they work together. The establishment of a mentoring relationship will facilitate the development of the proposal, implementation of the project, and the evaluation of the outcomes.

### Writing the Proposal

The development and completion of the proposal are complex processes that include input from each of the committee members. Attention must be given to the format and structure of the proposal, along with the writing style. Each DNP program sets the criteria for the development of the proposal, depending upon the purpose of the scholarly work. This information should be made available to the student prior to the development of the proposal.

Once the PICO(T) question has been developed, systematic review has been completed, and plan for the capstone project finalized, work can begin on the proposal. In many programs, the development and approval of the proposal is accomplished in the first capstone project course. Important points for the student to consider are (1) read and follow carefully the proposal guidelines; (2) seek the recommendations of your capstone committee and content experts; (3) incorporate the correct components of the style of writing such as the American Psychological Association so that headings and reference formats are correct; (4) review the proposal for ethical issues or evidence of bias; and (5) meticulously prepare for the review by knowing the content well and anticipating any questions. Students should anticipate several revisions of their proposal based on the committee's feedback.

According to Nebiu (2000), a project proposal is a description of activities that are focused on solving a specific problem. Components of the proposal should include (1) rational for the project, (2) activities or plan for the project with a timeline, (3) methodology, and (4) resources needed to complete project such as participants, materials, and costs. Phases of a project cycle are (1) assess the literature or research studies, (2) identify the focus of the project, (3) design the project, (4) consider costs and resources to implement the project, (5) implement the project activities, and (6) evaluate the results of the project (Nebiu, 2000). These elements should be considered when developing the proposal according to the guidelines established by the school. The proposal guidelines may differ according to whether the focus is a clinical practice guideline, practice protocol, health policy change, or practice inquiry. Exhibit 4.1 provides an example of one school's outline for the proposal.

### Institutional Review Board

The Institutional Review Board is convened to protect human subjects. The IRB is composed of at least five members representing experience and expertise in research and diversity in race, gender, and culture. The IRB will also have members knowledgeable in and experienced with subjects in vulnerable categories, including children, prisoners, pregnant women, and the handicapped or mentally disabled. The IRB may also require documentation of informed consent or may waive this requirement.

Quality improvement projects do not require IRB approval but research studies do. Research is defined as "a systematic investigation, including research development, testing, and evaluation, designed to develop or contribute to generalizable knowledge" (United States Department of Health and Human Services, 2009). The functions of the IRB are to review and approve, make recommendations for modifications, or disapprove an IRB application. The IRB is also responsible for the continuing review of approved research at least once annually.

There are three different categories of review for research. Full review is required of research, including those subjects in the vulnerable category. Research involving minimal risk or with minor changes to approved studies may be in the category of expedited review.

*EXHIBIT 4.1*

Capstone Project Proposal Paper

## I. Introduction and Outline of the Proposed Project

- Introduction should contain two or three paragraphs at the most
- Tells the reader what is being proposed and why
- Clearly states the purpose of the project

## II. Background

- This section provides the reader with the set and setting of the project, as well as the rationale for why it is important. Often included in this section are related articles, professional opinions, statistics, supporting data, and the theoretical construct of the project (introducing your nursing theory)
- The Background section may be substantial—especially if there has been little empirical research

## III. Synthesis of the Literature

- Discuss which databases were searched, terms and descriptors used in the search, studies yielded (number, types)
- Group the articles by categories

Refer to: Galvan, J. L. (2009). *Writing literature reviews: A guide for students of the social and behavioral sciences*, 4th ed. Glendale, CA: Pyrczak Publishing.

## IV. Theoretical Framework

- All papers need a theoretical grounding
- The theoretical piece needs to be identified by name (middle range or other)
- The theoretical piece needs to be integrated throughout the paper—not just mentioned and then forgotten, show how the theory fits in, the theory drives your issue, guides your examination of the varied questions, and helps to develop any intervention and evaluation you are doing

## V. The Project Description

- Outline the project (the actual project is part of the Appendix)
- Discuss the methods, tools, and techniques that will guide implementation
- Identify your committee members, how they were chosen, and the roles they have agreed to play
- Formulate a plan for eliciting system involvement in implementing the project

- Describe the fiscal, ethical, political, legal, and legislative facets related to implementation of the project in a selected clinical/organizational context
- Address any potential constraints for facilitating a successful project
- Develop a plan for critically evaluating the project using a multi-dimensional framework (see evaluation rubric below)

**Project Evaluation Rubric**

| Objectives | What evidence-based measures/instruments will be applied to the evaluation plan? | What method of analysis will you use for each objective? | In what ways will you evaluate the success of your project? |
| --- | --- | --- | --- |
|  |  |  |  |

**VI. Discussion**

- Written Discussion due with final paper
- Relate the project's purpose to the background and literature review
- Discuss what is missing in the area you are addressing and how your project will contribute to the reader's knowledge development about this topic
- Discuss the development of the project
- Often the actual project is part of the Appendix (such as a teaching tool) and will be referred to in this section

**Conclusion**

- Due with final proposal
- Tell the reader what was done
- Apply project to nursing by referring to any nursing theory used or by discussing application to nursing practice

**References**

**Appendices**

This review may be conducted by the IRB chairperson or by one or more IRB members appointed by the chairperson. The IRB will have a procedure for notifying all members of the status of approval for research in this category. Research in the exempt review category is identified in Exhibit 4.2.

Students, in concert with their committee, need to discuss whether or not they will need to have IRB approval early on. Most institutions have a contact person who can review the student's ideas and help negotiate the process, whether the project is exempt, expedited, or full review. Attention must be paid to IRB submission deadlines and meeting dates in order not to extend the timeline that the student anticipates. When two institutions are involved (the school and a hospital for example), the first reader can help the student identify how the process will work. In some institutions, first readers need to be the Principal Investigator.

***EXHIBIT 4.2***

**Categories of Exempt Research**

Research conducted in established educational settings that may include regular or special education instruction;

Research using educational tests such as cognitive, diagnostic, aptitude, achievement tests. The research may also use surveys, interviews, or observations of public behavior;

The subjects can not be identified or linked to the research;

The subjects can not be public officials or candidates for public offices and confidentiality of subjects must be maintained;

Research consisting of existing data, documents, records, or specimens.

Research or projects investigated by or requiring approval of department or agency administrators which are designed to evaluate or examine public benefit or service programs, procedures for having benefits or services from these programs, changes or alternatives to these services, and changes in methods or levels of reimbursement for benefits or services;

Research involving taste and food quality and evaluation of consumer acceptance.

*Source:* United States Department of Health and Human Services, 2009.

■ CAPSTONE PROJECT IMPLEMENTATION AND EVALUATION

Once the committee has approved the capstone project proposal, the next important step is the implementation of the capstone project within the specified time frames and evaluation of the results. The final step is the dissemination of the information collected during the implementation of the capstone project.

## Capstone Project Implementation

The capstone project implementation involves a detailed plan that is a component of the proposal. The more detailed the plan with approval of stakeholders, the more likely the direction of the proposal will have minimal variations. Important competencies for the student that lead to the successful completion of the project include the ability to manage and collaborate with the team, manage the integral tasks of the project, and implement leadership skills for the team and key stakeholders (Balch, John, Reynolds, & Rick, 2011). Expertise at achieving these competencies is honed during the development, implementation, and evaluation of the capstone project.

The institutional stakeholders within the organization where the project is being carried out should be consulted at this point about the process that the student plans in the implementation of the project, collection of data, or other methods of conducting the project. Their endorsement is important to limit any challenges and facilitate the implementation of the project. The key stakeholders can also facilitate the implementation of the capstone project through endorsement of the project and setting the stage for approval by the employees. They should be involved from the beginning, receive updated progress reports, and have the opportunity to address concerns throughout the implementation (McElmurry et al., 2009).

Once approval is received from the Institutional Review Board, if needed, the implementation of the capstone project may commence. Not all capstone projects require IRB approval, for example, quality improvement projects. It is important to request a letter from the IRB stating that capstone project was quality improvement. Many journal editors require documentation that the capstone project either has IRB approval or that it is quality improvement project. The capstone project implementation must follow the plan as identified in the proposal. Any changes to the plan will require the filing and approval of an amendment for those capstone projects having oversight of the IRB. If the project underwent a full or expedited review process, as the capstone project was implemented, there may be changes to the plan that require approval of the IRB through the submission of an amendment form.

It is important to develop the team prior to the implementation of the capstone project. A model by Tuckman (2001) includes the stages of team development. The stages are forming, storming, norming, and performing. A fifth state was added in 1977 called adjourning (Tuckman, 2001). The evolution of the team may progress through these stages depending upon their communication and cohesiveness. The student should focus on using their leadership and management skills to guide the team through these stages. The components of this model are identified in Table 4.8.

### Project management

The implementation of the capstone project should follow the detailed plan. The capstone project team, including the faculty, should have regularly scheduled meetings. The key stakeholders should also have periodic updates about the status of the capstone project. Communications at all levels are important to the success of the project.

Project management is the use of knowledge, skills, instruments, and personnel to plan and implement a project within identified timelines and specified budgets while addressing stakeholders' expectations (Nicholas, 2001). Any risks or challenges encountered should have a plan in place to address these issues and keep the capstone project on track.

The student is in a role similar to project manager's. This role involves planning, organizing, and completing the capstone project within the identified time frame and costs. The risks and issues associated with the capstone project should also be a consideration for the student who is managing the project. This role is also important to guide or lead the members and stakeholders through the different stages of team development so that the project will be successful (Williams & Murphy, 2005).

## Capstone Project Evaluation

The project has been implemented according to plan and the activities have been completed. Some projects may have ongoing processes, or formative evaluation, while others may evaluate the outcomes of the project once completed (summative evaluation) while others use both processes. There are several approaches to evaluating the success of the capstone project.

**TABLE 4.8  Team Development**

| Stage | Team Members | Obstacles |
|---|---|---|
| Forming | Forming the team<br>Establishing project objectives<br>Identifying common interests<br>Developing trust<br>Bonding of team members | Disagreement on project objectives<br>Resistance to the group dynamics<br>Inability to develop trust<br>Team members unable to work cohesively |
| Storming | Identifying power issues<br>Improving communication skills among the team<br>Identifying resources for the project<br>Discussing differences in team members | Power imbalance between team members that are not resolved<br>Team members unable to communicate effectively<br>Conflict with roles and responsibilities |
| Norming | Agreeing on team members' roles<br>Developing processes for problem solving<br>Facilitating trust between team members | Inability to assume role responsibilities<br>Problem solving processes are not effective<br>Team members do not trust each other |
| Performing | Establishing an identity for the group<br>Working collaboratively on the project<br>Achieving effective outcomes | Team members are not able to establish a group identity<br>Not all members are able to work together<br>Outcomes for the project are not achieved |

### Data analysis

The data analysis approach was identified in the plan for the project. Taking into account any modifications in the information collected, there may be some changes on how the outcomes are evaluated. Once data are analyzed, the results can be compared to the aims or objectives of the capstone project.

The ability to evaluate the implications of the results of the data analyses requires knowledge of statistical processes. The student may need guidance from the DNP capstone committee and/or consultants. It is important that the conclusions of the findings are accurate. Some of this expertise comes from knowledge gained in the DNP program and the experience of conducting a capstone project. It is important to base conclusions on the evidence rather then making erroneous recommendations.

### Benchmarking the outcomes

After the data are analyzed, the outcomes of the project are compared with current benchmarks or outcomes of other projects. These benchmarks may be based on standards of practice or best practices identified by institutions and national professional organizations. The outcomes of the project are compared with these other standards to determine the success of the project in translating evidence from systematic reviews to practice. If the project experienced outcomes different from other benchmarks or information in the literature, an exploration of the reasons for these results is indicated. There may have been a problem with the design of the capstone project methodology, data analyses procedures, or interpretation of the outcomes. If the project is successful in improving practice and patient safety, then strategies should be developed to incorporate this change into the organization or other organizations. This process would entail the development of a new plan and potentially a new group of team members and key stakeholders. In the meantime, the student should share the outcomes with team members, key stakeholders, and organizations at local, regional, state, national, and international levels.

## ■ VENUES FOR DISSEMINATION

The old adage *if it's not written down it didn't happen* can be applied to knowledge development in nursing. It is our professional responsibility to share knowledge—knowledge generated from practice. Publishing in peer-reviewed journals has the highest prestige in the hierarchy of scholarship dissemination. DNP students and graduates who plan on teaching in academics will want to build their scholarship portfolio. Therefore, aiming for peer-reviewed venues is encouraged. Conferences generally do peer review for podium presentations or poster sessions and are a much faster way to get project outcomes out to professional colleagues. Certainly the capstone can be shared in a variety of ways.

### Poster Presentations

Presenting the capstone project as a poster is an effective venue for the dissemination of the capstone project outcomes. A poster presentation is a widely accepted strategy used for conferences sponsored by nursing and other disciplines. Scholarship can be shared in a more timely fashion, although with a more limited audience than when published in a journal.

Conference committee members often post notices of the meeting with a request for abstract submissions for poster and/or podium presentations. There are usually specific instructions for the abstract submissions, including format, blinded or not blinded, and total word count. The focus of the abstract should be congruent with the goals of the conference and/or professional organization. The abstract submission is usually due by a specific date, with the decision to accept or not accept made by a committee who usually does a blinded peer review.

The software program often used for developing posters is PowerPoint® (Microsoft Corporation, Redmond, Washington). The advantage of using this media is that presentations utilizing graphs, clip art, and photographs can be developed using PowerPoint® (Stein, 2006). There are specific considerations in developing the poster including title, names of those involved with project, and institutional affiliation at the top of the poster. The next step is determining the format of the poster. This format may be identified in the poster instructions for the conference or by the presenter. It is important to lay out the components before designing the poster using a software program. Make sure the poster is easy to read and the components flow in a logical sequence (Block, 1996). There are a number of Internet sites that have suggestions for making good PowerPoint® slides.

Many presenters include handouts of their abstract during the poster session. This session gives the audience the opportunity to review the posters at the conference. Some individuals will speak with the presenter to discuss their similar projects or ask advice on future projects. These sessions provide presenters and the audience time to network during the conference. Finally, some conferences recognize posters in specific categories such as projects or research.

## Podium Presentations

C. Oster (personal communication, August 18, 2011) suggests four issues to consider when preparing a podium presentation: (1) the type of presentation that is expected, (2) the audience, (3) time allotment, and (4) and the purpose of the presentation. The setting of the presentations, such as a unit-based meeting, a roundtable conference, or a formal local, national, or international conference, will set a different tone for the kind of presentation and the amount of audience participation.

Understanding the audience is critical in any presentation and will make or break the session. Content should be aimed in a voice that the participants will understand. For example, using heavy theoretical content without tying it to practice will put nonlicensed nursing personnel to sleep! Practicing staff nurses or advanced practice nurses expect the latest information and that the presenter is knowledgeable and current in practice. Take into consideration the size of the audience, the composition (generalists vs. specialists), and the demographics (age, ethnicity, level of education); these are important factors in order to reach the level of the audience (C. Oster, personal communication, August 18, 2009).

Timing is also crucial; when given 20 minutes, including questions and answers session, the presenter must finish on time. This requires practice, practice, and practice. On the other hand, if one is giving an hour keynote address, it is also important to time the session appropriately and not finish early, leaving the audience to wonder why they are paying to hear you! Finally, the purpose of the presentation should be foremost on your mind, and will guide the session and development of the topic.

Other things to consider when conducting your presentation include how you will "grab" the audience (C. Oster, personal communication, August 18, 2011) and get them interested in your subject. The use of body language is also important; many speakers practice in front of a mirror or with colleagues to help critique their presentation style. Simple rules apply: do face the audience, look individuals in the eye as if you are talking to them, smile, use different kinds of vocal inflection, use your hand gestures judiciously; do not read your notes or pace back and forth across the podium. At the end of the session, summarize your talk if it is a long one, and if short, give a clinical "bottom line" to allow the audience to focus on the purpose of the talk.

## Preparing Manuscripts for Publication

Consult your author guidelines for your selected journal. In some cases, a letter of inquiry to the editor can assist in establishing whether that particular journal is a good venue for your work. Texts such as *Writing for Publication in Nursing* by Oermann and Hays (2011) walk an author through the steps from selecting a journal to the publishing process. Software applications such as EndNote X4® are very helpful in formatting various journal styles and creating a reference list.

Publishers of peer-reviewed journals will send your manuscript for peer review, which can take a matter of a few months to complete. Do not be disheartened by the publishing process; it can take months and many revisions before your manuscript is actually published. The final product is worth the wait!

## ■ REFERENCES

American Association of Colleges of Nursing. (2006). *The essentials of doctoral education for advanced nursing practice.* Retrieved from http://www.aacn.nche.edu/DNP/pdf/

APRN Consensus Work Group & National Council of State Boards of Nursing APN Advisory Committee. (2008). *Consensus Model for APRN Regulation: Licensure, accreditation, certification, and education.* Chicago, IL: National Council of State Boards.

Balch, M., John, R., Reynolds, M., & Rick, C., (2011). Requisite competencies and skills for effective project planning and program management. In J. Harris, L. Roussel, S. E. Walters, & C. Dearman (Eds.), *Project planning and management a guide for CNLs, DNPs and nurse executives.* Sudbury, MA: Jones & Bartlett Learning.

Block, S. M. (1996). The dos and don'ts of poster presentations. *Biophysical Journal, 71n*(6), 3527–3529.

Cook, D. J., Mulrow, C. D., & Haynes, R. B. (1997). Systematic reviews: Synthesis of best evidence for clinical decisions. *Annals of Internal Medicine, 126*(5), 376–380.

Eldridge, C. R. (2011). Nursing science and theory: Scientific underpinnings for practice. In M. E. Zaccagnini (Ed.), *The doctor of nursing practice essentials: A new model for advanced practice nursing* (pp. 3–36). Sudbury, MA: Jones and Bartlett Publishers.

Galvan, J. L. (2009). *Writing literature reviews: A guide for students of the social and behavioral sciences* (4th ed.). Glendale, CA: Pyrczak Publishing.

Gardenier, D., Stanik-Hutt, J., & Selway, J. (2010). Point counter-point. Should DNP students conduct original research as their Capstone projects? *Journal for Nurse Practitioners, 6*(5): 364–365.

Greenhalgh, T. (1997). How to read a paper: Getting your bearings (deciding what the paper is about). *British Medical Journal, 315*(7102), 243–346.

Guyatt, G., & Rennie, D. (2002). *Users guide to the medical literature.* Chicago, IL: American Medical Association.

Kenney, J. (2006). Theory-based advanced practice nursing. In W. K. Cody (Ed.), *Philosophical and theoretical perspectives for advance nursing practice* (pp. 295–310). Sudbury, MA: Jones and Bartlett Publishers.

McElmurry, B. J., McCreary, L. L., Parke, C. G., Ramos, L., Martinex, E., Parikh, R. . . Fogelfeld, L. (2009). Implementation, outcomes, and lessons learned from a collaborative primary care health program to improve diabetes care among urban Latino populations. *Health Promotion Practice, 10*(2), 293–302.

McEwen, M. W., & Wills, E. M. (2007). *Theoretical basis for nursing* (2nd ed.). Philadelphia, PA: Lippincott, Williams & Wilkins.

McKenna, H. (1997). Choosing a theory for practice. In Hugh McKenna (Ed.), *Nursing theories and models* (pp. 158–189). New York, NY: Rutledge.

Meleis, A. I. (1997). *Theoretical nursing: Development and progress* (3rd ed.). Philadelphia, PA: Lippincott.

Melnyk, B. M., & Fineout-Overholt, E. (2011). *Evidence-based practice in nursing & healthcare: A guide to best practice* (2nd ed.). Philadelphia, PA: Wolters Kluwer Health/Lippincott Williams & Wilkins.

National Organization of Nurse Practitioner Faculties. (2007). *NONPF recommended criteria for NP scholarly projects in the practice doctorate program.* Washington DC: NONPF. Retrieved from: http://www.nonpf.com/associations/10789/files/ScholarlyProjectCriteria.pdf

Nebiu, B. (2000). *Project proposal writing*. Szenendre, Hungary: The Regional Environmental Center for Central and Eastern Europe.

Nicholas, J. (2001). *Project management for business and technology: Principles and practice* (2nd ed.). Saddle River, NJ: Prentice Hall.

Nollan, R., Fineout-Overholt, E., & Stephenson, P. (2005).Asking compelling clinical questions. In B. M. Melnyk & E. Fineout-Overholt (Eds.), *Evidence-based practice in nursing and healthcare: A guide to best practice*. Philadelphia, PA: Wolters Kluwer Health/Lippincott Williams & Wilkins.

Oermann, M. H., & Hays, J. C. (2011). *Writing for publication in nursing* (2nd ed.). New York, NY: Springer Publishing Company.

Olsen, L., Aisner, D., & McGinnis, J. M. (2007). *The Learning Healthcare System: Workshop Summary*. Washington, DC: National Academies Press. Retrieved from http://www.nap.edu/catalog.php?record_id=11903

Oster, C. A. (2011). *How to prepare a podium presentation*. Retrieved August 6, 2011, from http://www.centuraconferences.org/Podium+Presentation+Boot+Camp+Handout+3+22+Post+Final-3.pdf

Peterson, S. B. (2009). *Middle range theories: Application to nursing research* (2nd ed.). Philadelphia, PA: Walters Kluer Health/Lippincott Williams & Wilkins.

Reed, P. G. (2011). The spiral path of nursing knowledge. In P. G. Reed, *Nursing knowledge and theory innovation: Advancing the science of practice* (pp. 1–35). New York, NY: Springer Publishing Company.

Rios, P. L., Ye, C., & Thabane, L. (2010). Association between framing of the research question using the PICOT format and reporting quality of randomized control trials. *Biomedical Central Medical Research Methodology, 10*(1), 2010.

Roy, C., &. Jones, D. (2007). *Nursing knowledge development and clinical practice*. New York, NY: Springer Publishing Company.

Smith, M., &. Liehr, P. R. (2008). *Middle range theory for nursing* (2nd ed.). New York, NY: Springer Publishing Company.

Stein, K. (2006). The dos and don'ts of PowerPoint presentations. *Journal of the American Dietetic Association, 106*(11), 1745–1748.

Stillwell, S., Fineout-Overholt, E., Melnick, B., & Williamson, K. (2010). Evidence-based practice, step by step: Asking the clinical question, a key step in evidence-based practice. *The American Journal of Nursing, 110*(3), 58–61.

Terry, A. J. (2012). *Clinical research for the doctor of nursing practice*. Sudbury, MA: Jones and Bartlett Learning.

Tuckman, B. W. (2001). Developmental sequence in small groups. *Group Facilitation: A Research and Applications Journal, 3*, 66–81.

United States Department of Health and Human Resources. (2009). *Cold of Federal Regulations, Table 45 public welfare, Part 4 protection of human subjects*. Retrieved from http://www.hhs.gov/ohrp/humansubjects/guidance/45cfr46.html#46.108

West, S., King, V., Carey, T. S., Lohr, K. N., McKoy, N., Sutton, S. F., & Lux, L. (2002). *Systems to rate the evidence of evidence*. Rockville, MD: Agency for Healthcare Research and Quality.

Williams, J., & Murphy, P. (2005). Better project management: Better patient outcomes. *Nursing Management, 36*(11), 41–47.

# CHAPTER 5

# Nurse Executive and Administration Views of Capstone: System Change

Teresa Kuta Reske, Maureen Sroczynski,
Lisa Colombo, Patricia Lussier-Duynstee,
Marianne Ditomassi, Jeanette Ives Erickson, and Elaine Bridge

We invited nurse executives and administrators to write about capstones involving leadership. Authors in this chapter address how to do a systematic review, consultation, organizational analysis, program evaluation, practice change initiative, and quality improvement project. These are but a few of the possibilities that nurse executives and administrators can use in designing a capstone project that will influence nursing practice.

## ■ SYSTEMATIC REVIEWS OF THE LITERATURE

### TERESA KUTA RESKE

An approach to critical appraisal of the literature is a scholarly systematic inquiry. A *systematic review* is a scientific approach using a compilation of similar and existing studies that address a specific clinical question by way of a detailed, comprehensive search strategy and rigorous appraisal method. It is the research of research focusing on a clinical topic and to answer a specific question (Cook, Mulrow, & Haynes, 1997; Whittemore & Knafl, 2005). The DNP's investigative focus is to critically appraise available research findings through development of practice-oriented actionable nursing knowledge to improve health outcomes and initiate intraorganizational change (Dahnke & Dreher, 2011).

The purpose of a systematic review is to search primary and original research through a structured and systematic process based upon a narrowly defined topic and following the rigorous standards of primary research for clarity, rigor, and replication (Centre for Reviews and Dissemination, 2009; Cook et al., 1997). A quality systematic review requires substantial preparation and planning, including a considerable amount of effort to search the literature, appraise the study quality, and reach thoughtful, appropriate conclusions applicable to practice (Wright, Brand, Dunn, & Spindler, 2007). To advance practice knowledge, the findings from a systematic review may have an immediate implication as translational when applied with relevancy to practice, as a practice recommendation to improve outcomes, or to test a specific existing intervention or propose future nursing research (Dahnke & Dreher, 2011; Houser, 2008).

Systematic reviews are being explored in depth not only to guide and inform practice about the prevalence of problems but also to justify reimbursement in the cost effectiveness of health care interventions and services (Murphy, Robinson, & Lin, 2009). Evidence-based health care decisions require the integration of the best possible research evidence and based upon the patient and their significant family/member's values, concerns, and choices in order to improve practice (Melnyk & Fineout-Overholt, 2011).

Under the umbrella of systematic reviews is a *narrative review*. A narrative review is a summary of research evidence that lacks an explicit description of an organized methods approach to identify and critically appraise the literature. Its value may support an author's point of view as expert opinion and give a broader awareness on a particular issue with no statistical measures (Duffy, 2005).

Systematic reviews may require the doctoral student in her/his thoroughness to examine qualitative evidence or quantitative evidence. A *meta-analysis* synthesizes results of quantitative studies into a statistical summary measure that may be complex in communicating contradictory results or unmanageable amounts of research. Individual studies become the unit of analysis, rather than individual people. A meta-analysis offers two advantages: objectivity and power (Polit & Beck, 2012). From a meta-analysis, a nurse may conclude with a great deal of certainty that patient care improvements and interventions can be expected or that the findings can be used with confidence (Houser, 2008). A *meta-synthesis* is the development of over-arching themes about the meaning of human events based upon the synthesis of multiple qualitative studies and characteristics of methods that elevate evidence by the outcome. Replication of qualitative studies enhances trustworthiness and the confidence that one can generalize the results (Houser).

An *integrative review* follows the same detailed search strategy except it does not apply summary statistics to the results due to the limitations in the studies (Fineout-Overholt, O'Mathúna, & Kent, 2008). Integrative reviews are broader reviews including experimental, nonexperimental, and theoretical research to explore a wider range of goals, such as to define concepts more broadly, review evidence holistically, analyze methodology from diverse perspectives, and provide a comprehensive understanding of the human condition to change or advance practice (Houser, 2008; Melnyk & Fineout-Overholt, 2011; Whittemore & Knafl, 2005).

Systematic reviews (Figure 5.1) are observations of previous research, and similar to other retrospective observations, they are open to systematic error (publication bias and/or researcher bias) or when the influence of other variables may be related to the outcome being measured (confounding variables) (Montori, Swiontkowski, & Cook, 2003). The goals in conducting a systematic review are using an objective and unbiased, rigorous method that can be replicated; this is especially important when there is a substantive question to be used to generate practice knowledge (Salmond, 2012).

## Why Conduct One?

A systematic review is considered the strongest evidence in practice because findings provide the foundation for evidence-based nursing interventions, clinical practice guideline development, and recommendations for practice improvements (Center for Reviews and Dissemination, 2009; Holly, Salmond, & Saimbert, 2012). The complexity of nursing practice requires the search for in-depth answers through evidence to discover new relationships between concepts, nursing theory, and practice (Marrs & Lowry, 2006).

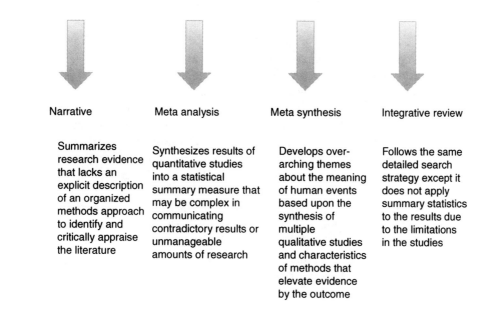

**FIGURE 5.1** Systematic reviews.

A systematic review for a doctoral nursing practice capstone will address a specific clinical question and determine its value for practice (Table 5.1).

### TABLE 5.1 Hierarchy of Steps in Performing a Systematic Review

1. Formulate the research question
2. Organize and search efficiently for the best available evidence
3. Critically assess the quality of the studies and evidence
4. Synthesize the evidence
5. Interpret the results
6. Communicate the results

## Hierarchy of Steps in Writing a Systematic Review

### Step 1—Formulate research question

To help formulate a researchable question, begin by using the *PICO(T)* format to clarify and focus interests by specifying a *patient* or *problem, intervention, comparison* intervention (if relevant), *outcome* (Glasziou, Irwig, Bain, & Colditz, 2001; Institute of Medicine, 2008) (See Chapter 4 Capstone Project). This format guides question formulation, so it is neither too broad to reach conclusions, nor too narrow to limit generalizability to populations, yet it is researchable (Whittemore & Knafl, 2005). A well-developed question is the primary building block to the methodology used to translate the research into practice (Purdy & Melwak, 2009).

- What do you expect to discover and answer from your research question?
- What systematic review is the best way to research your question?
- Do preliminary decisions need statistical integration? (Polit & Beck, 2008)

At the outset, the capstone committee will make recommendations to guide the inquiry so that the student's question is defined clearly and minimizes bias when read by two reviewers.

### Step 2—Organize and search efficiently for the best available evidence

A distinguishing characteristic of systematic reviews is describing the criteria for searching and selecting studies to avoid bias in article selection, evaluation, or reasons for elimination from consideration (Purdy & Melwak, 2009; Polit & Beck, 2012; Lin, Murphy, & Robinson, 2010; Salmond, 2012). Library electronic databases are more comprehensive when searching for and retrieving topics relevant to the subject being explored. The objective of the literature search is to be exhaustive enough to develop a comprehensive list of potentially relevant studies, and for its quality conducted by scientific review methods to minimize error and bias (McGowan & Sampson, 2005).

Accessing electronic databases may include Cochrane controlled trials register, *Cochrane Handbook for Systematic Reviews of Interventions* (Higgins & Green, 2011) (see references for web version), Best-Evidence 3, and MEDLINE, while including other databases such as PsycINFO and Cumulative Index of Nursing and Allied Health Literature. Other methods of retrieval include hand-searching bibliographies of articles within journals, conference proceedings, and unpublished and ongoing studies including searches without language restrictions (Houser, 2008).

Searches are limiting when you reach "saturation," that is, finding the identical articles and authors using different key words, or when you can no longer locate relevant evidence (Polit & Beck, 2012). Keep asking the research question during the literature search: does the evidence answer the clinical question?

### Step 3—Method to critically assess the quality of the studies and evidence

Planning the search strategy and protocol may involve a sequence of carefully constructed questions to document the search criteria, appropriateness, and validity of the results. Table 5.2 uses a table format with subentries (Houser, 2008; Melnyk & Fineout-Overholt, 2011; Wright et al., 2007) which is helpful to organize your findings. Importantly, include a rating scheme based upon the GRADE system to identify key elements in the quality, quantity, and consistency of the research evidence (high quality, moderate quality, low quality, and very low quality) to support practice recommendations (Jones, 2010).

### TABLE 5.2  Rating the Literature

Reference: journal, title, author, volume, issue, page numbers

Objective: the study objective as stated by the authors

Population: demographics of the participants in the study

Study design: type of trial or method of research

Intervention: description of the intervention

Control: description of the control group or alternative intervention

Outcome: results of the intervention and how measured, including statistics used. Were the primary studies of high methodological quality?

Comments and details regarding the study quality: is the intervention applied for a clinical practice setting?

### Step 4—Synthesizing the evidence

Data synthesis consists of tabulation of the study characteristics, quality acceptable versus not acceptable levels of research, and the statistical methods for exploring differences between studies when combining their effects (Houser, 2008). Guidelines for critiquing systematic reviews are well presented in Holly, Salmond, and Saimbert's text, *Comprehensive Systematic Review for Advanced Nursing Practice* (2012).

Synthesizing the articles and summaries involves identifying what was and was not discovered during searches and whether or not there is a connection to the research question (Purdy & Melwak, 2009). Does this mean there are no answers to the questions and further study is required? Systematic reviews may identify a variety of weaknesses during this step if a less than thorough literature search missed important studies, which may affect conclusions (Wright et al., 2007).

### Step 5—Interpreting the results

Synthesis is not just about reporting findings; it is about combining, contrasting, and interpreting a body of evidence to reach a conclusion that may be common and unique across studies (Melnyk & Fineout-Overholt, 2011). To rate the strength of the evidence and support practice recommendations, Jones (2010) developed the following evaluation table to maximize control over factors that may interfere with the validity of findings (Table 5.3).

Once studies have been defined for inclusion, synthesis occurs based upon what the ratings provide as key information concerning the quality of evidence, the magnitude of effect of the interventions examined, and the main outcomes for understanding the diverse research evidence (Duffy, 2005; Higgins & Green, 2011; Jones, 2010).

### TABLE 5.3 Evaluation Questions to Maximize Control Over Factors That May Interfere With the Validity of Findings

Were the sources critically analyzed?

Were the studies assessed for strengths and weaknesses?

Were the results similar from study to study?

How precise were the results?

Do the outcomes measured answer the research question?

Do the study questions identify if the interventions can be replicable?

Are specific directives for new research proposed?

*Source:* Jones, K. R. (2010). Rating the level, quality, and strength of the research evidence. *Journal of Nursing Care Quality, 25*(4), 304–312.

### Step 6—Communicating knowledge and results

The validity of study findings depends on how well researchers use study design principles and how different designs best match the clinical question under investigation to improve practice. High-quality systematic reviews recognize that all studies have limitations. To determine if the appraisal addresses the highest quality of studies is to justify conclusions by answering the clinical question (Melnyk & Fineout-Overholt, 2011):

- Do the recommendations include the nursing professionals for practice improvements?
- Are the benefits worth the costs and potential risks?
- Do the findings have a direct impact in quality patient care? (Duffy, 2005)

Systematic reviews can improve patient care by summarizing areas that have been adequately investigated while identifying deficient areas to focus future research efforts and resources (Wright et al., 2007). Searching evidence from a well-formulated research question will provide valuable information for practice, whereas a search based on a weaker clinical question may yield vague conclusions, limiting its applicability in practice (Onady & Raslich, 2003).

This has been an introduction to systematic review. If DNPs are going to pursue conducting a review, they are referred to Holly, Salmond, and Saimbert's (2012) text for an extensive discussion and tool kit for conducting systematic reviews. By publishing a systematic review in a professional journal, the DNP student contributes to nursing knowledge and clinical practice. If you intend to submit your review to a nursing journal, obtain the journal's author guidelines which will provide instructions and procedures for submitting your review, from how to organize your ideas and thoughts to writing style format.

## ■ CONSULTING AS CAPSTONE

### MAUREEN SROCZYNSKI

Consulting is a process in which an individual shares knowledge and expertise to assist other individuals, groups, or organizations to solve problems or achieve change. This change can be structural, procedural, or the interpersonal change that arises from the shared learning that occurs during the process of consultation. Schein (1969) was one of the earliest authors to describe the value of consultation to organizational development and change. He described both the expert and collaborative role of a consultant. In either role, the recipients of the consultant's advice are called clients and the major goal of the consultation is sustained change or improvement. The role of the consultant is determined by (1) the needs of the client, (2) the nature of the work, and (3) the skill and expertise of the consultant. Although in a position of influence, the consultant has no direct power to make changes or implement programs (Block, 2000). The consultant relies on strong interpersonal skills, technical knowledge, skills in facilitation, and the process of consultation to effectively engage with the client to create new solutions and sustain change.

### The Consultant Role

Consultation is an interactive, synchronistic process that occurs in the relationship between the client and the consultant. Depending on the nature of this relationship, the consultant role can encompass those of expert, theoretician, advocate, teacher, fact finder, adviser, and bridge builder (Block, 2000; Ciampi, 2009; Jacobson, Butterill, & Goering, 2005). The consultant works to give the client insight into what is going on within the individual, the organization, or group. For the purposes of a capstone experience, the consultant role can provide an opportunity for practical application of both theory and research to problem identification, intervention, and evaluation. Working in collaboration, the agency mentor (client) and the consultant can engage in exchange of ideas to define the problem to be studied and the outline the evidence-based approach for analysis and development of innovative solutions that benefit the organization and meet the requirements for a capstone experience.

The process of consulting involves both quantitative and qualitative analysis to fully define the problem and propose solutions. The stages of a consulting process reflect the phases of the nursing or problem-solving process and include (1) contracting, (2) assessment, (3) design, (4) implementation, and (5) follow-up (Bens, 2005; Block, 2000). Engagement with the client begins in the contracting phase, when the project is defined and the limits and boundaries of the work are established. The assessment phase involves the collection of personal information, objective data, and emerging best practices. The design phase includes a focus on the feasibility (what is possible), the viability (what is likely for sustaining the work), and the desirability (what makes sense for people) as criteria for the framing of successful, innovative outcomes (Brown, 2009). In the implementation phase, the consultant provides the client with preliminary interpretations of data or ideas for change or innovation. This phase encompasses feedback from the client, the negotiation of the ways the recommendations should be framed, and the planning of action steps for implementation. The evaluation phase focuses on the evaluation of the outcomes and can cycle back to the assessment phase for another view of the data and information used to shape the recommendations for change. Within each of the phases, the consultant focuses on developing and maintaining a collaborative, open-ended, and open-minded dialogue with the client. This dialogue fosters the trust that is essential to the mutual learning and development that occurs in the consultant/client relationship. This relationship lies at the heart of a successful and authentic consulting engagement and can be applied to a variety of settings and projects.

## Consulting as Knowledge Transfer

Knowledge transfer has been defined as the "exchange, synthesis, and ethnically sound application of knowledge within a complex system of relationships" (Jacobson et al., 2005, p. 299). From a nursing perspective, the mutual process that occurs between persons and their environments provides the framework for both the discovery and the confirmation of knowledge (Reed, 2009). The consultant both creates and disseminates knowledge and, through this process, links practice and scholarship. In the relationship between the consultant and client there is a bidirectional transfer of knowledge. Both the client and the consultant benefit from the exchange of ideas and the purposeful dialogue. The consultant role serves as a vehicle to link the theoretical and the observable to create innovative solutions.

### The nursing theory perspective

The transactions that occur between the nurse and the client in King's systems theory can be applied to the transactions that occur between the consultant and the client within a consulting engagement. According to King (Austin & Champion, 1983), the practice of nursing takes place through interpersonal relationships and purposeful interactions. King's theory is a systems approach that links the personal, interpersonal, and social systems to create an interactive framework as the foundation for goal attainment (Sieloff & Frey, 2007). The personal system refers to the individual and includes the concepts of self perception, growth and development, and time and space (King, 1981). The interpersonal system involves individuals interacting with one another and encompasses the concepts of interaction, transaction, communication, role, and stress. The third system is the social system and involves the concepts of community or society, shared goals, interests and values, a framework for interaction, relationships, and courses of action (King, 1981). These three open interacting systems serve as the conceptual framework for the theory of goal attainment. The major elements of goal attainment are found in the interpersonal system where the interaction between the nurse and the client, and their individual perceptions, judgments, and action, lead to a transaction that forms the framework for mutually agreed upon goal attainment (Austin & Champion, 1983). Application of King's theory to the relationships within a consulting engagement recognizes the unique knowledge and skills of the nurse consultant and the value of the personal, interpersonal, and social systems in the development of strong relationships and success in achieving mutually agreed upon goals in the consulting engagement.

### The scholar perspective

The expectation for DNP graduates is to act as clinical scholars and develop a new body of practice-oriented knowledge. From this perspective, the concept of evidence in the practice setting is complex and may differ from the traditional scientific explanation. This practice-based evidence has been categorized as (1) evidence of feasibility, (2) evidence of appropriateness, (3) evidence of meaningfulness, and (4) evidence of effectiveness (Dahnke & Dreher, 2011). The consultant uses expertise and a rigorous process of inquiry to generate practice-based learning for improvement in practice or educational settings. This process must be feasible, appropriate, meaningful, and effective. At the center of the process is an authentic partnership with an agency, school, or organization that is in need of change and/or innovation to improve their environment. Each consultation engagement is unique and requires a custom-designed approach. Breakthrough ideas emerge from the rigorous application of knowledge and challenging accepted patterns and trends. In the complex health care environment, nurse leaders and educators are continually searching for the creativity, innovation, and efficiency in patient care and nursing education (Fralic, 2010). The experience of consultation can provide a new generation of nurse leaders with the knowledge and skills needed to meet these challenges.

## ■ ORGANIZATIONAL ANALYSIS

### LISA COLOMBO

Organizational analyses are done to compare organizational performance against established evidence-based standards. Examples include assessing organizational culture and the impact on patient safety and quality, assessing compliance with regulatory standards such as Centers for Medicare and Medicaid (CMS) conditions of participation, or accreditation standards, such as The Joint Commission, Magnet, or Baldrige criteria. The overarching purpose of analyzing organizational performance against such established standards is to support the delivery of safe and effective care. Generally, the result of an organizational analysis identifies gaps between the organization's performance and the established standards. The results of these analyses are then used to develop organizational action plans, which are then used to drive organizational process improvement. Organizational process improvement is intended to result in desirable patient outcomes that are both safe and effective.

### Examples

An organizational assessment can be done to evaluate an organizational culture. In health care, the highest strategic order for any organization is the provision of safe and effective care. The Agency for Healthcare Research and Quality (AHRQ), as part of its goal to support a culture of patient safety and quality, sponsored the development of a survey tool for hospitals, nursing homes, and ambulatory practices. The survey tool is designed to assess aspects of an organization's culture that support quality and safety. AHRQ (2010) suggests that these tools can be used in organizations to:
- Raise staff awareness about patient safety
- Diagnose and assess the current status of patient safety culture

- Identify strengths and areas for patient safety culture improvement
- Examine trends in patient safety culture change over time
- Evaluate the cultural impact of patient safety initiatives and interventions
- Conduct internal and external comparisons

Links to the survey can be found on AHRQ's web site: http://www.ahrq.gov/qual/patientsafetyculture/

A capstone project using this survey can be structured in several different ways. In an organization that has used this survey and has baseline data, the survey could be administered for the purpose of comparing results over time. The survey is constructed with a Likert scale, which makes it adaptable to quantitative statistical analysis, specifically analysis of variance (ANOVA). This allows the organization to identify statistically significant variances from internal benchmarks. Additionally, organizations that use the AHRQ Culture of Safety Survey have access to comparative databases for all other hospitals in the United States that use the survey. If an organization wishes to understand its results as compared to both internal and external benchmarks, a multivariate analysis of variance could be used. The results of the statistical analyses can then be used to identify areas where performance improvement initiatives should be implemented to support the culture of safety and recommendations for an action plan can then be developed.

An organizational assessment can also be done to assess an organization's compliance with established evidence-based standards. In 1987, the U.S. Department of Commerce developed the Malcolm Baldrige National Quality Award, which was intended to encourage companies to adopt principles of total quality management to improve competitiveness based on quality (Borawski & Brennan, 2008). Recognition in this award program distinguishes an organization as one that has been innovative in improving products and services in a way that allows them to deliver world-class results. An organization that achieves the award is more likely to achieve quality outcomes that will support the success and sustainability of the organization (Baldrige National Quality Program, 2011).

The Baldrige Healthcare Criteria for Performance Excellence encompasses seven domains: (1) leadership; (2) strategic planning; (3) customer focus; (4) measurement, analysis, and knowledge management; (5) workforce focus; (6) process management; and (7) results. Assessment of organizational congruence with the performance elements under each of these categories is a first step in assessing an organization's compliance with the Baldrige criteria (Baldrige National Quality Program, 2011).

The National Institute for Standards and Technology, which administers the Baldrige Criteria, provides organizations with self-assessment tools for both leadership and staff (National Institute of Standards and Technology, 2004). The goal of using these two companion questionnaires is to assess if the perceptions of the staff and leadership are similar as they relate to organizational performance. Discordant perceptions help organizations to identify areas that need the most attention and for which performance improvement activities can be directed (Colombo, Perla, Carifio, Bernhardt, & Slayton, 2011). This survey is also constructed with a Likert-type scale, which makes it conducive to quantitative statistical analysis. Analysis of variance at the category level will identify which of the seven domains is most in need of attention. Further analysis at the item level can help to zero in on specific contributing factors to the discordance at the category level. All of this information can then be used to make recommendations for an action plan aimed at closing the gap between staff and leadership perceptions.

The above are two examples of organizational assessments that can be constructed as part of a DNP capstone project. There are many more opportunities for using organizational analysis in the context of a capstone project. Any time an organization aspires to comply with established evidence-based standards, an organizational analysis can be used to assess the organization's compliance. A standard gap analysis, which assesses a current state as compared to a desired future state, identifies areas when "gaps" exist and need to be filled to achieve compliance with the established standards. The gaps are areas where performance improvement initiatives can be developed to help the organization achieve the desired future state.

In the changing health care environment, where organizations strive to meet quality and safety requirements, data from organizational analyses to assess an organization's ability to deliver results have become important drivers of improvement. This makes the organizational analysis an important focus to consider for DNP students when selecting capstone projects.

## ■ PROGRAM EVALUATION

### PATRICIA LUSSIER-DUYNSTEE

Evaluation skills are essential for nurse leaders as they advocate for, support, and adjust organizational programs. Without an evaluation process, there is no way to see if what one set out to do was ever accomplished. An evaluation answers the questions, "Did we do what we wanted to do?" and "Can we do this in a different way?" Evaluations provide feedback for improvement and measure success. Nurse leaders use evaluation to determine program effectiveness in delivery, efficiency in time and money, target group coverage and bias, and program improvement.

There was a time when it was enough to fund and start programs that simply made sense based on the norms of the time. Programs were interventions that leaders *thought* should work. Evaluations were not part of the planning process. Without evaluation, it was individual experiences and values that measured the worth of the project, neither of which was objective or necessarily valid. Funded and long-lived programs *seemed* useful and felt like the right thing to do. The risk of wasting time and money was high.

Purposeful, well-constructed program evaluations gather the evidence that allows improvements in program design and eliminates financial waste. The risk of wasting time and money and not meeting goals is reduced as evaluation design is included in program planning and as programs are evaluated for efficiency and effectiveness.

### Types of Evaluators

Evaluators may come from inside or outside of an organization, and they may be involved during the program planning process or called in at a later time, during implementation of a program. Insiders and outsiders have their own advantages and challenges.

#### Inside evaluators
Inside evaluators may have a clear, valid understanding of what the goals of a project are, but may be already biased and will need to be certain that the evaluation design has objective measurements, reducing or eliminating the influence of that bias. Determining clear goals and objectives upfront during the planning process allows the inside evaluator to have the best possible objective process of evaluation.

### Outside evaluators

Outside evaluators consult on programs. While it is most ideal for outside evaluators to be involved in the planning process, they may be called in once a program is up and running. The first step in focusing the evaluation is gaining an understanding of *who* is asking for the evaluation. Interest in evaluating an ongoing program comes either from within or outside of a program. The organization may want to question a program's goals, improve a program, or document need. An outside funder may want justification of program costs. The outside evaluator determines the usefulness of the evaluation and its purpose—what the program/ organizations want to learn through an evaluation process. As a true consultant, the outside evaluator *listens* to the interests of the program and determines the best evaluation design and the best measures of the desired objectives. The program objectives determine evaluation design. Caution avoids applying a favorite design for evaluation whether or not it fits the program and its objectives.

## Types of Evaluations

Program evaluations can be formative or summative, that is, identifying process or determining outcomes. Formative evaluation monitors the implementation of a program. It answers the question "Are we doing what we said we would do?" and relies on identifying and monitoring the activities that are integral to the program and the level of participation of the intended target population. Process evaluations explain if and how a program should be adjusted.

Summative evaluations focus on the effectiveness, efficiency, and impact of the program. Unexpected outcomes, both desired and undesired, may be uncovered.

Use of theory in the project design helps to define the parameters of an evaluation. But there is oftentimes not a theory present in ongoing projects. With or without theory, a logic model can be applied to determine the expectations and the measurements of both process and outcome. Logic models provide clarity and usefulness in both process and outcome evaluations of programs.

> The program logic model is defined as a picture of how your organization does its work—the theory and assumptions underlying the program. A program logic model links outcomes (both short- and long-term) with program activities/ processes and the theoretical assumptions/principles of the program. (W. K. Kellogg Foundation, 2004, p. III)

> A logic model draws a visual picture of what a program is all about. It defines the resources/inputs, the activities, the outputs, outcomes, and impact of a program (W. K. Kellogg Foundation).

There are three approaches to logic models: theory, activities, and outcomes. When a logic model is used in the program planning process, it focuses the evaluation and leads to a systematic approach to implementation and a rationale for evaluation. A logic model to monitor implementation offers insight into activities and allows for program adjustment to better meet the expected outcomes. Evaluations that utilize an outcome and impact approach model clearly outline the expected results of a program that emerge from planned resourced activities (W. K. Kellogg, 2004).

Guba and Lincoln (1992) encourage stakeholder participation in designing an evaluation, to ensure that the evaluation is meaningful. Stakeholders may be varied and multiple, creating a challenge for the evaluator to fully appreciate who is invested in the program and the evaluation results (Rossi and Freeman, 1993).

Gathering and generating data for evaluation may utilize both quantitative and qualitative methods. Both types are useful in providing rigor and validity to the evaluation. It is essential that the methods utilized are reflective of the evaluation questions rather than the evaluator's expertise. Formative data may come from qualitative methods and are useful in redesigning programs. Impact data are generated by quantitative methods and suggest impact of the program (Rossi and Freeman, 1993). There may be limitations in the methodology due to organizational resources. Lack of financial resources for large surveys, staffing limitations for gathering data, and availability of data may impact what methods are used for gathering and generating data. Nurse leaders must be creative in determining the most useful and feasible evaluation design that clearly answers the questions, "Did we do what we said we did?" and "Did it matter?"

## ■ PRACTICE CHANGE INITIATIVE: EVALUATION/APPLICATION OF A NEW PRACTICE MODEL

### MARIANNE DITOMASSI AND JEANETTE IVES ERICKSON

In today's health care environment, ensuring that the professional practice environment for nurses and other members of the health care team is supportive and responsive to clinicians is more important than ever. In fact, today's nurse leaders are poised to chart a new direction for nursing. The articulation or refinement of a professional practice model provides the roadmap for practice to drive patient and family-focused outcomes and provides a rich area for study.

A professional practice model provides a framework that allows nurses to clearly articulate their contributions. With a well-designed framework, nurses feel connected within the context of their own practice and the work of the institution, and can establish specific strategies and goals. With a framework, nurses can better plan for and manage change. The model gathers the pieces of nurses' contributions and fits them together to reveal the whole or essence of nursing at a given institution. It is an effective strategy for making the often-invisible work of nurses visible.

The importance of a professional practice model has been well known since the first Magnet Hospital Study (McClure, Poulin, Sovie, & Wandelt, 1983) that articulated the salient elements of professional practice as autonomy, control over practice, and collaborative relationships with physicians. At the Massachusetts General Hospital, our model (Figure 5.2) builds on that foundation and incorporates additional research on collaborative decision making, clinical recognition and advancement, care delivery models, research and evidence-based practice, innovation, professional development, and the importance of a narrative culture.

To evaluate our professional practice model over time, we developed and administered the Staff Perceptions of the Professional Practice Environment survey (RPPE) to nurses and clinicians throughout Patient Care Services every 12 to 18 months since 1997. This tool provides an assessment of eight organizational characteristics (Table 5.4) determined to be important to nurse and clinician satisfaction, allows clinicians the opportunity to have a voice in setting the strategic direction for Patient Care Services, trends key information, and identifies key opportunities to improve the environments for clinical practice.

This psychometrically sound tool has been implemented locally, nationally, and internationally (Ives Erickson, Duffy, Fitzmaurice, Ditomassi, & Jones, 2004; Ives Erickson, Duffy, Ditomassi, & Jones, 2009). The MGH survey results and the data from other organizations

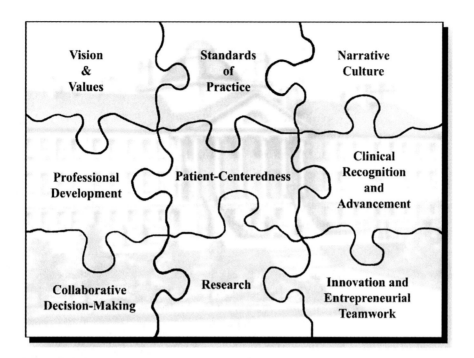

**FIGURE 5.2**  MGH professional practice model—2006.

that have administered the survey provide a rich opportunity for data mining and further study, as illustrated by the following two capstone projects.

The first example focuses on the student's curiosity about how selected demographic variables and organizational characteristics as measured by the RPPE scale and the additional characteristics measured by the Practice Environment Scale of the Nursing Work Index (PES-NWI) by Lake (2002) explain MGH nurses' work satisfaction. To accomplish this, the 2010 Staff Perceptions Survey was augmented to include the PES-NWI scale, so data were simultaneously collected for both scales to answer the research question: To what extent do the demographic variables of age, years in the profession, and years at MGH and the RPPE organizational characteristics of autonomy, control over practice, RN-MD relations, communication, teamwork, conflict management, internal work motivation, and cultural sensitivity, plus the PES-NWI organizational characteristics of nurse participation in hospital affairs, nursing foundations for quality of care, nurse manager ability, leadership and support of nurses, staffing, and resource adequacy, and collegial nurse–physician relations explain registered nurses' work satisfaction? These variables are measured by using a one-item, four-point Likert scale asking respondents to rate their overall sense of satisfaction working on their primary unit. We anticipate that the results of this capstone project will provide key information about the influence of demographics and the organizational characteristics of both the RPPE and PES-NWI scales on MGH nurses' sense of overall work satisfaction, and will inform future evaluation processes of MGH's professional practice environment.

The student of the second capstone project example is particularly interested in the Chief Nurse's role in improving the environment in which health care is delivered. According to Adams and Ives Erickson (2011), the Chief Nurse must influence others to achieve positive patient/organizational outcomes. In short, the Chief Nurse is accountable for the professional practice environment. In this study, the student is not only asking questions of the

**TABLE 5.4 MGH Patient Care Services, Organizational Characteristics, and Definitions**

| Organizational Characteristic | Definition | Source |
|---|---|---|
| Autonomy | The quality or state of being self-governing and exercising professional judgment in a timely fashion | Aiken, Sochalski, & Lake (1997) |
| Clinical–physician relations | Relations with physicians that facilitate exchange of important clinical information | Aiken, Sochalski, & Lake (1997) |
| Control over practice | Sufficient intraorganizational status to influence others and to deploy resources when necessary for good patient care | Aiken, Havens, & Sloan (2000) |
| Communication | The degree to which patient care information is related promptly to the people who need to be informed through open channels of communication | Shortell, Rousseau, Gillies, Devers, & Simons (1991) |
| Teamwork/leadership | A conscious activity aimed at achieving unity of effort in the pursuit of shared objectives | Zimmerman, Shortell, Rousseau, Duffy, Gillies, Knaus, et al. (1993) |
| Conflict management/ handling disagreements | The degree to which managing conflict is addressed using a problem-solving approach | Zimmerman, Shortell, Rousseau, Duffy, Gillies, Knaus, et al. (1993) |
| Internal work motivation | Self-generated motivation completely independent of external factors such as pay, supervision, and coworkers | Hackman & Oldham (1976) |
| Cultural sensitivity | A set of attitudes, practices, and/or policies that respects and accepts cultural differences | The Cross Cultural Health Care Program |

MGH RPPE data, but also looking at what the RPPE data collected in other national and international sites tell us about the transferability of the RPPE tool into practice sites outside of MGH. Thus, the following three questions will be studied:

*(1)* To what extent do the demographic variables of age, highest level of earned education, gender, and the eight organizational characteristics of the RPPE explain work satisfaction for nurses at MGH?

*(2)* To what extent, if any, is there a difference in responses from the various sites utilizing the RPPE?

*(3)* To what extent, if any, do demographics influence the responses to the eight characteristics of the RPPE across practice sites?

Responses to these three questions will enhance the nurse leaders' understanding of the key levers involved in improving the work environment to ensure it is supportive of the nurse–patient relationship and addresses any barriers to quality and safety.

Lastly, both of these capstone projects will contribute to the literature and nurses' understanding of essential elements of a professional practice environment and resultant models. The study results will also advance the ultimate goal of developing a common definition of "professional practice environment," which is lacking in the literature.

## ■ QUALITY-IMPROVEMENT PROJECT

### ELAINE BRIDGE

The IOM report, *Crossing the Quality Chasm* (IOM, 2001), raised national awareness of concerns about the quality of health care and called for providers to refocus and recommit to six dimensions of quality care, including that the care be safe, effective, patient-centered, and efficient. This report was considered a call to action for health care providers across the country. Additionally, the report emphasized the importance of having senior nurse leaders placed in key leadership positions, thus providing nursing with the opportunity to participate in and influence quality decisions impacting patient care.

Following the release of the IOM report, the AHRQ (2003) released a set of patient-safety indicators and identified that nurses are key to ensuring that patient care is of the highest quality and is provided in the safest environment. Subsequently, the IHI proposed that there be a transformation of health care leadership with a renewed commitment to organizational improvement in order to accomplish the challenge of delivering ideal care set forth by the IOM (IHI, 2006).

Meanwhile, the term *nurse-sensitive indicator,* which correlates to nurse-sensitive care outcomes, was redefined by Needleman, Buerhaus, Mattke, Stewart, and Zelevinsky (2001) as patient outcomes which are potentially sensitive to nursing care. Nurses, whose central role is to provide patient surveillance and intervention, are believed to have a unique opportunity to impact patient outcomes. It is reasonable, therefore, to conclude that nurse leaders have significant responsibility and opportunity to influence patient care and patient outcomes as they lead and direct frontline staff.

What is the role of the DNP-prepared nurse leader in these quality efforts? As nurse leaders, we review and reflect on the overall nursing practice continuously within our domains of practice. We have an over-arching goal of ensuring the delivery of the highest quality patient care. We are obligated and accountable to ensure that the practice environment fosters the delivery of that high-quality, safe, effective patient care.

According to AACN, DNP study requires the student to identify a practice-oriented final project in order to achieve the goal of the practice-focused program of study (AACN, 2006). It follows that the focus of a capstone project might be to explore an aspect of quality improvement while considering how to translate, evaluate, and apply new science to practice.

Quality improvement capstone topics might include evaluating the environment, human factors, and/or individual competence against patient outcomes. Exploring the practice environment may uncover structural barriers to care. It may also uncover systems issues that prevent practitioners from achieving desired patient outcomes. Exploring human factors related to patient outcomes might include evaluating interpersonal communication, the use/adoption of technology, or issues related to health care hierarchy. As the complexity of the practice environment increases and clinicians are challenged to maintain skills and knowledge required to care for complex patient populations, studying or evaluating individual practioner competence as it relates to patient outcomes might also be considered.

Case studies, analyses of trended data, recurrent complaints/concerns, or less quantitative issues such as those that causes you to wonder "What was he/she thinking?" might be the burning question you seek to answer. Although quality improvement is every practitioner's obligation and evidence as the basis for practice has become the norm in health care, the nurse leader is ultimately accountable and responsible for ensuring that safe, high-quality, evidence-based care is provided to every patient.

As a nurse leader, there comes a point when an outcome trend no longer makes intuitive sense; at such time, you might feel at a loss to understand how poor outcomes occur, sometimes repeatedly. When that question arises, the leader needs to explore the circumstances and develop interventions to improve outcomes. Understanding how to study such a question is an essential skill of nurse leaders. For a doctorally prepared nurse leader, the obligation and responsibility to explore quality issues will grow in importance. This is the essence of clinical scholarship defined by Palmer (1986) as "knowledge derived from analysis and synthesis of observations of clients/patients" (p. 318).

## ■ REFERENCES

Adams, J. M., & Ives Erickson, J. (2011). Understanding influence: An exemplar applying the Adams influence model (AIM) in nurse executive practice. *Journal of Nursing Administration, 41(4),* 186–192.

Agency for Healthcare Research and Quality. (2010, November). *Surveys on patient safety culture.* Retrieved January 2, 2011, from http://www.ahrq.gov/qual/patientsafetyculture

Agency for Healthcare Research and Quality (2003). *AHRQ quality indicators—Guide to patient safety indicators.* Rockville, MD: Agency for Healthcare Research and Quality. Retrieved from http://www.qualityindicators.ahrq.gov/psi_overview.htm

Aiken, L., Havens, D., & Sloane, D. (2000). The Magnet nursing services recognition program: A comparison of two groups of Magnet hospitals. *American Journal of Nursing, 100*(3), 26–36.

Aiken, L., Sochalski, J., & Lake, E. (1997). Studying outcomes of organizational change in health services. *Medical Care, 35*(suppl.)11, NS6–NS18.

American Association of Colleges of Nursing (AACN). (2006). *Essentials of doctoral education in advanced nursing practice.* Washington, DC: Author.

Austin, K. A., & Champion, V. L. (1983). King's theory for nursing: Explication and evaluation. In Chin (Ed.), *Advances in nursing theory development* (pp. 49–61). Rockville, MD: Aspen.

Baldrige National Quality Program. (2011). *2010–2011 health care criteria for performance Excellence* [Brochure]. Retrieved August 22, 2011, from www.quality.nist.gov/healthcare_criteria.html

Bens, I. (2005). *Advanced facilitation strategies: Tools and techniques to master difficult situations.* San Francisco, CA: Jossey-Bass.

Block, P. (2000). *Flawless consulting: A guide to getting your expertise used.* San Francisco, CA: Jossey-Basss/Pfeiffer.

Borawski, P., & Brennan, M. (2008). The Baldrige model: An integrated and aligned systems approach to performance excellence. *Journal of Association Leadership.* Retrieved from http://www.asaecenter.org/Resources/JALArticleDetail.cfm?ItemNumber=35717

Botwinick, L., Bisognano, M., & Haraden, C. (2006). *Leadership guide to patient safety.* IHI Innovation Series White Paper. Cambridge, MA: Institute for Healthcare Improvement. Retrieved from www.IHI.org

Brown, T. (2009). *Change by design.* New York, NY: Harper Collins.

Centre for Reviews and Dissemination. (2009). *Systematic reviews: CRD's guidance for undertaking reviews in health care.* Retrieved from http://www.york.ac.uk/inst/crd/SysRev/!SSL!/WebHelp/SysRev3.htm

Ciampi, F. (2009). Exploring knowledge creation pathways in advanced management consulting. In A. Buono (Ed.), *Emerging trends & issues in management consulting: Consulting as a Janus-faced reality* (pp. 3–40). Charlotte, NC: Information Age Publishing.

Colombo, L., Perla, R., Carifio, J., Bernhardt, J., & Slayton, V. (2011). Organizational and leadership perceptions assessment: Opportunities and challenges using the Baldrige companion surveys. *Journal for healthcare quality, 33*(1), 14–21.

Committee on Quality of Health Care in America, Institute of Medicine. (2001). *Crossing the quality chasm: A new health system for the 21st century.* Washington, DC: National Academies Press.

Cook, D. J., Mulrow, C. D., & Haynes, R. B. (1997). Systematic reviews: Synthesis of the best evidence for clinical decisions. *Annals of Internal Medicine, 126*(5), 389–391.

Dahnke, M. D., & Dreher, H. M. (2011). *Philosophy of science for nursing practice: Concepts and application.* New York, NY: Springer Publishing Company.

Duffy, M. E. (2005). Systematic reviews: Their role and contribution to evidence-based practice. *Clinical Nurse Specialist, 19*(1), 15–17.

Fineout-Overholt, E., O'Mathúna, D. P., & Kent, B. (2008). How systematic reviews can foster evidence-based clinical decisions. *Worldviews on Evidence-Based Nursing, 5*(1), 45–48.

Fralic, M. (2010). Contemporary nurse executive practice: One framework, one dozen cautions. *Nursing Clinics of North America, 1*, 33–38.

Glasziou, P., Irwig, L., Bain, C., & Colditz, G. (2001). *Systematic reviews in health care: A practical guide.* Cambridge, UK: Cambridge University Press.

Guba, E. F., & Lincoln, Y. S. (1992). *Effective evaluation: Improving the usefulness of evaluation results through responsive and naturalistic approaches.* San Francisco, CA: Jossey Bass.

Hackman, J., & Oldman, G. (1976). Motivation through the design of work: Test of a theory. *Organization of Behavioral Human Performance, 16*(2), 250–279.

Higgins, J. P. T., & Green, S. (eds.). (2011). *Cochrane handbook for systematic reviews of interventions* Version 5.1.0 [updated March 2011]. The Cochrane Collaboration, 2011. Retrieved from http://www.cochrane-handbook.org/

Holly, C., Salmond, S. W., & Saimbert, M. K. (2012). *Comprehensive systematic review for advanced nursing practice.* New York, NY: Springer Publishing Company.

Houser, J. (2008). *Nursing research: Reading, using, and creating evidence.* Sudbury, MA: Jones and Bartlett Publishers.

Institute of Medicine. (2008). *Knowing what works in health care: A roadmap for the nation.* Washington, DC: National Academies Press.

Ives Erickson, J., Duffy, M., Fitzmaurice, J., Ditomassi, M., & Jones, D. (2004). Development and psychometric evaluation of the professional practice environment (PPE) scale. *Journal of Nursing Scholarship, 6*(3), 279–285.

Ives Erickson, J., Duffy, M., Ditomassi, M., & Jones, D. (2009). Psychometric evaluation of the revised professional practice environment (RPPE) scale. *Journal of Nursing Administration, 39*(5), 236–243.

Jacobsen, N., Butterill, D., & Goering, P. (2005) Consulting as a strategy for knowledge transfer. *Milbank Quarterly, 83*(2), 299–321.

Jones, K. R. (2010). Rating the level, quality, and strength of the research evidence. *Journal of Nursing Care Quality, 25*(4), 304–312.

King, I. (1981). *A theory for nursing: Systems, concepts, process.* New York, NY: John Wiley & Sons.

Lake, E. T. (2002). Development of the practice environment scale of the nursing work index. *Research in Nursing & Health, 25*, 176–188.

Lin, S. H., Murphy, S. L. & Robinson, J. C. (2010). Facilitating evidence-based practice: Process, strategies, and resources. *The American Journal of Occupational Therapy, 64*(1), 164–171.

Marrs, J., & Lowry, L. W. (2006). Nursing theory and practice: Connecting the dots. *Nursing Science Quarterly, 19*(1), 44–50.

McClure, M. L., Poulin, M. A., Sovie, M. D., & Wandelt, M. (1983). *Magnet hospitals: Attraction and retention of professional nurses.* Washington, DC: American Nurses Publishing.

McGowan, J., & Sampson, M. (2005). Systematic reviews need systematic reviewers. *Journal of the Medical Library Association, 93*(1), 74–80.

Melnyk, B. M., & Fineout-Overholt, E. (2011). *Evidence-based practice in nursing and healthcare* (2nd ed.). Philadelphia, PA: Lippincott Williams & Wilkins.

Montori, V. M., Swiontkowski, M. F., & Cook, D. J. (2003). Methodological issues in systematic reviews and meta-analyses. *Clinical Orthopaedics and Related Research, 413,* 43–54.

Murphy, S. L., Robinson, J. C., & Lin, S. H. (2009). Conducting systematic reviews to informoccupational therapy practice. *The American Journal of Occupational Therapy, 63*(3), 363–368.

National Institute of Standards and Technology. (2004). *Are we making progress as leaders (Brochure).* Retrieved August 22, 2011, from www.baldrige.nist.gov/Progress_leaders.htm

Needleman, J., Buerhaus, P., Mattke, S., Stewart, M., Zelevinsky, K. (2001). *Nurse staffing and patient outcomes in hospitals.* Final Report: US Department of Health and Human Services, Health Resources and Services Administration Contract. Retrieved from 10.1056/NEJMsa012247346/22/1715 [pii]

Onady, G. M., & Raslich, M. A. (2003). Evidence-based medicine: Asking the answerable question (question templates as tools). *Pediatrics in Review, 24*(8), 265–268.

Palmer, I. S. (1986). The emergence of clinical scholarship as a professional imperative. *Journal of Professional Nursing, 2*(5), 318–325.

Polit, D. F., & Beck, C. T. (2008). *Nursing research: Principles and methods* (8th ed.). Philadelphia, PA: Lippincott Williams & Wilkins.

Purdy, I. B., & Melwak, M. A. (2009). Implementing evidence-based practice: A mantra for change. *Journal of Prenatal Neonatal Nursing, 23*(3), 263–269.

Reed, P. (2009). Nursing reformation: Historical reflections and philosophic foundations. In P. Reed & N. Crawford Shearer (Eds.), *Perspectives on nursing theory* (pp. 100–107). Philadelphia, PA: Wolters Kluwer/Lippincott Williams & Wilkins.

Rossi, P. H., & Freeman, H. E. (1993). *Evaluation—A systematic approach.* Newbury Park, CA: Sage Publications.

Salmond, S. W. (2012). Steps in the systematic review process. In C. Holly, S. W. Salmond, & M. K. Saimbert (Eds.), *Comprehensive systematic review for advanced nursing practice* (pp. 13–31). New York, NY: Springer Publishing Company.

Schien, E. (1969) *Process consultation: Its role in organization development.* Reading, MA: Addison-Wesley.

Sieloff, C. L., & Frey, M. (Eds.). (2007). *Middle range theory development using King's conceptual system.* New York, NY: Springer Publishing.

W.K. Kellogg Foundation. (2004). *Evaluation handbook.* Battle Creek, MI: Author.

Whittemore, R., & Knafl, K. (2005). The integrative review: Updated methodology. *Journal of Advanced Nursing, 52*(5), 546–553.

Wright, R., Brand, R., Dunn, W., & Spindler, K. (2007). How to write a systematic review. *Clinical Orthopaedics and Related Research, 455,* 23–29. Retrieved from http://www.externarelationer.adm.gu.se/digitalAssets/1273/1273271_How_to_write_a_systemaic.pdf

Zimmerman, J., Shortell, S., Rousseau, D., Duffy, J., Gillies, R., Knaus, W., ... Draper, E. (1993). Improving intensive care observations based on organizational case studies in nine intensive care units. *Critical Care Medicine, 21*(10), 1443–1551.

## ■ APPENDIX

Supportive websites when preparing to conduct and write your systematic review:

Cornell University. (2011). Critically analyzing information sources. Retrieved from http://olinuris.library.cornell.edu/ref/research/skill26.htm

George Washington University. (2006). Preparing scholarly reviews of the literature: A webtorial. Retrieved from http://www.gwu.edu/~litrev/

Dalhousie University. (2010). Paraphrasing. Retrieved from http://academicintegrity.dal.ca/Student%20Resources/Paraphrasing.php

### Textbooks

Salmond, S. W. (2012). Steps in the systematic review process. In C. Holly, S. W. Salmond, & M. K. Saimbert (Eds.), *Comprehensive systematic review for advanced nursing practice* (pp. 13–31). New York, NY: Springer Publishing Company.
Webb, C., & Row, B. (2007). *Reviewing research evidence for nursing practice: Systematic reviews/edition 1*. New York, NY: John Wiley and Sons.

# CHAPTER 6

# The Capstone Project: Students' Experiences

Susan Jacoby, Judith L. Webb,
Nancy Ann Kelly, Daisy Goodman, and Richard Ahern

This chapter centers on the student experience of the capstone project. It is written by former students in a variety of advanced practice roles, who were able to talk about the challenges and obstacles they faced and the mentoring and progress they made throughout the course of their doctoral work. Their work exemplifies *clinical scholars who do practice inquiry to produce practice knowledge* (see Chapter 3). They came into the doctoral program with *burning questions* from their practices, honed their ideas in various courses, and strategized with classmates, colleagues, and mentors to develop their projects. These examples demonstrate how doctors of nursing practice (DNPs) are changing the face of nursing practice.

## ■ CERTIFIED NURSE MIDWIFE LOOKS AT OBSTETRICAL CARE FOR WOMEN WITH INFIBULATION

### SUSAN JACOBY

In my clinical practice as a certified nurse midwife, I realized that there was a critical need to improve the childbirth experiences of African immigrant women who were infibulated (the most severe form of female genital cutting). One particular experience crystallized this need.

I was on call for obstetrical triage, when a young Somali woman was brought to the maternity unit by ambulance in advanced labor. When I arrived in the patient's room, I could see that she was still infibulated and that the scar tissue was preventing the delivery of her baby. She was thrashing around wildly on the bed and did not have anyone with her for support or to interpret. She appeared to be in a dissociative state of fear and pain, with her eyes rolling back in her head and she was trying to escape over the back of the headboard. Her baby's heart rate was in the 80s, a terminal bradycardia.

I explained to her, through the telephone interpreter, that I needed to cut her scar tissue to open her vagina and allow the baby to be born. I explained that I would numb the skin so she would have no pain, but that I needed to deliver the baby as soon as possible due to the low heart rate. As I approached her, she lashed out with her leg and kicked me in the stomach. I told the nurse to get the physician stat, and when she arrived, she immediately sized up the situation, climbed on top of the woman, and told her "I'm going to cut you," and proceeded to do so. I then delivered the baby, who needed to be resuscitated. I was shaking as I delivered the placenta because the situation had been so traumatic with everyone yelling, from the interpreter to the nurses and the physician, and I was really worried about her baby. However, the woman was calm once she was no longer in pain.

The next day, I interviewed both the nurses and physicians about their birth experiences with women with infibulation. Everyone had a different traumatic birth story to tell, and the most expressive of them literally threw up his hands and walked away, saying, "What are you going to do? They're all like that!" Well, I thought, someone should do something! We as obstetric health care providers must do a better job or suffer dire consequences.

This experience inspired my *burning question*, how to provide culturally appropriate maternity care for women with infibulation, and guided my scholarly work and research for the next 2 years. I wanted to try to understand what the experience of childbirth is like for them, to try to see it through their eyes.

## Cultural and Institutional Obstacles

Challenges I faced while completing my capstone included both institutional and cultural difficulties. Resources for immigrant women in general are lacking in scope, and the needs are great. One of the critical parts of providing good care is having a female interpreter present for every prenatal visit. This was challenging, as there are many more male interpreters than female. It is difficult to have an antepartum discussion through a male interpreter about deinfibulation when cultural mores prohibit this. I learned that the staff and administration needed to be educated about the culture of the Somali immigrants and the patients needed to be educated about the difficulty in having a vaginal birth while still infibulated.

## Step-by-Step Progression to a Completed Capstone

The DNP program allows for exploration of a scholarly question in a step-wise fashion. As each course unfolds, there is an orderly progression of knowledge learned by the student, so that by the end of the program, students have already written and refined their chosen topics. This logical progression allowed me to explore my research question thoroughly from conception, background, review of the literature, theoretical framework, implementation of the educational program, and statistical analysis of the final product. The final culmination was my capstone project entitled *Certified Nurse Midwives' Obstetrical Management of Women with Type III Female Genital Mutilation/Cutting (FGM/C)* (Jacoby, 2009).

Nursing theory taught me the importance of using a theoretical framework for my capstone. Nursing research helped me to frame my study and learn how to research my topic. From epidemiology to health care economics and statistics, each course was tailored to assist in the exploration of my chosen course of research. The more I learned, the more my project came together into a cohesive scholarly work.

My capstone was designed to help midwives learn to care for Somali women with type III infibulation in a culturally competent manner. I combined a didactic educational course with simulation technology using pelvic models into a one-day workshop, educating midwives to provide culturally appropriate care and deinfibulate type III FGM/C scar tissue during second-stage labor. Using a comparison measure of confidence, I was able to assess the midwives' self-reported confidence in caring for infibulated women, both before and after the educational session. This approach uses translational research to guide evidence-based practice. Ultimately, the goal is to provide culturally competent maternity services for infibulated women and to prevent obstetric trauma for both mothers and babies.

## ■ PALLIATIVE CARE NURSE PRACTITIONER CONCERNED WITH THE CARE OF PATIENTS' LOVED ONES

### JUDITH L. WEBB

My clinical practice as a palliative care nurse practitioner stirred many clinical questions and launched my inquiry into a capstone project. My patients were in the terminal stages of illness, and I developed a deep commitment to alleviation of their suffering at the end of their lives. My work usually included the people around the patients. I often initiated discussions about end-of-life decision making with the families and loved ones of my patients. As I worked more and more with them, I heard similar themes emerge. They had had experiences in the past—and sometimes many years before—that still caused them varying degrees of emotional distress. It was not uncommon for me to hear comments such as:

> My mother died 20 years ago and I still wonder if I made the right decisions for her.

> My brother died 2 years ago and I can't get the picture of his pained expressions out of my mind.

> I took care of my elderly neighbor and I am haunted by the rattling sounds of her breathing.

> I know he didn't want heroic measures, but I don't know if a feeding tube was heroic.

My clinical questions surrounded these frequent observations of long-term distress and uncertainty among the loved ones of the dying. My practice was aimed at relieving the suffering of my patients. Yet, I realized that the suffering of their loved ones was not as well understood. In particular, I wondered if the experience of making end-of-life decisions compounded their suffering.

### Challenges of an Inaccessible Population

I had to overcome several obstacles as I refined my clinical question, but the most formidable obstacle I faced was access to the population I wanted to study. Technically, the patients in my clinical practice were the terminally ill. However, I interacted on a daily basis with many family members and friends of my patients, and that was the population I hoped to study. I weighed several methods of reaching the loved ones of deceased patients. Patient health records did not always capture information about the loved ones. Typical retrospective reviews of the health records of deceased patients would not consistently identify this population. If I relied on the patient record, I would likely have access only to the next of kin. And, once the patient had died, often the address and phone numbers were no longer accurate. This was especially true over long periods of time. My clinical observations had suggested that the apparent distress I had noticed endured for years and often for decades.

Not only did I want to study loved ones, I wanted to focus on a subset within that group. I wanted to know more about end-of-life decision makers. I considered a variety of means to contact decision makers by finding the people named as health care proxies in the patient records, but those documents were also inadequate and would have required a lengthy review. Further, even if I had discovered a way to locate people who had made end-of-life decisions for others, I had another confounding problem. How would I determine if their level of distress was different from any other person who had experience the death of a loved one? My clinical questions seemed unanswerable.

## Reaching a Population Through Social Networks

Through the progression of courses that lead to the capstone project, I had anchored my questions in theory, identified a population, and examined various clinical research methods. My independent study in a mentored practicum channeled my final steps. In the process of refining a methodology with my mentor, I realized that I needed to maneuver away from health records and look for access to my population in the village streets. I decided to use social networks and apply an informatics strategy. This was the turning point in my journey toward answering my clinical question.

With the guidance of my mentor and my committee, I constructed an online survey using a previously validated instrument to measure self-identified distress following the loss of a loved one. I posted the link to the survey on Facebook. Within 2 weeks, over 300 people responded to my survey. To my surprise and delight, I had gathered twice the needed sample. And, more importantly, I had reached respondents who were both decision makers and non-decision makers. I was then able to compare these two groups statistically.

My capstone project shed light on this rather inaccessible population. In clinical practice, I am now able to apply the knowledge gained from my capstone project to better care for loved ones of the terminally ill, especially those who make end-of-life decisions for others. I was able to share my findings at two national conferences and also in a nursing publication (Webb & Guarino, 2011).

## ■ GERIATRIC NURSE PRACTITIONER CONCERNED WITH PATIENT SAFETY DURING HANDOFF COMMUNICATION

### NANCY ANN KELLY

The basis for my capstone project was planted in my experience as a geriatric nurse practitioner (GNP). In my practice, in both skilled nursing facilities and acute care, I realized that communication between providers in these settings was inconsistent. At times, crucial information was lost when patients transitioned from one level of care to another.

As a GNP, my experience included primary care, skilled nursing facility transitional care, skilled nursing long-term care, and acute care. When I worked in the skilled nursing facilities, I did my best to ensure communication between settings. Still, communication between settings was inconsistent and at times, dangerous. This was evident in discrepancies between medication lists as patients were transferred from one level of care to another. Patients' baseline cognitive and functional statuses were often poorly communicated. It seemed that patients with hearing deficits were mistakenly assumed to be "confused," and bed rest was a commonly listed functional level. Without knowing a patient's medications or functional and cognitive status, the risk for medical complications and prolonged hospital stay was high because the patient's baseline status was not known. Communication remedies, such as calling from the acute setting to a nursing facility, were fraught with challenges. A call to the nursing facility often resulted in reaching someone who was unfamiliar with the patient. My concern about ineffective communication gave me the impetus for my capstone project.

## Challenge: Narrowing a Broad Topic

I met with my academic advisor on the first day of the program with a vague idea that my capstone would focus on transitions of care from skilled nursing facilities to acute care. With that vague idea, I chose my capstone topic. In my next meeting with her, I discussed the need for communication between care settings, the possible benefits of improved communication to decrease avoidable hospital admissions, the cost savings in preventing hospitalizations, and, finally, how length of stay would be decreased with improved understanding of a patient's baseline functional and cognitive status. Her response: "Whoa!" That wasn't exactly what I wanted to hear, thinking I had the best-laid plan for a superior quality improvement project with implications across all settings. The problem was that I had focused too widely on my topic.

## Mentorship Helped Refine the Capstone

With support and guidance from my advisor, professors, and colleagues, refinement of my burning question took a few months. I learned that before affecting cost and outcomes, there had to be a standardized method of communication. Therefore, my burning question was narrowed, and my capstone focused on how and what information should be communicated from the skilled nursing facility to the hospital.

The course work of the doctoral program supported why my project was important in the health care system. Course work provided opportunity to research the effects of communication on individual patients and providers, and outcomes related to poor communication on costs of health care. Each course allowed me to focus on a different aspect of the capstone project, ranging from epidemiology to costs of care and health care system issues. Although, one course brought it all together: nursing theory. This course provided an opportunity for critical reflection on my burning question and clarifying questions from my student colleagues. I believe this course was most helpful because the focus was on how we are nurses, and helped me examine my practice using Carper's ways of knowing (Carper, 1978). This was the cornerstone for my growth as a doctorally prepared nurse: I am foremost a clinician.

I was fortunate that my advisor told me at our first meeting to focus course work research on my burning question, the capstone topic. Heeding her advice was wise, and my papers and research contributed to supporting the quality focus and system need for improving communication between skilled nursing facility and hospital providers. If I had not done this, I am not sure if I would have been prepared to carry out the project in a timely fashion. Also, I enlisted help from leadership in one skilled nursing facility, where the project was done, and the director of Quality and Safety at the Department of Public Health. Both leaders were eager to have a standardized communication tool for the skilled nursing facility staff to use for patients transferred to the emergency room. Without this background work and leadership support, it would have been an arduous task to complete the project timely, if at all.

## Another Challenge: Writing the Paper

A major challenge was writing the capstone paper that was to be submitted for publication (Kelly, Mahoney, Bonner, O'Malley, 2012). My capstone committee members were coauthors for the paper; this meant that four people needed to agree upon the content and the writing style. At low times, I felt that I was not writing in my words, I was writing what other people wanted. I understood that we were all authors and there was a need for consensus, but this posed great challenges to reconcile four points of view and writing styles. Although this was a low point, it was a learning experience for future scholarly projects to keep the number of authors for one paper to the minimum number necessary for scholarly work. My confidence to defend my voice during edits was affected by my status as "student." Confidence improves with three letters—*DNP*—after your name!

Reflecting on my student experience, one year after finishing the doctoral program, I recall a great deal of good luck, a strong advisor, wonderful faculty, and outstanding colleagues. It took a village for me to develop my burning question, formulate the capstone project, and carry it out. I believe the greatest step toward success was my willingness to ask for help and speak up when I was unsure of action plans. This has helped in my role as a clinician to always ask questions when uncertain. Enlisting the help of others will help achieve the desired outcome.

## ■ NURSE PRACTITIONER TACKLES OPIOID DEPENDENCE IN RURAL PREGNANT WOMEN

### DAISY GOODMAN

My capstone consisted of the development and validation of an evidence-based clinical guideline for the obstetrical care of rural, opioid-dependent women. Over the past decade, addiction to prescription painkillers and heroin has developed as a significant public health problem among women of childbearing age in rural New England. Chronic opioid exposure during pregnancy poses serious risk for mother and fetus, due both to the physiologic effects of exposure and the chaotic lifestyle associated with illegal drug use, poor maternal nutrition, homelessness, and inadequate prenatal care. Obstetrical providers in rural community hospitals struggle to prevent preterm delivery, placental abruption, fetal death, and neonatal withdrawal requiring prolonged hospitalization, all adverse outcomes associated with maternal opioid dependence. Intimate partner violence and antenatal and postpartum depression and anxiety are also strong correlates of perinatal drug abuse, contributing further to poor obstetrical outcomes. The high cost of caring for fragile newborns and providing services for older children is overwhelming the resources of rural health systems.

In the 1970s, methadone maintenance became the standard of care for treatment of perinatal opioid dependence. The goal of therapy is prevention of in-utero withdrawal, premature birth, and other adverse outcomes and stabilization of a woman's social situation, allowing her to receive prenatal care and other services. Unfortunately, access to methadone treatment in rural communities is extremely limited. Programs specializing in perinatal addiction are located exclusively in urban settings. Rural obstetrical providers often lack knowledge regarding the management of opioid dependence during pregnancy, and their patients lack the resources to travel to obtain treatment. As a result, rural women do not receive the support needed to initiate and sustain recovery, or participate in obstetrical care addressing their special needs. Lack of access to adequate prenatal care contributes to poor obstetrical outcomes, placing additional burden on rural health care systems least able to absorb additional cost.

### Challenge: Perinatal Addiction Treatment for Low-Resource Rural Population

Given the lack of access to methadone treatment, what alternatives exist for pregnant women in rural, low-resource communities? The challenge of the capstone project was to define the scope of the problem to be addressed. Review of literature on perinatal opioid dependence supports what clinical experience implies: that depression, anxiety, and intimate partner violence are interwoven with maternal substance abuse, and that the vast majority of opioid-dependent women experience posttraumatic stress. Programs that integrated obstetrical care with addiction treatment and intensive social support were associated with the best outcomes for both mothers and infants. However, published data were collected at perinatal addiction centers in urban areas. Discussion of rural women's experience was entirely lacking.

Minimizing obstetrical risks for pregnant women with opioid dependence requires not only managing addiction, but also addressing the social and psychological stressors linked to drug abuse. Creative use of local resources is necessary to put together a treatment program that is both comprehensive and accessible to rural women. Fortunately, the elements of such a program are identifiable in the literature, including the use of buprenorphine, an office-based, accessible opioid maintenance therapy appropriate for use during pregnancy. The capstone project, therefore, focused on outlining a rural-centered practice guideline for addressing the multiple needs of opioid-dependent pregnant women in the rural community setting.

### Developing Evidence-Based Guidelines for Buprenorphine Maintenance Therapy

During the first phase of the capstone project, relevant theoretical, methodological, and clinical components were gathered and synthesized, and an evidence-based guideline for the care of rural pregnant women using buprenorphine maintenance therapy developed. During the second phase, content and face validity of the guideline were tested through a survey of both content expert and naïve clinicians. Specific sections, about which clinical evidence was equivocal, or which addressed areas of variation in practice, were selected for content validation using techniques described by Polit and Beck (2006). Open-ended questions addressed the usefulness and readability of the guideline, allowing respondents to comment on face validity.

Ten members of the American College of Nurse Midwives, the American Academy of Family Practice Physicians, and/or the American College of Obstetricians and Gynecologists responded anonymously to the 25-item survey, at a 50% response rate. The approach outlined in the guideline was validated. Respondents supported the use of buprenorphine during pregnancy as an alternative to methadone in rural, low-resource settings and found the guideline relevant to practice. The format chosen was found to be readable and useful. Two of the guideline recommendations were deemed invalid through the survey and were marked for revision (Goodman, 2010).

Advanced practice nurses (APNs), including nurse-midwives and nurse practitioners, have been a driving force for improving services for drug-dependent pregnant women and their families in Maine. Translation of the current evidence into practice with a rural underserved population was initiated through this capstone project. Since completion of the project, a multidisciplinary statewide task force has been developed in Maine to address the issue of perinatal substance abuse. The stated goal of the task force is the development of evidence-based recommendations for providers of perinatal care and to facilitate appropriate use of rural resources to meet the special needs of this patient population.

### ■ ADULT NURSE PRACTITIONER FOCUSES ON NURSING THEORY APPLIED TO CLINICAL PRACTICE

#### RICHARD AHERN

My experience as an APN has taken me from a community health center, to home care of people infected with human immunodeficiency virus (HIV), to an outpatient infectious diseases (ID) clinic. Throughout my nursing career, I have always felt that the contributions of the APN were significant.

In my master's program in nursing, I took the required course on nursing theory but never really gave it much thought afterward. However, when I entered the DNP program, the significance of nursing theory in informing my clinical practice was reinforced through the courses on knowledge and inquiry and population health. Whether I realized it or not, nursing theory shapes all my interactions. This realization raised a burning question about the impact that nursing has on the patient encounter in my current practice.

The ID clinic follows many patients infected with HIV. Part of the routine evaluation of both female and male patients is to screen for anal abnormalities caused by human papilloma virus (HPV) through cytology (analogous to cervical papanicolaou cytology). It is believed that oncogenic strains of HPV are associated with an increased risk of developing anal cancer. Many of our patients had positive "pap" tests, including high-grade dysplasia. We decided that the clinic needed to establish an anal dysplasia clinic using with high-resolution anoscopy (HRA), which uses colposcopy and biopsy. Therefore, a physician in the practice and I traveled to San Francisco to attend a course conducted by the American Society for Colposcopy and Cervical Pathology. On our return, the logistics of costs related to the use of clinic personnel, equipment, and the like, were assessed; this information was enhanced by the health care economics course in my doctoral program. Eventually, the first HRA session was conducted. However, I noticed that the model that was implemented in the clinic was more medically based. The patients' experience of this invasive procedure, including their physical and psychological needs, was not addressed, which was concerning to me.

## Challenges: Integrating a Nursing Focus Into a Medical Model Clinic

I addressed this perceived deficiency with several of the doctors involved in the anal dysplasia clinic. However, there seemed to be a lack of understanding of how the experience of the patient could be enhanced through a different model. The institution where I practice is very medically focused, so there is a greater emphasis on giving the patient some written information prior to and after the procedure. Nonetheless, I was encouraged in my quest by a doctorally prepared APN colleague. This spurred the topic of my capstone project about the impact of nursing on the patient's experience and, in particular, the development of a nursing-centered model of care that could enhance the patient's experience in this specialty clinic.

## The Process: Clinical Application of Caring Theory

To address this issue, with the assistance of faculty and APN colleagues, I first reviewed numerous nursing theories and concluded that a theory of caring, a central tenet of nursing, was most appropriate, and chose Kristen Swanson's theory of caring, which seemed most applicable. I initially planned to develop a general APN guideline for any anal dysplasia practice; however, conversations with APN experts in the field of anal dysplasia suggested the uniqueness of each practice setting. Consequently, I decided to focus instead on applying this nursing theory to this particular ID clinic in which I practice.

I then conducted a thorough review of the literature focusing on this population, a process that was reinforced by my population health and research courses in the doctoral program. This did not yield any previous literature on the population from this nursing perspective. Then, I reviewed the current medical model through the nursing perspective of caring using Swanson's theory. The nursing model that was developed was subsequently reviewed by APN experts in the field as well as faculty advisors and was revised several times. The patient-centered model that was developed includes engaging patients in their own care, educating them, acknowledging their feelings, advocating for them, and providing a therapeutic milieu. The final capstone project was entitled *Infusing Swanson's Theory of Caring into an Advanced Practice Nursing Model for an Infectious Diseases Anal Dysplasia Clinic* (Ahern, 2010).

My doctoral program shaped the development of my capstone project and the nursing theoretical foundation of my clinical practice. My hope is to eventually implement this nursing model into the current anal dysplasia clinic at this institution and to evaluate whether it enhances patient satisfaction and well-being.

## ■ REFERENCES

Ahern, R. L. (2010, April). *Infusing Swanson's theory of caring into an advanced practice nursing model for an infectious diseases anal dysplasia clinic.* Capstone Project paper presented in completion of requirements for Doctor of Nursing Practice degree at MGH Institute of Health Professions, Boston, MA.

Carper, B. A. (1978). Fundamental patterns of knowing in nursing. *Advances in Nursing Science, 1,* 13–23.

Goodman, D. (2011). Buprenorphine for the treatment of perinatal opioid dependence: Pharmacology and implications for antepartum, intrapartum and postpartum care. *Journal of Midwifery and Women's Health, 56,* 240–247.

Jacoby, S. D. (2009, December). *Certified nurse midwives' obstetrical management of women with type III female genital mutilation/cutting.* Capstone Project paper presented in completion of requirements for Doctor of Nursing Practice degree at MGH Institute of Health Professions, Boston, MA.

Kelly, N. A., Mahoney, D. F., Bonner A., & O'Malley, T. (2012). Use of a transitional minimum data set (TMDS) to improve communication. *Journal of the American Medical Directors Association, 13,* (85.e9e85.e15).

Polit, D., & Beck, C. (2006). The content validity index: Are you sure you know what's being reported? Critique and recommendations. *Research in Nursing and Health, 29,* 489–497.

Webb, J., & Guarino, A. J. (2011). Life after the death of a loved one: Long-term distress among surrogate decision makers. *Journal of Hospice & Palliative Nursing, 13,* 378–386.

# PART III

# Application of the Essentials to APRN Role Development

Doctors of nursing practice (DNPs) function in a number of distinct advanced practice roles. The evolution of the role will be explored, and in the process, we will begin to define the role in health care delivery today. Seven practicing DNPs—working as clinician, educator, administrator, midwife, nurse anesthetist, medical science liaison, and in the field of global forensics—will share their experiences. Lessons learned as the DNP is integrated into different sectors of health care are valuable and provide useful information as the role for the DNP is being defined.

Holding the terminal practice degree in nursing, DNPs will be required to be strong leaders. As DNPs move into these roles, the process of acquiring the specific skills needed for strong leadership is important. Advanced practice nurses may be new to the leadership role and need to seek out leadership opportunities. Practical steps to develop leadership skills in the clinical setting are useful and provide a roadmap for beginning leaders.

The executive nurse leaders play a critical role in improving health care systems and must be innovative and flexible and have practice driven by evidence-based knowledge. An organizational commitment to executive nurse leadership to develop knowledge-based practice (KBP) nurse executives, directors, and managers is explored. This example highlights the development and integration of research into the practice environment.

# CHAPTER 7

# A Degree Is Not a Role: DNP Education and Role Implementation

Lynda Tyer-Viola and Sheila M. Davis

*Knowing is not enough; we must apply. Willing is not enough, we must do.*
—Goethe (IOM, 2011)

Nursing is a profession of continual evolution. This dynamic state has provided both opportunities and challenges, and the introduction of the doctorate of nursing practice (DNP) degree also follows this trajectory. In accordance with the 2004 DNP position statement, the DNP degree has been proposed as the entry-level degree for advanced practice registered nurses (APRN) beginning in 2015 (AACN, 2004). As we navigate the infancy stages of this degree, it is critical that we define and closely direct the integration of the DNP into today's health care systems.

Gardner et al. (2010) eloquently discuss the historical expansion and contraction of nursing's scope of practice in response to political, societal, theological, and theoretical forces. Modern day nursing, as we know, began in the early 1900s in response to the poor living conditions of the influx of immigrants, and necessitated nurses taking on a social justice approach to care and advocacy based in the communities. The United States' entry into modern day warfare in World War I and later World War II highlighted the role of nursing, and this in conjunction with a nursing shortage led to the initial national investments in nursing education.

The rapid rate of scientific discovery and technological advances that began and accelerated through the mid-century (and continues to be happening at breakneck speed) necessitated a shift to a more educated nurse capable of critical thinking and applying scientific theories. Nurses who had worked primarily in the community shifted into the hospital setting and were immersed into the medical model. Observing the medical model "take over," visionary nursing leaders during this time began to more purposefully explore, define, and articulate the unique contributions of nursing.

Knowledge generation through development of conceptual frameworks and theoretical foundations for nursing practice remains an active component of the nursing discipline today. The ability of the profession to continually adapt while maintaining a strong and articulated nursing identity remains our strength and our biggest challenge. This is also true for the integration of the DNP-prepared APRN into practice. It is important to monitor how the DNP role is conceptualized, ensuring that the fundamentals of nursing and foundations of our discipline are maintained while at the same time DNP-prepared practitioners practice to the scope of their education. This chapter reviews how APRN practice will be transformed with the integration of the doctorally prepared practitioner.

## ■ INCREASING DEMANDS OF THE HEALTH CARE ENVIRONMENT

Society's changing needs and demands of the health care environment and the advancements in health care delivery have necessitated a more educated nurse professional. In 1996, the American Association of Colleges of Nursing (AACN) called for a baccalaureate degree in nursing to be entry level into the profession, "BSN nurses not only provide more complex aspects of daily care and patient education, but also design and coordinate a comprehensive plan of nursing care for the entire length of a patient's stay" (AACN, 2000, p. 1). Evidence in the literature strongly supports the need for baccalaureate-prepared nurses. Aiken, Clarke, Cheung, Sloane, and Silber (2003) showed that there was a decrease in the risk of patient death and failure to rescue by 5% for every 10% increase in the proportion of nurses holding Bachelor of Science in Nursing (BSN) degrees in the hospital. In a later study, Aiken, Clarke, Sloane, Lake, and Cheney (2008) corroborated the findings, showing that for every 10% increase in the proportion of BSN nurses on the hospital staff, there was a 4% decrease in the risk of death. These studies and others demonstrate a clear correlation between higher levels of education of nurses and improved patient outcomes. Although called for by the AACN in 1996 and supported by strong evidence of better patient outcomes in the literature, approaching the end of 2011, the BSN as entry level for nursing remains elusive.

Recognizing the need for a more experienced care provider, the Carnegie Foundation and Benner, Sutphen, Leonard, and Day (2009) took the recommendations to the next level, calling for the preparation for all entry-level registered nurses at the baccalaureate level and a master's degree within 10 years of initial licensure. The trend toward BSN as entry level, although not without controversy, is evident. Many hospitals, particularly major academic medical centers, have BSN as minimum entry, and there are traditional and accelerated BSN programs graduating students to fill this niche. Whether or not the recommendation for a master's degree for all nurses within 10 years of entry into practice will be embraced by the nursing profession is yet to be determined. Historical precedent of educational mandates (i.e., the BSN as entry level to practice) leads one to believe that it will be a slow process.

## ■ ADVANCED PRACTICE NURSING

The journey to advanced practice is discussed at length by Wolf and Ahmed in Chapter 1. Nursing's journey to the current iteration of advanced practice nursing has contained a fair amount of struggle, discourse, and ambiguity. The four currently recognized advanced practice roles in nursing designated by insurers are certified nurse midwife (CNM), certified registered nurse anesthetist (CRNA), clinical nurse specialist (CNS), and nurse practitioner (NP). As described by Wolf and Ahmed, other roles emerging, such as nurse executives, nurse educator, and case manager, reflect the growing specialization of advanced knowledge within the practice of nursing. Current APRN practice has demonstrated valuable contributions to the health and well being of the society. Care by NPs and CNMs has been shown to be more efficacious, satisfactory, and cost effective (Kennedy, 2000; Mundinger et al., 2000; Naylor et al., 1999; Naylor & Kurtzman, 2010; Pohl, Hanson, Newland, & Cronenwett, 2010; Turnbull et al., 1996). CRNA practice has been highly supervised by physicians, yet no difference in care has been demonstrated between supervised and unsupervised care (Dulisse & Cromwell, 2010). In 2001, the Centers for Medicare and Medicaid Services (CMS) began allowing states to not require physician supervision of care, and to date, 15 states have allowed this expansion of practice (AANA, 2011). Allowing APRNs to practice to their full education scope will allow for new models of care delivery.

The NP role gained credibility and expansion when in 1978 the Institute of Medicine (IOM) supported the revision of state regulations to include a broader scope of practice for NPs to include prescription authority under a physician's supervision (Mason, Vacarro, & Fessler, 2000). The NP and other APRN roles, although borne out of need for increased access and demand for care, continue to be challenged by other medical providers. The integration of a doctorally prepared APRN practitioner will require strong nurse leaders and advocacy for acceptance. This support will remain critical and current efforts include diligence to stop restriction in scope of practice, reimbursement equity, and a prominent place in health care reform.

## ■ HIGHEST LEVEL OF NURSING PRACTICE

The DNP is a degree, not a role. This is an important distinction to make, as the negative response by many physicians and other medical providers to the DNP is fueled by this confusion. The acquisition of the degree does not change licensure or credentialing as an advanced practice nurse. As previously stated, in analysis of master's APRN education, it is evident that the time spent in education is not congruent with the degree earned, and in today's changing health environment, new knowledge is needed to practice (AACN, 2004). In the primary clinical role as NPs, DNPs will practice within the current scope of clinical care dictated by clinical practice standards. However, in recognition of the quality chasm that exists, the need for expanded knowledge, including leadership, stronger analytical skills, and understanding of informatics, ethics, and policy to design, implement, and assess health systems will be needed.

Nursing has been plagued by lack of clear delineation and lack of clarity of scope of practice and knowledge. The DNP, as the terminal or highest level of advanced practice degree, has inherited this ambiguity and confusion. The outcome of many decades of "reinvention and reinterpretation" in nursing is evident in the "alphabet soup" of letters after our names and leads to sometimes negative intraprofessional, interprofessional, and public perceptions of the profession. To avoid this, in the face of numerous changes in our health system, it is important that when DNP practice occurs and new roles are defined, the advances in nursing are communicated with the society. To avoid more confusion on the role of nursing in health care, we must clearly articulate the need for the degree as in the *AACN Position Statement on the Practice Doctorate in Nursing* (2004). The curriculum in the *DNP Essentials for Doctorate Education* (2006) is evident of the educational preparation of the DNP graduate and the role the DNP-prepared APRN can play in our health care systems.

Integrating the role of the DNP into the current scope of practice is a challenge. When NPs were negotiating for a place in health care in the 1990s, they had to generate and preserve role boundaries by cultivating, bargaining, confronting, and disengaging (Martin & Hutchinson, 1997). They used these techniques to create a symbolic space in health care that was necessary for them to become, as they stated, "part of the national consciousness"

(p. 89). Today, DNPs will have to create this same symbolic space to ensure recognition within the health care system and, more importantly, the ability to practice to the full extent of their education.

It is clearly stated in the IOM report, *The Future of Nursing: Leading Change, Advancing Health*, that removing barriers and allowing nurses to practice to their full potential and education will benefit society (IOM, 2010). However, they explicitly state that although the committee fully supported the transition to the DNP for entry into advanced practice nursing, this did not define the potential role of DNP nurses for lack of evidence. This gap in knowledge is currently being addressed as more new graduates develop their roles and share their experiences.

Most important though for the patient, the agency, the health care system, and society is to understand that the DNP is not a "super-charged" APRN. A doctorally prepared nurse is an APRN who, through his/her education, has mastered the essentials of DNP education. The AACN adopted a resolution that, by 2015, the educational preparation for entry into APRN practice is the DNP degree (AACN, 2009). As discussed above in relation to BSN as entry practice, nursing has a long history of being slow to adopt proposals to education mandates. APRN practice has evolved with the support of integration into health care systems and acceptance by the medical community as partners in care. As previously stated, NP practice has become increasingly more visible due to the economics of utilizing APRNs within hospital settings to ensure quality of care by highlighting their ability to support and work more collaboratively with nursing professionals. The DNP APRN will focus on a wider scope of practice and view their influence in the profession from a wider lens. The current health system in the United States is acknowledged by many to be "broken." The continual escalation of costs, in a setting of 47 million uninsured Americans, dictates an overhaul of the complex health delivery system (Kaiser Family Foundation, 2010). Approaching innovation from a systems approach to health care via a clinical lens allows the DNP to fill a critical role within our new health system.

## ■ CURRENT APRN PRACTICE

If we meet the IOM challenge, due to workforce issues and national health care reform, we will continue to have APRNs with differing educational preparation during a time of tremendous change in health care (Cronenwett et al., 2011). History tells us that those who are practicing will be grandfathered into the APRN role. How will the DNP role be defined and what are the expectations of DNP practice beyond that of a master's-prepared APRN? The DNP role should be developed distinctly from the current APRN role with expectations that this cadre of nurses exhibit the DNP essentials to meet the goals set forth by the IOM.

In 2006, the AACN DNP Roadmap Task Force recommended as specialty nursing education transitions to the doctoral level, "that institutions consider reconceptualizing their master's degree programs to prepare generalists." The AACN endorsed the task force's recommendations, and this is consistent with an AACN member-endorsed position statement, "As the education of the generalist nurse is elevated to the master's degree level, it is reasonable to assume that specialty education and the education of those individuals prepared for the highest level of nursing practice would occur at the practice doctoral level" (AACN, 2009). The assumption by the task force was that the advanced date of 2015 would allow time for the issue of the master's degree to be addressed. As 2011 is ending, there continues to be no lack of consensus on if and when to close master's programs.

To meet the IOM challenge and the pending demands of health care reform, both master's-prepared NPs and doctorally prepared APRNs will be needed. Health care reform, as well as the 2008 World Health Report from the World Health Organization (WHO, 2008), calls for a renewed focus on the provision of primary care. To fill this chasm of care, APRNs will be in demand and highly integrated into our new health care delivery systems. Clinton and Sperhac (2006) discuss the potential mechanisms for this process, including application of prior experience in the advanced practice role as part of the educational requirements. As with all transitions, the window of opportunity to take advantage of this option will be time limited, thereby making clarification about the proposed date of 2015 for DNP as entry-level requirement even more critical. This is important to note, as the integration of DNP-prepared APRNs is not meant to displace the practicing professionals. The intent is to ensure that all facets of nursing practice, wherever it occurs, are evaluated and executed from the lens of the highest level of nursing education and executed by those with the most knowledge of specific populations. That said, master's-prepared APRNs will be needed for focused, specialty practice, whereas doctorally prepared APRNs will understand these populations yet view their needs in a broader context involving thorough review of best evidence for care and implementing collaborative delivery systems.

■ ROLE DEFINITION AS DEFINED VIA THE DNP ESSENTIALS OF DOCTORAL EDUCATION

Integrating the DNP role into our health care system is the next challenge for nursing. There was overwhelming support from specialty nursing organizations that a newly defined practice doctorate was essential in meeting the quality gap identified in *Crossing the Quality Chasm* (IOM, 2001). The 2004 *DNP Position Statement* outlined nine benefits to a clearly defined practice doctorate in nursing education that would be integral to improving our health care system (see Exhibit 7.1).

---

### EXHIBIT 7.1

#### Benefits of a Practice Doctorate in Nursing

---

1. Development of needed advanced competencies for increasingly complex practice, faculty, and leadership roles
2. Enhanced knowledge to improve nursing practice and patient outcomes
3. Enhanced leadership skills to strengthen practice and health care delivery
4. Better match of program requirements and credits and time with the credential earned
5. Provision of an advanced educational credential for those who require advanced practice knowledge but do not need or want a strong research focus (e.g., practice faculty)
6. Parity with other health professions, most of which have a doctorate as the credential required for practice
7. Enhanced ability to attract individuals to nursing from nonnursing backgrounds
8. Increased supply of faculty for clinical instruction
9. Improved image of nursing

*Source:* AACN, 2004, pp. 7,8

These benefits were aligned closely with the agenda to redesign our health care delivery system and quality improvements necessary in educating our future health care work force (IOM, 2001, 2003). To ensure that nursing was adequately prepared, the *DNP Essentials for Doctoral Education* was crafted (see Exhibit 7.2). These essentials are not mastered as individual competencies but are woven within the curriculum. Mastery of the essentials includes the ability to ebb and flow between and within these competencies in practice. DNP practice occurs with distinct populations and settings. In defining the DNP role, emphasis should not be on one essential of education but how these essentials will create a competent practitioner. As the DNP role emerges, how these essentials define it and are supportive of it in diverse settings is yet to be determined. The following is a review of each essential and how it may be articulated in practice. Key to role clarity is the ability for our profession to clearly articulate doctorally prepared APRN practice and its contribution to overall health and the profession.

### *I.* Scientific underpinnings for practice

Mastering the scientific underpinnings for practice is mandated for nursing practice due to the complexity of today's health care delivery systems (AACN, 2006). The call for increased rigor of educating health care professionals was recommended by the IOM in the 2001 report, *Crossing the Quality Chasm* (IOM, 2001). The committee recognized that additional skills will be needed to "manage a continually expanding evidence base and technological innovations ..." (IOM, 2001, p. 208). To prepare for this role, the DNP masters an understanding of the foundations of nursing and the etiology of nursing science. Nursing practice is based on the interaction of the person with the environment, with the DNP effectively and efficiently translating science into knowledge for practice to benefit nurses and patients (Porter-O'Grady, 2003). The role of the DNP is to view problems at the patient and system levels in reference to how nursing can intervene and collaborate with the interdisciplinary team. The foundations of nursing knowledge have expanded beyond nursing science to include those sciences relevant to the human experience, such

---

### *EXHIBIT 7.2*

#### The Essentials for Doctoral Education for Advanced Practice

1. Scientific underpinnings for practice
2. Organizational and systems leadership for quality improvement and systems thinking
3. Clinical scholarship and analytical methods for evidence-based practice
4. Information systems technology and patient care technology for the improvement and transformation of health care
5. Health care policy for advocacy in health care
6. Interprofessional collaboration for improving patient and population health outcomes
7. Clinical prevention and population health for improving the nation's health
8. Advanced nursing practice map for success

*Source:* AACN, 2006.

as psychology and sociology, all functioning within a complex system of health and well being. The competent DNP practitioner will be able to synthesize this complex knowledge, translate it for application to specialty populations, and articulate it in a way that will integrate it into nursing practice.

### II.   Organizational and systems leadership for quality improvement and systems

Improving access to and quality of care for diverse populations requires that health care leaders adjust and redefine health care delivery systems. Health care agencies need now more than ever to "accelerate efforts to redesign their approaches to interacting with patients, organizing services, providing training, and utilizing the healthcare workforce" to their utmost potential (IOM, 2001, p. 112). DNP curriculum stresses the need for doctorally prepared nurses to be experts in assessing care delivery systems, designing interventions, facilitating organization change, and monitoring quality of care (AACN, 2006). The role of the DNP is to drive continuous quality improvement with stakeholders by utilizing their sophisticated expert knowledge of populations, health systems, and communities of interest. Their in-depth knowledge of patient populations and health systems will assist organizations in targeting those patient populations that are most vulnerable and implementing interventions and changes to those that are patient-centered. The DNP advanced practice nurse will drive policy that is equitable, economic, and efficient by tapping into other health care sectors and science disciplines.

### III.   Clinical scholarship and analytical methods for evidence-based practice (EBP)

The cornerstone to improving the quality of health care and patient outcomes is applying best evidence to patient care. EBP is the "the conscientious and judicious use of current best evidence in conjunction with clinical expertise and patient values to guide health care decisions" (Sackett, Rosenberg, Gray, Haynes, & Richardson, 2007; Titler, 2011, p. 1). Alarming though is the gap between research and integration into practice. In previous years, the lag between the identification of best practice and integration into clinical practice was found to be between 15 and 20 years (Balas & Boren, 2000). Cutting-edge interventions once considered a luxury found only in academic medical centers now must be integrated within and between health care systems (Titler, 2011). A key role of the DNP-prepared APRN is the synthesis, translation, and integration of a plethora of data into clinical practice. The foundation to excellent nursing care is the ability for nurses to gather data, identify needs, and apply best evidence and interventions to achieve patient outcomes. The case for efficiency as well as effectiveness is much more acute in times of great change in our health care systems (Rycroft-Malone, 2010).

Doctorally prepared nurses will be in increased demand as both PhD and DNP curricula emphasize finding solutions to complex nursing problems. However, the purpose of the DNP is to take knowledge generated by their colleagues and integrate it into practice by designing new care delivery systems and teaching new knowledge to nurses (Edwardson, 2010). A vital role of the DNP nurse is competence both in integrating evidence into health care delivery and promoting how to translate and adopt evidence into health care. DNP prepares nurses to understand the nature of the evidence, how it is communicated to the health care workforce, and the context of practice as well as what evidence is the most effective for specific populations (Titler, 2011). The competent DNP is an expert in and values the attention that must be afforded to the adoption process and implementation of analysis to ensure EBP is a continuous quality process. The DNP practitioner will excel in the role of mentor for clinical scholars who continually question what is the best care for patients (Fineout-Overholt, Melnyk, & Schultz, 2005).

### IV. Information systems technology and patient care technology for the improvement and transformation of health care

Within the Patient Protection and Affordable Care Act (PPACA) of 2010 will be a growing dependence on and expectation that nursing care will be supported by health care information technology (HIT) (United States, 2010). To practice at the level of a doctorally prepared nurse, DNP graduates need to be proficient in the practical application of innovative patient care technology. In many instances, these two sophisticated areas of science will blend and APRNs' knowledge will be critical in evaluating clinical support systems and computerized patient care equipment that will enhance decision making and clinical care to improve patient safety. In the 2003 IOM report, *Health Professions Education: A Bridge to Quality*, utilizing informatics to support patient care was viewed as one of the essential core competencies of health care providers, yet many are not trained in how to access the expanding data base of evidence (IOM, 2003). Competency includes not only personal knowledge but also knowing which sciences best inform innovative practice. As experts in practice, doctorally prepared nurses understand the needs related to HIT and care innovations from the multiple stakeholder perspectives. The role of the DNP practitioner will be to analyze the needs of stakeholders, to assess available technologies, to evaluate the economics of acquisition and implementation with an interdisciplinary team, and to measure the impact of these systems/equipments on patient outcomes.

### V. Health care policy for advocacy in health

DNP practitioners provide the needed interface in health care between practice, research, and policy, as they are knowledgeable about and represent several layers of the health care system (AACN, 2006). Their position within and between the patient and nurse, nurse and management, and research and administration provides them with the opportunity to view and advocate for policy to improve health. Translating the needs of diverse populations and crafting policy and guidelines to meet those needs during the implementation of health care reform will require the competencies of APRNs. Nurses are viewed as knowledgeable yet are not seen as opinion leaders. This is the opportunity for DNP nurses to expose their knowledge and be more influential in health care reform. Through their expert practice knowledge, they have the ability to inform policy makers at the local, community, state, and national levels. Furthermore, as nurses, these practitioners will advocate for health with a social justice perspective and place value on the need for health equity for all (Boutain, 2005).

### VI. Interprofessional collaboration for improving patient and population health outcomes

The IOM (2001, 2003) has made a strong case for establishing a new environment of care and improving the quality of health care providers. Current care environments continue to have silos of care; medical specialists make rounds without their nursing colleagues, support professionals make policies without seeking input from those who are closest to the patient, and the nurses and administrators responsible for product purchases do not consult those who will use equipment in daily care. The future of health care reform lies within the ability for all professionals to work in teams and to communicate effectively throughout the care environment. With education viewed as the bridge to quality, it is mandated that all health professionals "cooperate, collaborate, communicate, and integrate care in teams to ensure that care is continuous and reliable" (IOM, 2003, p. 45). The competent DNP will possess these skills and strive to seek first to understand while being able to cultivate and mentor the skills within other nursing professionals (Covey, 2004). The role of the DNP is to be a cooperative team member as well as an advocate for and support to other nursing members. As team leaders, DNP practitioners will lead interdisciplinary teams in analyzing complex patient care problems and ensure that nurses as participants in care teams have the skills and supports to be effective.

### VII. Clinical prevention and population health for improving the nation's health

Clinical prevention and health promotion are critical to preserving our nation's health. DNP curriculum focus will include a shift toward including science from those disciplines that promote behavior change, nutrition, exercise physiology, and an array of other sciences that will support primary care (Burman et al., 2009). *Healthy People 2020*, the national road map for health initiative, has a renewed focus on people attaining a level of wellness and achieving health equity by eliminating disparities and understanding preventable disease and disability, injury, and premature death (DHHS, 2011). The competent DNP practitioner will address care at the patient, system, and community level, focusing on four foundational health measures: general health status by providing high-level primary care; health-related quality of life and well-being by promoting and educating populations on preventable diseases; determinants of health by increasing community awareness on how the ecosystem and the environment affect health; and disparities by ensuring that quality care is available to all. The DNP role will exhibit a renewed focus on population health including disparities related to age, gender, and disease. As specialists, the DNP will apply individualized care with a renewed focus on social determinants to health. As trusted members of the community, nurses have the capacity to mobilize, assess, plan, implement, and track framework (otherwise known as MAP-IT) for healthy people (DHHS, 2011). The DNP-prepared APRN is an ideal leader to facilitate this framework to meet our nation's health goals.

### VIII. Advanced nursing practice

Specialization and expert practice is the cornerstone of APRN practice. DNP graduates are expected to achieve competency in areas that span all specialty settings such as advanced assessment, pharmacology, and pathophysiology with an understanding of the legal and regulatory issues associated with care. Many DNP candidates will have expertise in a specialized field of nursing. Health care in the twenty-first century requires those nurses to integrate new knowledge, to be open to visionary thinking, and to actively seek out best nursing practice. DNP preparation includes multiple experiential opportunities to cultivate advanced levels of clinical judgment, systems thinking, and accountability (AACN, 2006). The APRN practice of a DNP graduate will be defined by a wider understanding of specialized care; a commitment to educate and guide individuals, communities and nursing colleagues through complex physical care; and the multiple transitions present in health care today. The role of the DNP will be to provide expert specialized care while understanding the implications of care provision in a wider context.

### ■ RECOMMENDATIONS FOR ROLE DEFINITION AND INTEGRATION

These are the recommendations related to the multitude of roles that DNP APRN will be prepared to fulfill in the current and future health care systems. The 10 essentials of DNP education are not discrete, and each DNP will be required to incorporate aspects from all 10 essentials to provide quality health care:

- The DNP-prepared APRN is the catalyst for the synthesis, translation, and integration of a plethora of data into clinical practice.

- Master's-prepared APRN are needed to fill a significant gap in health care access and will need close collaboration with doctorally prepared APRN's, who will be responsible for implementing best evidence for practice. The future of the master's-prepared APRN needs to be assessed on an ongoing basis for their ability to apply innovations and clinical guidelines in practice.
- DNP practitioners will translate complex knowledge and apply it to the clinical context of nursing practice at the local, community, and national levels.
- The role of the DNP is to drive continuous quality improvement with stakeholders by utilizing their sophisticated expert knowledge of populations, health systems, and communities of interest.
- The DNP role will include application of practical innovative patient care technology and steward these innovations into a variety of health care settings.
- The role of the DNP to advocate for policy to improve health hinges on the key position of the DNP within and between the patient and nurse, nurse and management, and research and administration.
- The DNP role will include the sophisticated translation of the needs of diverse populations to craft policy and guidelines to meet those needs during the implementation of health care reform.
- The DNP practitioner's role will include leadership of interdisciplinary teams in analyzing complex patient care problems and ensuring that nurses as participants in care teams have the skills and supports to be effective.
- The DNP practitioner role is critical in addressing care at the patient, system, and community levels, exhibiting a renewed focus on disparities related to age, gender, and disease with an emphasis on the social determinants of health.
- The DNP will provide expert specialized care while understanding the implications of care provision in a wider context.

## ■ REFERENCES

American Association of Colleges of Nursing (AACN). (2000). *The baccalaureate degree in nursing as minimal preparation for the profession.* Washington, DC: AACN. Retrieved from http://www.aacn.nche.edu/publications/positions/baccmin.htm

American Association of Colleges of Nursing (AACN). (2004). *DNP position statement.* Washington, DC: AACN. Retrieved from http://www.aacn.nche.edu/dnp/dnppositionstatement.htm

American Association of Colleges of Nursing (AACN). (2006). *Essentials of doctoral education for advanced nursing practice.* Washington, DC: AACN. Retrieved from www.aacn.nche.edu

American Association of Colleges of Nursing (AACN). (2009). *Frequently asked questions of the position statement of the doctorate of nursing practice.* Washington, DC: AACN. Retrieved from http://nursing.cua.edu/graduate/dnp/faq.cfm

AANA. (2011). *Study in health affairs confirms quality and safety of nurse anesthesia care.* Washington, DC. Retrieved from http://www.aana.com/newsandjournal/News/Pages/080310-Study-in-Health-Affairs-Confirms-Quality-Safety-of-Nurse-Anesthetist-Care.aspx

Aiken, L. H., Clarke, S. P., Cheung, R. B., Sloane, D. M., & Silber, J. H. (2003). Educational levels of hospital nurses and surgical patient mortality. *Journal of the American Medical Association, 290,* 1617–1623.

Aiken, L. H., Clarke, S. P., Sloane, D. M., Lake, E. T., & Cheney, T. (2008). Effects of hospital care environment on patient mortality and nurse outcomes. *Journal of Nursing Administration, 38*(5), 223–229.

Balas, E. A., & Boren, S. A. (2000). Managing clinical knowledge for health care improvement. In: J. Bemmel & A. T. McCray (Eds.), *Yearbook of medical informatics 2000: Patient-centered systems* (pp. 65–70). Stuttgart, Germany: Schattauer Verlagsgesellschaft mbH.

Benner, P., Sutphen, M., Leonard, V., & Day, L. (2009). *Educating nurses: A call for radical transformation* (The Carnegie Foundation for the Advancement of Teaching). San Francisco: Jossey-Bass.

Boutain, D. (2005). Social justice as a framework for professional nursing. *Journal of Nursing Education, 44*, 404–408.

Burman, M. E., Hart, A. M., Conley, V., Brown, J., Sherard, P., & Clarke, P. N. (2009). Reconceptualizing the core of nurse practitioner education and practice. [Review]. *Journal of the American Academy of Nurse Practitioners, 21*, 11–17.

Clinton, P., & Sperhac, A. (2006). National agenda for advanced practice nursing: The practice doctorate. *The Journal of Professional Nursing, 22*, 7–14.

Covey, S. (2004). *Seven habits of highly effective people.* Franklin Covey. Retrieved from https://www.stephencovey.com/7habits/7habits-habit5.php

Cronenwett, L., Dracup, K., Grey, M., McCauley, L., Meleis, A., & Salmon, M. (2011). The doctor of nursing practice: A national workforce perspective. *Nursing Outlook, 59*, 9–17.

DHHS. (2011). *Healthy People 2020.* Washington, DC: Author. Retrieved from http://www.healthypeople.gov/2020/default.aspx

Dulisse, B., & Cromwell, J. (2010). No harm found when nurse anesthetists work without supervision by physicians. *Health Affairs, 29*, 1469–1475.

Edwardson, S. R. (2010). Doctor of philosophy and doctor of nursing practice as complementary degrees. *Journal of Professional Nursing, 26*, 137–140.

Fineout-Overholt, E., Melnyk, B. M., & Schultz, A. (2005). Transforming health care from the inside out: Advancing evidence-based practice in the 21st century. *Journal of Professional Nursing: Official Journal of the American Association of Colleges of Nursing, 21*, 335–344.

Gardner, G., Gardner, A., Middleton, S., Eella, P., Kain, V., & Doubrovsky, A. (2010). The work of nurse practitioners. *Journal of Advanced Nursing, 66*, 2160–2169.

Institute of Medicine (IOM). (2011). *The future of nursing: Leading change, advancing health.* Washington, DC: U.S. Government Printing Office.

Institute of Medicine (IOM). (2001). *Crossing the quality chasm.* Washington, DC: National Academy Press.

Institute of Medicine (IOM). (2003). *Health professions education: A bridge to quality.* Washington, DC: National Academy Press.

Institute of Medicine (IOM). (2010). *The future of nursing: Leading chance advancing health.* Washington, DC: Author. Retrieved from http://www.iom.edu/Reports/2010/The-Future-of-Nursing-Leading-Change-Advancing-Health.aspx

Kaiser Family Foundation. (2010). *U.S. health care costs.* Retrieved from http://www.kaiseredu.org/Issue-Modules/US-Health-Care-Costs/Background-Brief.aspx

Kennedy, H. P. (2000). A model of exemplary midwifery practice: Results of a Delphi study. *The Journal of Midwifery & Women's Health, 45*, 4–19.

Martin, P. D., & Hutchinson, S. A. (1997). Negotiating symbolic space: Strategies to increase NP status and value. *Nurse Practitioner, 22*, 89–91.

Mason, D., Vacarro, K., & Fessler, M. (2000). Early views of nurse practitioners: A Medline search. *Clinical Excellence for Nurse Practitioners, 4*, 175–183.

Mundinger, M. O., Kane, R. L., Lenz, E. R., Totten, A. M., Tsai, W.-Y., Cleary, P. D., et al. (2000). Primary care outcomes in patients treated by nurse practitioners or physicians. *JAMA: The Journal of the American Medical Association, 283*, 59–68.

Naylor, M. D., Brooten, D., Campbell, R., Jacobsen, B. S., Mezey, M. D., Pauly, M. V., et al. (1999). Comprehensive discharge planning and home follow-up of hospitalized elders. *JAMA: The Journal of the American Medical Association, 281*, 613–620.

Naylor, M. D., & Kurtzman, E. T. (2010). The role of nurse practitioners in reinventing primary care. *Health Affairs, 29*, 893–899.

Porter-O'Grady, T. (2003). Nurses as knowledge workers. *Creative Nursing, 9*(2), 6–9.

Pohl, J. M., Hanson, C., Newland, J. A., & Cronenwett, L. (2010). Analysis & commentary unleashing nurse practitioners' potential to deliver primary care and lead teams. *Health Affairs, 29*, 900–905.

Rycroft-Malone, J. (2010). Evidence-based practice in an age of austerity. *Worldviews on Evidence Based Nursing, 7*, 189–190.

Sackett, D. L., Rosenberg, W. M., Gray, J. A., Haynes, R. B., & Richardson, W. S. (2007). Evidence based medicine: What it is and what it isn't, 1996. *Clinical Orthopaedics and Related Research, 455*, 3–5.

Titler, M. G. (2011). Nursing science and evidence-based practice. *Western Journal of Nursing Research, 33*, 291–295.

Tumbull, D., Holmes, A., Shields, N., Cheyne, H., Twaddle, S., Gilmour, W. H., et al. (1996). Randomised, controlled trial of efficacy of midwife-managed care. *The Lancet, 348*, 213–218.

United States. (2010). *The Patient Protection and Affordable Care Act. H.R. 3590.* Retrieved from http://democrats.senate.gov/pdfs/reform/patient-protection-affordable-care-act-as-passed.pdf

World Health Organization (WHO). (2008). *World health report—Primary health care; Now more than ever. World report.* Geneva: WHO. Retrieved from http://www.who.int/whr/2008/en/index.html

CHAPTER 8

# Personal Perspectives on Role Integration

Sheila M. Davis, Richard Ahern, Dawn Carpenter, Lisa J. Hogan,
Susan Jacoby, Amanda D. Jojola, Thomas J. McQuaid, and Joyce P. Williams

Due to the relative newness of the doctor of nursing practice (DNP) degree, many students who begin their educational journey do so without the ability to envision how the terminal degree impacts their professional career. Recent DNP graduates are often the trailblazers in their workplace as the new DNPs integrate into all sectors of health care. The DNP degree neither expands the legal scope of practice nor does it add additional clinical credentialing—but graduates leave their programs having completed a rigorous course of study and many will approach their practice differently. Many DNP graduates stay in the same positions they were in before or during school and, therefore, their external work environment often does not change, but they have. In this chapter, DNPs who are working in different areas were asked to reflect upon how obtaining the DNP degree has affected them and their current position. Different paths and expertise brought the seven nurses that are highlighted below to a number of different DNP programs throughout the Unites States. Included are recent graduates and others who have been out for a few years. Through their lived experience, we gain glimpses about the growth, challenges, opportunities, and disappointments experienced by DNPs working today.

## ■ CLINICAL

### RICHARD AHERN

I enrolled in a DNP program at the same nursing school from which I graduated with a master's degree, not so that I could use the title "doctor" (neither of interest nor of importance to me), but rather as the natural progression in my pursuit and acquisition of knowledge through inquiry as an advanced practice nurse in clinical practice. I was encouraged in this endeavor by my advanced practice nursing (APN) colleague who had graduated from the first DNP class.

Since graduation more than 1 year ago, my role and responsibilities have not changed at all in the specialty clinic in which I practice, a large academic medical center. I believe this is due to the lack of understanding of the significance of this degree on the part of my physician colleagues. For example, during my studies for this degree, I recall discussing with one of the physicians some issues related to heath policy and the economics of health care and his astonish-ment at the depth of the complexity of the issues that we DNP students were considering. In addition, I also practice in an institution that is very physician-focused; hence, the opportuni-ties available for advanced practice nurses are somewhat "traditional," and therefore, limited.

However, I believe that the DNP degree has significantly changed me both as a per-son and as an advanced practice nurse professional. It has increased my sense of inquiry—particularly, in what constitutes best practice. It has also enhanced my nursing identity in the delivery of care and fostered my desire to evaluate how this holistic perspective can enhance the care and outcomes of patients in our practice setting. I likewise look at my practice in a broader perspective, for example, by incorporating the knowledge gained about systems and processes, so that I can recommend how operations may be modified to optimize the efficiency and quality of care that is delivered.

The challenge remains as to whether the impact and importance of the DNP degree will be acknowledged in my current clinical practice and more broadly in the health care institution as a whole. My belief is that as more nurses pursue this degree, the more the health institution will "open its eyes," become familiarized with the competencies that DNPs bring, appreciate their value, and open up opportunities for them to use the knowledge and skills they have acquired.


## ■ EDUCATION

### DAWN CARPENTER

The process of obtaining the DNP degree changes each and every one of us. Changes occurred in very subtle, almost imperceptible ways. However, the changes of my views, thought pro-cesses, and interactions were far more prominent to those with whom I worked most closely. When I finally arrived on the other side of the DNP educational process and had time to reflect, I found that my perceptions had changed dramatically.

Upon graduating with the DNP degree, I noticed a distinct change in how other educa-tors and health professionals perceived the DNP-prepared faculty. They seemed to view my faculty role as having significantly more credibility than prior to obtaining the DNP degree. As a result, they more readily listened to ideas, suggestions, and concerns. I was perceived as the expert in my respected field, and others now eagerly sought information, guidance, and input. This change in perception has led to multiple opportunities for my growth as DNP faculty.

Since graduation a little over a year ago, DNP preparation has provided many oppor-tunities as an invited speaker, author, and with interprofessional collaboration. As a DNP faculty, I was asked to speak at the annual American College of Chest Physician (ACCP) conference in Hawaii for the fall 2011 conference. I was asked to be part of a four-person podium presentation, and the topic to be covered involved strategies to retain nurse practi-tioners (NP) and physician assistants in acute and critical care settings.

Having the DNP degree, along with clinical and educational expertise, has assisted in obtaining an invitation to become an item writer for one of the national NP certifying exams. Invitations to write and publish have occurred as well. One example is being asked to par-ticipate in writing this chapter on my DNP experience as a faculty member. It was through personal contacts combined with experience as an educator and having the DNP degree that opened this door.

Other opportunities as DNP faculty include multiple invitations to collaborate on interprofessional teams to develop clinical practice guidelines. In addition, a significant leadership opportunity was presented, leading me to make a very difficult decision about my career path. I chose to stay in education, my other true passion after patient care, rather than pursue a management position. As an educator, I can influence patient care more globally through preparing new Acute Care Nurse Practitioners (ACNP) for the workforce.

In my role as coordinator of an ACNP track, the DNP degree changed how I teach; not so much my teaching style, but rather by refocusing my content to include areas prominent in the DNP curriculum. Assignments have been modified to include a slightly different spin on certain areas, such as evidence-based practice (EBP) and case studies including diversity and underserved populations.

First and foremost, the DNP degree has engrained EBP into everything that I do in education related to NP practice. It is now of second nature, and thus, has become more integrated into each reading assignment, lecture, and assignment. Student-assigned EBP projects are evolving to help students more readily appreciate the process of identifying, synthesizing, integrating, and implementing EBP.

As a DNP-prepared faculty, I have changed two key areas of our case studies. First, more diversity and underserved populations are incorporated into our case studies. I have asked the students to differentiate how treatments or approaches may differ with different populations, ages, and socioeconomic status. These diverse populations are specific to our community, including non-English speaking patients with Latino backgrounds. Second, I have expanded the case study section where students explain what and how they would teach the patient and family about the diagnosis and treatments to include health literacy concerns.

Lastly, when I have assessed clinical placements during site visits with the students, I assessed the preceptors and sites to ensure they were adhering to EBP. In addition, I have provided each preceptor with evidence to augment their skills at precepting students. As one of the few DNP-prepared faculties at the school, I was asked to participate in teaching the capstone proposal course as well as being the faculty capstone mentor for one of the DNP students. This has been an honor as well as a bit unnerving. I thought: "I have only been out of the program for 1 year, I am not ready for this; I am not the expert." But then, in the classroom and in meeting with students individually, I realized I did, in fact, develop some areas of expertise.

Specifically, I found I had become adept at navigating organizational structure and politics and analyzing organizational priorities. I found I was able to help students navigate the clinical systems, identify key stakeholders, and state their proposal in such a way as to gain support from these key stakeholders. To parallel this concept, it became evident how truly engrained I had become in working within interprofessional teams. It was easy to see when students may not have grasped this importance in developing the proposal and I was able to coach them on building their interprofessional team to move their project ahead.

Throughout my DNP program, we routinely appraised fellow students' work, both oral presentations as well as written work. This process honed my ability to provide constructive feedback and augmented how I stated positive comments first and reframed criticisms into suggestions. The same is true for critically appraising student papers.

In summary, because of the DNP educational process, subtle but significant changes have been made to the curriculum incorporating EBP for acute care students. Having had time to reflect, I noticed the changes that have already occurred in adapting the curriculum because I had changed. In further contemplation, I can see many more changes that need to be made to the program. However, it remains a balancing act to provide the content students need to care for patients, along with content to ensure that they pass the certification exam, all while maintaining a manageable workload for the students.

## ■ NURSE ANESTHETIST

### LISA J. HOGAN

Nurse anesthesia is the oldest nursing specialty in the United States. Nurses have provided anesthesia care for nearly 150 years. In the late 1800s, the widespread use of diethyl ether came into use. Ether administration was a relatively simple procedure and Catholic nuns, who nursed, quickly mastered the technique and provided invaluable assistance to surgeons. Surgeons valued the work of the nurses, and the subspecialty of nurse anesthesia was developed (Fosburg & Kosh, 1995).

Nurse anesthetists today continue to provide safe high-quality anesthesia care in a variety of settings, administering 30 million anesthetics a year and providing more than 65% of the anesthesia care in the United States (AANA, 2010). Physician anesthesiologists over the years have made a number of attempts to undermine the creditability of nurse anesthetists using level of education as a point of contention. Historically, nurse anesthetists predate physician anesthesiologists by many years in the practice of anesthesia, and this may explain, in part, the adversarial relationship between the two groups. Many certified registered nurse ansthetists (CRNAs) see the transition to the DNP as giving more creditability to the profession and as an educational level of preparation that decreases disparities in education between physicians and other doctorally prepared health care professionals. The DNP does not change the scope of nurse anesthesia practice, but it enhances the leadership and the analytical skills of the CRNA to strengthen practice and the delivery of anesthesia care.

Over the years, nurse anesthesia educational programs have stayed in pace with other advanced practice nursing specialties requiring master's-level education for all accredited programs since 1998. The AANA supports the American Association of Colleges of Nursing's (AACN) move toward the clinical doctorate for advanced practice nurses and will mandate nurse anesthesia programs to offer doctoral preparation by 2025 for entry into practice (AACN, 2004; AANA, 2007). Many CRNAs embrace the move toward the DNP for entry into practice, realizing that health care is changing at an astonishing rate and the importance of keeping pace with these changes.

As the first CRNA DNPs emerge, there is enthusiasm and more participation in research and scholarly activities. CRNAs are coming out of their educational programs with a better understanding of research methods and translational research. These CRNAs are more confident in their skills to critically analyze the evidence and integrate this evidence into anesthesia practice. They are eager to share their knowledge of EBP and critical analytical skills with colleagues and are displaying this through informal discussions in the clinical arena, presenting at professional conferences, and taking on quality improvement initiatives.

CRNA DNPs have learned the importance of becoming active in professional organizations and have learned how to navigate through the complex health care system. They are quickly becoming more active participants in health care reform and contributing to health care policy. These activities may have an impact and shape the practice of anesthesia as health care evolves.

In nursing, there is an overall disparity in educational levels for registered nurses. For years, nursing has cultivated this disparity by accepting limited educational credentials to practice nursing. The profession has created a workforce with limited education, which contributes to lack of creditability within health care. These disparities hold true in nurse anesthesia as well. Since 1998, all nurse anesthesia educational programs are required to grant a master's degree. Unfortunately, only 60% of CRNAs have completed this level of education (Muckle, Apatov, & Plaus, 2009). Increasing the number of doctorally prepared nurse anesthetists and nurses in the workforce may boost the quality of nursing and the creditability of the nurse anesthesia profession within the health care arena.

The nurse anesthesia profession is demanding more clinical scholarship and curriculum in academic programs focusing on evidence-based medicine. There is a shortage of doctorally prepared full-time nursing faculty in nurse anesthesia programs. It is difficult to create clinical scholarship and teach EBP if the academic preparation of faculty is not adequate to meet these demands. The DNP does not prepare the nurse to be an educator any more than the PhD does, but the DNP provides a larger number of higher-educated and qualified nurses to assume academic roles that will foster clinical scholarship and cultivate an understanding of EBP.

It is difficult to say exactly what the DNP will bring to an individual's professional practice. It brings something different to each individual. Looking at the DNP from a broad prospective, the DNP may strengthen practice in many different ways. CRNAs may change the way they perceive themselves in their role in health care. The clinical doctorate may give CRNAs more confidence to take on leadership roles that they may not have assumed prior to the advanced education. Some CRNAs may assume academic appointments and take on administrative roles within nursing. Others may become more active in professional organizations. Many CRNAs may find themselves promoting clinical scholarship among colleagues and managing quality improvement initiatives in the clinical setting. Regardless of the direction, CRNAs will be presented with a number of opportunities to improve the quality of nurse anesthesia practice. There is no doubt that the clinical doctorate will overall strengthen nursing and the nurse anesthesia profession while elevating the profession to a higher level.

## ■ NURSE MIDWIFE

### SUSAN JACOBY

As a certified nurse midwife in full scope clinical practice for 12 years, I debated whether to return to school for a PhD. I ruled it out because I perceived that would be the path to a career in academics, and I wanted to remain in the clinical realm. I love to teach but my passion is taking care of women, babies, and their families during childbirth. The DNP seemed to me to be the best of both worlds. I could improve my care for women by learning research skills and methodology to critically review the literature and put it into practice. I could also identify a problem at the bedside, research it, and find an evidence-based solution that would translate into best practice. This linkage between the DNP and midwifery has served me well.

The problem, as many midwives and advanced practice nurses are aware, is where to find the money and time to pursue a graduate degree. Nurses are fortunate to have access to tuition reimbursement for school, and between that and a generous scholarship provided by my alma mater, I was able to finance my education. I have been fortunate to be able to work my way through school from an associate degree in nursing through a DNP, using various forms of tuition reimbursement. This is a benefit of the nursing profession that is not enjoyed by other professions.

Time for graduate education is also a problem for busy working professionals. Full-time employment, for a midwife who takes obstetric call, is between 48–96 hours/week. I was not able to decrease my work hours due to a critical staffing shortage. Factor in the obligations of children, family, and home responsibilities, and it does not leave much time for school. My four children, who were all born and raised during the time when I was completing my AD to MS degrees, were grown and living on their own at this time. I was fortunate to have an understanding husband who took over most of the home responsibilities such as cooking and cleaning. Initially, I tried to complete the DNP in 1 year; my first semester was 12 hours. This included a research course, which alone kept me busy. After that first semester, I scaled back to 9 hours and completed the DNP in four semesters. For every academic credit hour, one is required to complete 3 hours of homework. Imagine working 48–96 hours/week (for call weekends) and another 48 hours/week for school and you can begin to understand the scope of this endeavor.

The DNP has strengthened my role as a professional midwife and given me the tools necessary to keep abreast of the ever-changing health care arena. In addition to helping me to improve my role as a clinician, I am also engaged in ongoing clinical research for an immigrant Somali population of women with unmet needs for quality obstetric services. I was able to put these new tools into practice from the beginning of my research course throughout my educational program.

Many midwives and other obstetric care providers are not familiar with the practice of female genital mutilation or cutting (FGM/C). This is the term used to describe the practice of partial or total removal of the external female genitalia, or other injury to these organs, for nonmedical reasons (World Health Organization [WHO], 2008). Infibulation, also called type III FGM/C, is the most severe form. The neointroitus (i.e., new opening) will have a firm, fibrous band of tissue replacing the labia, obliterating the urethral and vaginal openings. The diameter of this new opening may be as small as or smaller than the size of a pencil, through which urine, menstrual blood, and, ultimately, the fetus, must pass. Infants born to women who have undergone FGM/C suffer a higher rate of neonatal death when compared with babies born to women who have not undergone type III infibulation (Banks, Meirik, Farley, Akande, Bathija, & Ali, 2008; WHO, 2008).

Midwives and other obstetric care providers who have never seen a woman with FGM/C may not understand how to provide culturally appropriate care for women with this type of scar tissue, how to safely perform the deinfibulation (removal of scar tissue), or how to prevent birth trauma for both mother and infant (Wall, 2008). My DNP capstone project, *Certified Nurse Midwives' Obstetrical Management of Women with Female Genital Mutilation/Cutting* (Jacoby, 2009), was designed to teach midwives how to perform deinfibulation during second-stage labor to prevent the complications of obstetric dystocia and trauma to infibulated women and their babies. It involved developing a culturally appropriate educational program that incorporated and implemented a clinical practice guideline for care of infibulated women (*Female Genital Cutting: Clinical and Cultural Guidelines*, Nour, 2004) and a hands-on skills workshop using pelvic models to teach midwives how to perform deinfibulation in the second stage of labor. My research demonstrated improved confidence levels among the midwives who attended the educational session and deinfibulation workshop in comparisons of pre- and postconfidence levels. I have since presented this information to family practice residents, nurses, and other health care providers.

As with many areas of research, the solution to one problem leads to further questions. My current research involves a mixed-methods multidisciplinary study, led by a certified nurse midwife that includes a physician, anthropologist, and Somali cultural broker. We are trying to determine the "what" with a quantitative and the "why" with a qualitative study of perinatal issues among immigrant Somali women, with an underlying theoretical framework of health literacy. Prior to obtaining the DNP, I would not have known how to ask the questions that we need to discern and how to provide the best care for this vulnerable population of women. This study, along with my capstone project, will assist my research career as a DNP clinician. I agree with Proctor and Renfrew (2000) that as midwives who aspire to be lead professionals in normal childbirth, the majority of all births, we must be willing to prepare to defend our profession rationally, through the critical examination of research. This will allow us to be an empowered profession that in turn empowers women (Proctor & Renfrew, 2000). Support for the excellence of midwifery outcomes have been demonstrated in the literature (Hatem, Sandall, Devane, Soltani, & Gates, 2009).

Another part of my practice that has changed since achieving the DNP is in the area of the business of midwifery. Like many young midwives, I just wanted to "catch" babies when I finished school. I had not taken any business courses or training during my career in either nursing or midwifery, and the *Health Care Economics* course opened my eyes to the business of health care. My practice was experiencing an acute shortage of midwives during the time that I was in school, and as lead midwife, I needed to completely reconfigure our practice. This course walked me through the mechanics of writing a proposal for a viable independent midwifery practice, which I presented to my hospital administration with excellent outcomes. We now have the kind of practice that makes me proud to work in, and it has been useful for marketing, recruitment, and retention of midwives. Other benefits have included recent changes made to the medical staff bylaws, removing supervisory language and giving midwives licensed independent practice (LIP) status with admitting privileges in our institution.

This past summer, my midwife colleagues and I lobbied our federal legislators to improve maternity care services for women in the United States, and we will continue to advocate for midwifery care for all women. We recently celebrated the passage of the midwifery Access to Care and Equity Act, part of the comprehensive health care reform bill, and increased the reimbursement of midwifery services under Medicare from 65% to 100% of a physician's fee schedule. This will ensure that we are viewed by third party insurers as a legitimate option for maternity care services for disabled women, and protect the future viability of the midwifery profession.

In summary, the DNP has allowed me to mature and grow as a midwife. It has "raised the bar" of professionalism within my practice and has helped to rejuvenate the attitudes and working conditions of the nurses and midwives with whom I work. Midwife meetings now incorporate peer review activities and ideas for research-based best practice patient care, rather than disagreement over the call schedule and vacations. We actively look for problems to solve within our department, not only in the area of patient care but also in the area of health care economics. As a midwife with the CNM, DNP credential, I am ready to take my place at the table, both locally and nationally, to help solve our health care crisis in the area of maternity care.

## ■ ADMINISTRATION

### AMANDA D. JOJOLA

There are many opportunities for change and growth as a professional in the discipline of nursing. After 22 years of working in various nursing fields, I decided that I needed to explore these opportunities once again. I worked in both urban and rural areas, and dabbled a bit in medical surgical nursing, ENT, neurology, and internal medicine as a baccalaureate-prepared nurse. As an advanced practice nurse, I worked in family practice and, most recently, nursing education. I quickly found that I loved the world of nursing academia. I have always valued higher education and witnessing others with similar values inspired me to look further into this area of nursing. Preparing individuals for the nursing role is an enormous responsibility. Thus, I somehow felt that I needed to be better prepared to take on this role. This was the catalyst that led me down the DNP path.

I knew that a master's of science in nursing (MSN) would only get me so far in academia. In most 4-year colleges and universities, a nurse with an MSN is not considered for tenure track teaching positions, let alone administrative positions. Typically, a doctoral degree is necessary, with the PhD being the preferred degree, especially for those seeking employment in research institutions. Those with a DNP credential are usually hired in clinical faculty positions. I knew deep in my heart that the research-focused curriculum of the PhD was not where I would thrive professionally, so I chose the DNP route. Honestly, I did not really know where it would take me at first. I was hoping that I would figure it out along my educational path. Moving forward "on the fly" is not in my character, so I was taking a huge risk, but something inside me told me I needed to pursue this avenue.

I remember that my fellow classmates were with high hopes that the DNP degree would help them become more advanced practitioners. I also remember a lot of confusion among my peers regarding the difference between doctoral degrees and the purpose of the DNP, myself included. Yet, I continued. I did not really meet many peers who were interested in academia. Generally, those interested in nursing education opted for the PhD path. I worried a bit more about my decision when my advisor told me that as a DNP I would have to practice clinically, otherwise I would be "... a doctor of what?" After all, the words nursing and practice are listed in the DNP credential. It makes sense, right? Still, as much as I enjoyed nursing practice, I enjoyed nursing academia more.

As the semesters passed, I began to see how the DNP role could easily meet my goals and I was able to breathe a bit easier. Core concepts such as leadership, quality improvement, EBP, and policy kept appearing and reappearing in the curricula, all concepts pertinent to nursing education. Therefore, I definitely began to see how the DNP role related to the faculty position.

In time, I was also able to see how important all these concepts were to the administrative role in nursing academia. Having served as the interim nursing department chair for 10 months prior to returning to school, I had a fairly good idea about the skills and knowledge necessary to fulfill the responsibilities of that position. I found that these foundational concepts were no different in practice than nursing education. For instance, as a leader, the academic nursing administrator continually solves problems, makes decisions, acts as an advocate, supports and initiates change, coaches others, and empowers members of the unit's team to reach a common vision. To accomplish this, quality improvement measures need to be established based on EBP. Action for improvement anywhere in health care often requires political activism. Of course, application of these concepts does vary, but the end result is improved outcomes, whether it is student, faculty, or patient outcomes.

I graduated with my DNP after 2½ years in a rigorous DNP program and was hired as the director of nursing in a rural liberal arts college within 2 months of graduation. As the interim director, only 3 years prior to completing the DNP program, I was unsure of my ability to adequately fulfill the responsibilities of that position. Today, because of my DNP educational path, I am confident that I can succeed in my current position and hope to be a role model for others pursuing similar professional paths. I no longer worry about being a "... doctor of what?" Now, I embrace being a DNP in an academic nursing administrative role because I know I am still making a difference and improving outcomes within the discipline of nursing. As I reflect on the past 3½ years of my life, I realize that I embraced the opportunity to change and grow as a professional. Therefore, I have accomplished what I initially set out to do.

## ■ PHARMACEUTICAL MEDICAL SCIENCE LIAISON

### THOMAS J. McQUAID

Excitement, disappointment, optimism—these common themes describe my emotional experience with the DNP and relate to my own view of my work as a doctorally prepared NP working in the pharmaceutical industry. I was lured out of clinical practice 7 years ago by a pharmaceutical company that was interested in better understanding the needs of patients around a specific disease state, a disease state where I had expertise and in which I had done some novel work. The appeal of a higher pay, better benefits, greater job flexibility, and in general, a better quality of life finally won despite my passion for patient care. As a master's-prepared NP, I was disappointed to find that certain positions within industry were closed to me because I did not have a terminal degree. In particular, I had an interest in moving from my initial industry position as a clinical specialist to that of a medical liaison or medical directorship. Medical liaisons generally function as technical expert spokespersons working in defined geographic fields to support a specific product or products manufactured by either a pharmaceutical or medical device company. The positions usually require a clinical doctorate or PhD in a field related to the product. The jobs are very competitive, requiring excellent communication and presentation skills and frequently a lot of experience. I found that doctors of pharmacy, even though many had never had patient contact, were being hired over me simply because they were doctorally prepared.

This probably should not have been surprising given the level of ignorance I faced from industry regarding the function, role, and scope of practice of nurses and NPs. I distinctively remember a discussion with a pharmaceutical company attorney who insisted that NPs were not responsible for what they prescribed. She went on to support her erroneous statement by stating that was why NPs did not receive drug recall or update warnings. She insisted that NPs in each and every state had to have a physician who would be held responsible for their decisions. I had to provide her with written evidence that she was incorrect and that the scope of practice varied from state to state. I additionally had to explain to her that supervising and collaborating physicians could only be held responsible for patients they saw, directed care for, or consulted on. Even when presented with evidence that she was incorrect, she seemed incredulous of the information and decided to prohibit NPs from participating in a Web site where they could offer treatment services for patients seeking a provider to treat them. This despite the fact that many NPs treated this disease autonomously. Other examples of role confusion pervaded. I recall one colleague asking me if an NP was similar to a licensed practical nurse (LPN). Though I excelled in industry at that time, won many awards, and was told by many colleagues, "you should really be a medical liaison" or asked "why did not you go to medical school?" I was repeatedly told that I did not have the correct academic credentials to be considered for the role.

I felt these somewhat negative experiences related to corporate perceptions of my abilities were based on my degree and what it meant regarding my preparation for certain positions. Thus, I was filled with excitement at the manifestation of a DNP program that would provide me with a terminal clinical degree. I explored a number of DNP programs and was sad to see criticism and controversy surrounding a number of the programs. This criticism appeared to be based on how closely aligned with the medical model of education they were. I view the role of NP as one that spans the disciplines between medicine and nursing and feel a great NP should be able to practice autonomously, with proficiency on both sides of this man-made divide. Based on my views of a more integrated view of nursing and medicine, I hoped that a DNP would level the playing field for me in competing for clinical jobs and open doors to positions that previously had been blocked to me. I felt it would allow me to compete in industry for positions that typically were given to terminal clinical degrees in medicine or pharmacy. I jumped at the first program that was flexible enough to allow me to work and pursue my DNP simultaneously and was thrilled.

While in pursuit of the degree and later in job-seeking interactions, I was disappointed. My disappointment was multifold. First, as mentioned previously, there was tremendous diversity in the curricula amongst the DNP programs, and this adds to the confusion within and outside of nursing about the degree. My experience of having my peers in industry not understand or have knowledge of my professional scope of practice forced me to realize my own feelings of ambivalence about the profession. It also forced me to ponder that nursing itself is responsible for much of the public's incorrect perceptions and ambiguity related to the roles in the profession. We have so many functions, variations in skills, and scopes encompassed under the same titles that it is confusing to anyone not immersed in the discipline. If we want to compete for positions in industry with the other terminal clinical degrees, we must demonstrate abilities to do what they do while at the same time keeping our dedication to our origins. We must not cling to our original definitions and boundaries with trepidation, thinking there is something wrong with having or developing the same skill sets as the other terminal clinical degrees do. Additionally, we need to give clear and meaningful titles to our individual roles and provide the public with clear messages about the functions related to these roles. Perhaps we could learn from nurse anesthetists in this regard.

With perseverance and networking, I finally obtained a job as a medical liaison. I look toward the future with tremendous optimism. I am working hard to make sure I perform as well as my medical doctor and pharmaceutical doctor peers. I strive to educate people about the DNP degree and its meaning, and I am seeing my colleague DNPs achieve and get recognition in new arenas everyday. I think a generation of DNPs that has practiced clinically as NPs is going to be able to transcend the boundaries of the tight definitions of nursing. It will be critical to let go of the fear of admitting that what we do as healers crosses the artificial boundaries created during an era of gender-based discrimination and overlaps with other clinical disciplines. I see the role of the DNP in industry continuing to grow in scope and depth, and defining the role clearly to the public and to ourselves as a terminal clinical degree is tantamount to this happening successfully.

## ■ GLOBAL FORENSICS

### JOYCE P. WILLIAMS

Following the completion of my master's education, an invitation via a colleague led me to a forensic injury analyst prevention position, where I was among a team of scientists who researched the proximal cause of death and how to transform body armor protection to improve individual and systems outcomes to decrease combat mortality. This position utilized advanced practitioners to provide comprehensive injury inquiry on individuals by investigating the environment surrounding the troops in combat, reviewing the person, mounted/dismounted, the surroundings, and all phases of fighting; this led to improvements in personal protective equipment as well as vehicle redesign and heightened situational awareness. The proposals were delivered to team members, stakeholders, and agencies with detailed findings and recommendations for improvising the protective methods to improve survivability.

Being involved in a surveillance position along with rigorous coursework expanded my entire philosophy of injury causation, how individuals and entire communities are affected, and the summative impact across the globe. Through my DNP education, each course carefully connected not only methodologies but also the relationships essential to influence policy and regulation. Safety has had a more profound presence in every aspect of my work since the initiation of the DNP degree.

Beginning in the first semester, the concepts contained in each forensic course amplified my comprehension of the economic impact of violence. Not only do we need to treat the physical aspects, but also, more importantly, the mental insults that are often lifelong.

This holistic approach is quite apparent when analyzing injury pathology, trauma, and the aftermath of a mass casualty event.

During my studies at the University of Tennessee, in my role as a specialist in the analysis of injuries, Johns Hopkins University approached me to expand the graduate-level clinical nurse specialist (CNS) program. Discussions continued, but I initially declined the request until I was closer to graduation. I finally accepted the offer to create a certificate with a forensic nursing focus, and it would consist of four courses that would advance the knowledge and practice of nurses engaging in injury prevention. I used my understanding and experience to develop elements significant in the practice of persons suffering from inflicted trauma. The modules consisted of in-depth injury identification pathology and subtleties across the lifespan, comprehensive physical and psychological trauma and violence assessment, legislative and policy opportunities for advanced practitioners, and the fundamental underpinnings pertaining to the health care needs of persons. Additional areas include global concepts of mass casualty and environmental events with efforts to better prepare communities to manage the consequences of an unexpected incident.

The academic role involves student mentoring incorporating real-life knowledge and personal experiences that translate EBP principles and practice. The strengths of a DNP-prepared person contribute significantly to teaching and preparing new professionals to provide and manage direct care to individuals and populations and to positively influence the quality of care and delivery of services.

During my nursing career, I placed great emphasis on providing direct care to individuals. As a trauma nurse, I became more attentive to the wounding mechanisms of the injured, resulting in the need to expand beyond the institutional setting. Professional involvement generated a new culture and emphasized the need for additional education. The development of more "whys" was apparent and the best place to accomplish this was graduate education. The educational venues I chose gave me the ability to expand on each theory by adding outreach experiences, where I created linkages within the forensic science community. I was able to draw on the expertise of subject matter experts who shared scientific principles and codes of ethics, paramount to the field.

In the clinical arena, DNP education is underscored in prevention and intervention activities targeted to individuals and populations. In concert with these initiatives, the development of advanced technology is plausible by working side by side with the injured, modeling and simulation specialists, and biomedical engineers to improve the quality of life with optimal outcomes for the injured. It is through the integration and collaboration of multidisciplinary research teams that we can address the paucities that exist, identify EBP interventions, and translate these into practice. I rank trauma and injury prevention as paramount at all levels.

I have had the opportunity to travel with a cohort of faculty to Australia to participate in a research conference. This allowed me to integrate among researchers and clinicians to discuss my roles as an expert in disaster forensic nursing. The combination of my work at disaster sites and my academic scholarship reinforced my credibility among my colleagues. My experience in working with the American Nurse Credentialing Center (ANCC) on portfolio recognition for the forensic nurse community has provided key elements necessary in the design of education content and rigor.

My areas of interest have concentrated on victims and populations sustaining injury due to violence. Traumatic injuries account for a significant burden to the health care system and impacts quality of life, including cognitive changes and complex comorbidities contributing to chronic disease conditions. Over the past few years, I have authored chapters in three textbooks, along with invited speaking engagements and consultations. Participating in research via community involvement assessments, and producing seminars and continuing education for practitioners and the community at large are important parts of my current role.

Professionally, in partnership with colleagues, we founded the DNP, LLC. I have been cochair of the annual Doctors of Nursing Practice Conference for the past 4 years. The value of an organization that coordinates practitioners and leaders in health care is vital to setting the pace for the future.

Membership in other forensic professional organizations as a DNP has afforded my ongoing engagement with colleagues and invitations for participation on various boards, such as vice president for the Forensic Nursing Certification Board. I have been an invited participant for the American Nurses Credentialing Center/International Association of Forensic Nurses as a collaborative member and have testified for Magnet status for one of our stakeholders.

The significance of the DNP was a personal investment that has enhanced my overall expectations as a clinical nurse. However, the journey was not only an achievement, but also, more importantly, it has helped me to see the world with more perceptiveness. I sense that I will be able to impact the lives of others in a positive way over the years.

My commitment lies in the study of the causal effects of injury and consequences of violence. This work will not only improve the lives of individuals and populations, but will also positively influence the quality of life and potential delivery of services to mankind. I have a special concern for risk assessment and potential health consequences of individuals with lack of regard for injury. Not only does this impact them personally but also places great economic burdens across the nation. The economic cost of motor vehicle crashes in 2000 was $230.6 billion (Blincoe et al., 2002). It is recognized that a 360° view of the impact can direct capacity building and change the culture of injury epidemiology. This is but one area critical to the delivery of effective responses to the short-, medium-, and long-term health needs of a population. My professional experience in trauma, emergency, and disaster services as well as graduate education in forensic science provides a relevant background specific to prevention services at all levels. I have witnessed the social determinants that impact the population and would like to offer global support to reduce the inequities that exist.

Maintaining active involvement in international and community organizations is important to me. As a member of the World Association for Disaster and Emergency Management, I have been appointed as chair to the education committee, where I have expertise working in complex events by responding to two mass fatality events. As a member of the Child Fatality Review Team for the past 8 years, I appreciate the aspects involved in unnecessary morbidity and mortality.

Is the DNP of value? Most certainly! The world cannot change without the allegiance and encouragement of DNP nurses who have the opportunity to close the gaps and transform the current burdens existing in the health needs of others by building capacity, creating linkages, and by working side by side to enable the abilities of others to sustain communities. The DNP role has begun to make a footprint in health care, a precedent that has the opportunity to be a profound change agent in the provision of health care and the reduction of violence and risk to all.

## ■ SUMMARY

The experiences of the seven DNP-prepared nurses highlighted in this chapter are diverse, although there are some common themes. No one in the group expressed regret over the time and expense of returning to school, although many mentioned the struggle of juggling work and family responsibilities with school workload. Respect for and acknowledgment of DNP peers were regarded as very important, and many were pleased with a growing DNP community. Despite disappointments noted by some with lack of recognition of the DNP degree by their colleagues, others felt that their contributions were more highly regarded because of the acquisition of the DNP degree. All of the contributors noted feeling optimistic about future opportunities. Although there are challenges ahead for the DNP integrating into health care systems, strides are being made in a number of diverse areas that highlight the contributions of DNP-prepared nurses. The breadth of experience, knowledge, and commitment as evidenced in the short pieces above reflect the strength of nurses who chose to pursue a practice doctorate in nursing and be the catalysts for change.

## ■ REFERENCES

American Association of Nurse Anesthetists (AANA). (2010). *Qualifications and capabilities of the certified registered nurse anesthetist.* Retrieved September 1, 2010, from http://www.aana.com/ceandeducation/becomeacrna/Pages/Qualifications-and-Capabilities-of-the-Certified-Registered-Nurse-Anesthetist-.aspx

American Association of Nurse Anesthetist (AANA). (2007). *AANA position on doctoral preparation of nurse anesthetists.* Retrieved September 2, 2010, from http://www.aana.com/ceandeducation/educationalresources/Documents/AANA_Position_DTF_June_2007.pdf

American Association of Colleges of Nursing (AACN). (2004). *AACN position statement on the practice doctorate in nursing, October 2004.* Retrieved April 6, 2012, from www.aacn.nche.edu/publications/position/DNPpositionstatement.pdf

Banks, E., Meirik, O., Farley, T., Akande, O., Bathija, H., & Ali, M. (2006). Female genital mutilation and obstetric outcome: WHO collaborative prospective study in six African countries. *Lancet, 367*, 1835–1841.

Blincoe, L., Seay, A., Zaloshnja, E., Miller, T., Romano, E., Luchter, S., & Spicer, R. (2002). *The economic impact of motor vehicle crashes, 2000.* Washington, DC: U.S. Department of Transportation, National Highway Traffic Safety Administration (NHTSA).

Fosburg, L. C., & Kosh, E. (1995). The AANA archives: Documenting a distinguished past. *AANA Journal, 63*, 88–93.

Hatem, M., Sandall, J., Devane, D., Soltani, H., & Gates, S. (2009). *Midwife-led versus other models of care for childbearing women* (Review). The Cochrane Collaboration. Retrieved June 21, 2009, from http://www.thecochranelibrary.com

Jacoby, S. D. (2009). *Certified nurse midwives' obstetrical management of women with female genital mutilation/cutting.* Unpublished Capstone Project in completion of Doctor of Nursing Practice, awarded by Massachusetts General Hospital Institute of Health Professions.

Muckle, T. J., Apatov, N. M., & Plaus, K. (2009). A report on the CCNA 2007 professional practice analysis. *AANA Journal, 77*, 181–189.

Nour, N. M. (2004). Female genital cutting: Clinical and cultural guidelines. *Obstetrical and Gynecological Survey, 59*, 272–279.

Proctor, S., & Renfrew, M. (Eds.). (2000). *Linking research and practice in midwifery: A guide to evidence-based practice.* Edinburgh: Bailliere Tindall.

Wall, L. L. (2006). Obstetric vesicovaginal fistula as an international public-health problem. *Lancet, 368*, 1201–1209.

World Health Organization (WHO). (2008). *Eliminating female genital mutilation: An interagency statement UNAIDS, UNDP, UNECA, UNESCO, UNFPA, UNHCHR, UNHCR, UNICEF, UNIFEM, WHO.* WHO Press. Retrieved November 2, 2008, from http://www.who.org

# CHAPTER 9

# Leadership Skill Set for the Advanced Practice Registered Nurse

Jeffrey Kwong

The doctor of nursing practice (DNP) graduate is faced with a wealth of new opportunities. For most registered nurses electing to pursue advanced practice roles, the DNP represents the first step in gaining a combination of both new clinical skills and a new identity as an advanced practitioner. For masters-prepared nurses who elect to complete the DNP, this new degree serves as a means of broadening one's clinical scope and refocusing on larger systems perspectives. As a result of this mix of nurses and the various paths to completion of the DNP (either post-master's or baccalaureate-to-DNP), the competencies and experiences of the DNP graduate will vary based on the individual's previous educational background and work history. Nonetheless, one of the core competencies and expectations of the DNP is that the DNP graduate will be able to serve as a clinical leader within their work environment and within the profession.

Not every DNP will choose to be the chief nursing officer, and not every DNP will rise to the ranks of an administrator or dean. However, being a leader does not necessarily mean that one must possess these titles as part of their job description. By having the title of advanced practice nurse, or by virtue of being a doctorally prepared nurse, it is implied that the individual who holds these degrees and titles has the ability and knowledge of higher level thinking, the ability to manage others, and the ability to serve in a leadership role in some capacity—be it taking on the responsibility of a working group, leading a special task force, or supervising other allied health professionals.

In 2010, the Institute of Medicine (IOM, 2010) published a report on the future of nursing, which emphasized the key role nurses play in the delivery, creation, and advancement of health care. The report places an emphasis on the leadership roles and responsibilities that nurses across the practice continuum (from nurses at the bedside to nurses in the executive office) possess and contribute to the health care environment. The report calls for nursing to "cultivate and promote leaders from within the profession" (IOM, 2010). The changing dynamic of health care is the ideal ground for nurses to demonstrate clinical expertise, leadership, and the ability to collaborate with other health professions in facilitating change. These requirements are also echoed in the competencies that are outlined in the essentials of the DNP curriculum.

According to the Merriam-Webster dictionary, a leader is "a person who has command-ing authority and influence" (Leader, n.d.). This definition applies to the role of the advanced practice nurse in the provision of patient care and in the hierarchical ranking among the vari-ous clinical nursing roles. By the mere definition of "advanced practice," one can assume that the nurse who holds this title is someone who has achieved a more in-depth level of educa-tion, has broader clinical acumen, and possesses the ability to envision the future. The role of the doctorally prepared nurse is one that requires further skills and leadership abilities, above and beyond those with master's degrees.

The American Association of Colleges of Nursing (AACN, 2006) emphasizes that the DNP-prepared nurse is a practice expert who possesses an array of knowledge as it applies to evidence-based practice, quality improvement, and systems-level thinking. As part of this practice-based role, the DNP graduate must be fluent in a broad base of general knowledge in addition to either a clinical focus or an organizational-aggregate focus, depending on the individual's specialty. Regardless of the specialty focus of the DNP, the AACN has articu-lated a core group of competencies expected of all DNP graduates. This provides the foun-dation from which DNP-prepared nurses are able to function and serve the organizations to which they belong, the patients they care for, and the students that they teach.

Exactly what are considered "leadership skills" and how does one develop these skills? The AACN has included *leadership* within several of the major core competencies. The com-petencies associated with leadership are listed in Exhibit 9.1. It is clear that the DNP graduate is expected to be competent in several areas of leadership—ranging from policy, to financial and cost-analysis, to quality improvement, and to general clinical leadership. However, as the saying goes, "Rome wasn't built in a day." Likewise, leaders and the skills of becoming a leader are not granted overnight. So the question remains, what can one do to develop these skills if you have never been a "leader" before?

It is assumed that academic programs will offer theory and education related to the foundational components of leadership. The study of leadership has roots in psychology and business. There are various theories on leadership, organizational strategy, and leadership style. To review and summarize these theories and principles of leadership are beyond the scope of this chapter. A number of DNP programs have specific nursing leadership courses as part of the standard curriculum, others may integrate leadership content into other courses, and some institutions may offer collaborative leadership courses with Schools of Business. Regardless of how leadership theory is taught, there still lies the challenge of gaining practical "hands-on" experience. Just as a nurse may be well versed in the pathophysiology of congestive heart fail-ure (CHF), it is not until the nurse has to care for a patient in acute CHF does the nurse learn to appreciate the nuances of the theoretical knowledge from the practical aspects of caring for someone experiencing the clinical manifestations of a disease. The focus of this chapter, there-fore, is to provide a brief guide on how to gain practical experience that will benefit the new DNP graduate in applying and developing the skills necessary to fulfill the role of DNP.

In reviewing the competencies of the DNP as established by the AACN, it would appear as though the DNP were an all-encompassing superhero, being able to accomplish the job of a dozen professionals—not just one single person. However, if one looks for broad themes within the DNP competencies, there are a few commonalities. The common themes that seem to arise as they relate to leadership include collaboration, communication, leading others, and evalua-tion. These domains seem self-explanatory, but learning or gaining experience in these areas can be challenging. This holds true especially for those with limited clinical experience or for those who may not view themselves as being in a leadership position in their current career.

### EXHIBIT 9.1

#### Leadership-Themed Competencies of the DNP

**Essential I: Scientific underpinnings for practice**

**The DNP program prepares the graduate to:**

- Use science-based theories and concepts to evaluate outcomes.
- Develop and evaluate new practice approaches based on nursing theories from other disciplines.

**Essential II: Organizational and systems leadership for quality improvement and systems thinking**

**The DNP program prepares the graduate to:**

- Develop and evaluate care delivery approaches that meet current and future needs of patient populations based on scientific findings in nursing and other clinical sciences as well as organizational, political, and economic sciences.
- Ensure accountability for quality of health care and patient safety for populations with whom they work.
  - Use advanced communication skills/processes to lead quality improvement and patient safety initiatives in health systems.
  - Employ principles of business, finance, economics, and health policy to practice initiatives that will improve the quality of care delivery.
  - Develop and/or monitor budgets for practice initiatives.
  - Demonstrate sensitivity to diverse organizational cultures and populations, including patients and providers.
- Develop and or evaluate effective strategies for managing the ethical dilemmas inherent in patient care, the health care organization, and research.

**Essential III: Clinical scholarship and analytical methods for evidence-based practice**

**The DNP program prepares the graduate to:**

- Design and implement processes to evaluate outcomes of practice, practice patterns, and systems of care within a practice setting, health care organization, or community against national benchmarks to determine variances in practice outcomes and population trends.
- Design, direct, and evaluate quality improvement methodologies to promote safe, timely, effective, efficient, equitable, and patient-centered care.
- Function as a practice specialist/consultant in collaborative knowledge-generating research.
- Disseminate findings from evidence-based practice and research to improve health care outcomes.

**Essential IV: Information systems/technology and patient care technology for the improvement and transformation of health care**

**The DNP program prepares the graduate to:**

- Design, select, use, and evaluate programs that evaluate and monitor outcomes of care, care systems, and quality improvement, including consumer use of health care information systems.
- Analyze and communicate critical elements necessary to the selection, use, and evaluation of health care information systems and patient care technology.
- Provide leadership in the evaluation and resolution of ethical and legal issues within health care systems relating to the use of information, information technology, communication networks, and patient care technology.
- Evaluate consumer health information sources for accuracy, timeliness, and appropriateness.

**Essential V: Health care policy for advocacy in health care**

**The DNP program prepares graduates to:**

- Critically analyze health policy proposals, health policies, and related issues from the perspective of consumers, nurses, other health professionals, and other stakeholders in policy and public forums.
- Demonstrate leadership in the development and implementation of institutional, local, state, federal, and/or international health policy.
- Influence policy makers through active participation on committees, boards, or task forces at the institutional, local, state, regional, national, and/or international levels to improve health care delivery and outcomes.
- Educate others, including policy makers at all levels, regarding nursing, health policy, and patient care outcomes.
- Advocate for the nursing profession within the policy and health care communities.
- Develop, evaluate, and provide leadership for health care policy that shapes health care finance regulation and delivery.
- Advocate for social justice, equity, and ethical policies within all health care arenas.

**Essential VI: Interprofessional collaboration for improving patient and population health outcomes**

**The DNP program prepares the graduate to:**

- Employ effective communication and collaboration skills in the development and implementation of practice models, peer review, practice guidelines, health policy, standards of care, and/or other scholarly products.

- Lead interprofessional teams in the analysis of complex practice and organizational issues.
- Employ consultative and leadership skills with professional and inter-professional teams to create change in health care and complex health care delivery systems.

**Essential VII: Clinical prevention and population health for improving the nation's health**

**The DNP program prepares the graduate to:**

- Evaluate care delivery models and/or strategies using concepts related to community, environmental and occupational health, and cultural and socioeconomic dimensions of health.

**Essential VIII: Advanced nursing practice**

**The DNP program prepares the graduate to:**

- Design, implement, and evaluate therapeutic interventions based on nursing science and other sciences.
- Develop and sustain therapeutic relationships and partnerships with patients and other professionals to facilitate optimal care and patient outcomes.
- Demonstrate advanced levels of clinical judgment, systems thinking, and accountability in designing, delivering, and evaluating evidence-based care to improve patient outcomes.
- Guide, mentor, and support other nurses to achieve excellence in nursing practice.
- Educate and guide individuals and others through complex health and situational transitions.
- Use conceptual and analytical skills in evaluating the links among practice, organizational, population, fiscal, and policy issues.

*Source:* Adapted with permission from the American Association of Colleges of Nursing (AACN). (2006). *The essentials of doctoral education for advanced nursing practice.* Retrieved from http://www.aacn.nche.edu/dnp/pdf/essentials.pdf

# ■ THE SKILLS: COLLABORATION

Collaboration and collaborative leadership describe a leadership style that involves working successfully between different parties or organizations. According to Archer and Cameron (2008), one of the key goals of the collaborative leader is being able to achieve value from inherent differences. This is especially true for the DNP graduate who is expected to work with key opinion leaders within an institution as well as those from partnering organizations who may not necessarily agree or have the same views. The DNP must be able to take the lead in balancing clinical outcomes with quality health care and the financial constraints of organizations. Being able to master collaboration will undoubtedly lead to successful outcomes for the DNP. Collaboration is more than being able to "get along well" or build consensus. Collaboration involves specific skills that require a global perspective of a situation, being able to recognize the barriers and facilitators to achieving a meaningful end, and being able to execute the steps necessary to attain a successful outcome.

## ■ COMMUNICATION

Another theme that is evident in the AACN essentials is communication. Effective communication is at the heart of leadership. As nurses, we have an advantage of having experience in communicating with others. The art of communication is inherent in the work we do with patients. As a nurse, one must be able to provide empathic care to the infirmed, provide education to someone who may be recently diagnosed with a life-altering diagnosis, or communicate the importance of preventive health screening to populations at risk for disease. The essence of nursing entails being able to effectively communicate with others, thus it makes sense that, as nurses, we all have the potential to be effective leaders.

James Clawson is a published author and professor of business administration at the University of Virginia. In his book entitled, *Level Three Leadership: Getting below the Surface* (2006), Clawson describes leadership as "managing energy…first in yourself and then in others" (2006, p. 3). He categorizes leadership on three different levels based on how the leader is able to view, understand, and communicate with others. *Level One* leadership is more of a superficial level of leading others. Leaders who practice at this level tend to make assessments based on others' visible behaviors. *Level Two* leaders require deeper-level understanding based on individuals' conscious thoughts. *Level Three* leaders lead and influence others by understanding the deep-rooted values, attitudes, behaviors, expectations (or as Clawson terms them, VABEs) of others and knowing how to influence individuals on this much deeper level. He goes on to state that effective level three leaders are able to "understand the basic assumptions and values of employees and to match them or educate them toward harmony with the goals and strategic directions of the firm" (2006, p. 60). He believes that new or potential level three leaders "must develop new skills, including the ability to view what people are thinking and feeling" (p. 60). The first step in being able to lead at level three begins with understanding and clarifying one's own VABEs.

As health care professionals, nurses are taught the importance of self-assessment and communication early on in their careers. Many will say that it is the nurse's ability to communicate with patients that sets them apart from other health professionals. Nurses develop strong listening skills, empathy, ways to recognize and manage personal emotions, and the ability to pay attention to others—the set of skills that Goleman (1998) refers to as *emotional intelligence*. Emotional intelligence is a concept and skill that allows leaders the ability to effectively lead and communicate with others. Nurses use emotional intelligence, or at least most components of emotional intelligence, as part of their everyday work and for most, it becomes second nature. The DNP is able to harness these skills and experiences and apply them to not only patients but also to others in the organization. It is this ability to transfer the basic skills of the clinical nurse to the broader scope of practice required by the DNP and advanced practice clinician that makes nurses ideal for leadership positions.

By being able to communicate effectively and by using both emotional intelligence and level three leadership techniques, the DNP-prepared nurse is able to work productively with other key personnel within organizations. The DNP is able to translate and share critical information regarding evidence-based practice with front-line clinical staff and researchers, and he or she is able to advocate for the needs of patients in the ever-changing and complex health systems.

## ■ LEADING OTHERS

Another theme stemming from communication and collaboration is the ability to lead others. This is the more traditional idea of what many people think of when they think "leader" or "leadership." However, it is important to remember that leading others is only one facet of a leader's role. The other two areas of communication and collaboration are used to enhance and make the job of leading others more effective. Many would argue that both collaboration and communication are components of what makes a good leader, but for the purposes of this chapter, the act of leading others is considered a separate domain and comprises a thematic area for the DNP graduate. The DNP graduate is expected to lead nurses, other health professionals, administrators, researchers, and populations. By utilizing the knowledge, training, and the other skills previously mentioned, the DNP serves a pivotal role as a change agent and a driving force between practice and research, between business and clinical care, and between patient care and technology.

## ■ EVALUATION

Finally, the DNP competencies emphasize the ability to evaluate and synthesize information critically as a means of being able to make effective change. In all DNP programs, the focus on evidence-based practice is universal. To be able to critically review and interpret data, to understand the implications both clinically as well as from a fiscal and quality improvement viewpoint, is one of the distinguishing characteristics of the DNP. Translating quality evidence into practice, being able to evaluate the outcomes of practice change, and identifying new and innovative interventions are ways that DNPs are able to lead organizational change and lead others in an effort to provide patients with the best care possible. Evaluation can be viewed as a skill that confers upon the DNP *expert power*. This is a concept that has been described in the theories of leadership by French & Raven (1959). Expert power has been associated with a form of leadership where others defer to a person based on their superior knowledge base or understanding of a subject matter. In essence, by having the skills and knowledge of a doctorally prepared nurse, you are viewed by others in the field, and in your organization, as being someone who has the skills and influence of being an expert. Having the ability to provide critical evaluation of practice recommendations or evaluating the overall cost-effectiveness of an intervention is highly valued by other health professionals and administrators. This is another area in which the DNP can find his or her niche and value to an organization.

## ■ DEVELOPING THE SKILLS

So how does one develop these essential skills, and what are the steps one must take in order to become competent in these skills? There are several ways in which one can develop and start on the "leadership path." Presented here is one example of a strategy that a new DNP may utilize.

### 1. Identify leaders you admire

One of the first steps in becoming a leader and developing the skills is to identify someone or a group of people who you feel embody or possess the qualities that you would like to develop. There is nothing better than seeing leadership in action. You can obviously pick one person, but since it is difficult for one individual to possess all of the skills that you see as ideal, you will probably need to find more than one person. The individuals you select could include a faculty member, a colleague, a boss, or someone that you know through your social network. Ideally, one (or more than one) of these individuals could mentor you in being a leader. This person or group of individuals you choose do not necessarily need to be a formal mentor in the classic sense of the term. More formal mentor–mentee relationships involve a mutually agreed-upon recognition of a formal relationship, a set of goals, and a long-term commitment of training and apprenticeship. You do not need to have this formalized relationship to identify someone or a group of persons who you would like to watch or learn from.

Once you have identified this person or set of individuals, it is important to observe and take note of exactly what it is they do in certain situations, particularly ones that involve collaboration, evaluation, conflict negotiation, communication, and leading or inspiring others. These situations do not have to be nursing or health care focused because the skills and the techniques that these individuals use can be adapted and applied to your work situation. You may find that you like how some leaders are able to take a visionary approach to motivating others, or how certain leaders approach a situation when they have made an error, or being at a meeting and watching how your boss is able to achieve consensus among two differing parties. When looking at these real-life examples, you will soon be able to identify the techniques that are successful and integrate them into your skill set.

### 2. Assess your skills and leadership style

Now that you have learned the leadership theory and have identified persons who possess the skills, the next step is to assess your current skill set—highlighting your strengths and challenges. There are various self-administered leadership inventories available—and many are available online. Much like a personality test, these self-assessments are one way to identify the type of leader you are, the type of leadership style that most closely resembles your personality and inherent strengths. It is important when interpreting these test results to remember that these tests are designed to give you a general sense of your traits, but it is important not to feel locked into the results. You can change or alter certain aspects of your leadership style if you feel that it does not mesh with your current organization or the organization you envision yourself leading. It is, however, a starting point that will provide a way to determine what areas you consider strengths and those that are opportunities for change.

### 3. Assess what leadership activities you are currently doing

Many individuals may not necessarily view themselves in a leadership role currently, but be sure to take a close look at the things you do in your everyday life. One of the first steps is to review your activities, accomplishments, and interests. This involves taking time to reflect on the things that you have done in life and what you enjoy doing. This is the time to once again "think outside the box," and not just focus on nursing. In reality, many of us may be leaders or use the same skills that are required of the DNP in other activities. For example, you may be someone who is active in your children's after-school activities, you may coach the soccer team, serve on the welcoming committee for your neighborhood association, you might be the type that likes to volunteer at the animal shelter, or you may be the person that organizes the fundraiser for the local homeless shelter. These may sound like "fun" activities (which they are), but they also provide a wonderful training ground for developing and practicing skills that you can use in your professional career.

Once you have identified the activities that you participate in, think about what types of skills you use in these activities and see if they fit into any of the main themes of the DNP competencies (e.g., communication, collaboration, evaluation, motivation, and leading others). Chances are you will find at least one or two things in your current activities that already include these skills, or at least will provide an opportunity for you to "practice" these skills in an environment or an organization that you already belong to and feel comfortable working in. Perhaps the tennis club that you belong to wants to know the most cost-effective way of increasing the budget without raising membership fees. (This task would require you to use your skills of evaluating data, looking at the financial objectives, and determining the best options). Or perhaps your homeowner's association is having difficulty with the landscaping company and they need someone to serve as a liaison and ensure that the company meets their requirements and completes the work that they were paid to do (this would involve communication, collaboration, and motivating others). Or perhaps your child needs extra assistance learning math skills and you do research on finding the best methods to teach kids geometry (you search and evaluate various techniques and you find the technique that has the best proven methods for tutoring adolescents on learning geometry). As you can see, there are a wide variety of ways to use the same skills and gain practical experience in building confidence to become a recognized leader.

### 4. Start small and then go big

If you find that you may still lack sufficient experience with certain skills, you can look for other opportunities to "try them out" on a small level. You may want to volunteer organizing the next bake sale for your child's school (this involves communication with others, leading and motivating the other parents, negotiating with the schools and other parents, etc.), or perhaps you have the opportunity to volunteer on a local political campaign (this involves working within a larger system, communicating with voters and the campaign office, negotiating with others who may have differing views, and inspiring or envisioning organizational change). Once you gain confidence or experience in these smaller or nontraditional venues, the next step involves applying the lessons learned to aspects of your professional career.

### 5. Seize the opportunity

If you are still completing your graduate studies and working as a staff nurse, most units within acute care settings have working groups or committees. These committees may be unit-based or they may be hospital-wide. Take (and make) the time to volunteer for these committees. Seize the opportunity to get involved and use your leadership skills. Even by serving as a working member of these committees, you automatically assume leadership responsibilities because you will represent your peers on these committees. Many times these committees may have a specific focus (e.g., patient safety), but, often, unit-based or hospital-based committees focus on issues related to quality improvement. This is the ideal setting for the DNP-in-training to gain first-hand knowledge of how organizational change occurs, how quality improvement opportunities are identified, and how strategies for improvement are implemented. By being involved in these work-based activities, you will undoubtedly be recognized as a valuable member of the committee because you will be able to share your knowledge gained from your DNP program with your colleagues. This is the first step in becoming an advanced practice nursing leader. Within these smaller committees, many times new ideas or projects are born—and this is where you may have the opportunity to create and lead a new working group or even perhaps a new program.

### 6. Create your own opportunities

If your unit or organization does not have existing working groups, then look at your work environment and see what areas or questions you have about your practice. This is actually the ideal way to find and identify a project for your capstone project, as well. If you are able to identify an area of interest, you can develop these smaller opportunities into larger projects. Perhaps you want to assess the patient discharge process on your unit to identify ways of making it more efficient, or you want to know how many patients attending your clinic received screening for tobacco use, or how many of your CHF home health clients required multiple in-home services. Be the impetus to drive or create change. Ask your supervisor or boss if you could look into these questions. Chances are they would be thrilled to have you look into these areas or perhaps they have had different projects on the "back burner" that they have needed to work on but have not had the opportunity. In some instances, you may get to complete these activities as part of your regular work, but be prepared to volunteer your time. Remember, you may be volunteering your time now, but you are gaining experience that will benefit you in the long run. Many of you probably worked as a nursing assistant or hospital volunteer before pursing your undergraduate nursing degree to gain exposure to the field of nursing. These are the same "practice" or experience-oriented opportunities that you need to seek as a leader-in-training.

### 7. Lead in the profession

Other areas to seek leadership opportunities include working with or joining professional organizations. Many major professional organizations have local affiliates or chapters. If you are not already a member of a specialty nursing organization, consider joining one. If you already are a member, consider volunteering for various committees or even running for a position as an officer. Professional organizations are a wonderful way to meet and network with nurses and nurse leaders outside of your place of employment. Within these organizations, you can exercise your skills of communication, collaboration, and leading others by working side by side with other recognized nurse leaders and advanced practice clinicians. This is another place where you may find your role models for leadership.

### 8. Reflect, review, and redirect

One of the components of learning a new skill is being able to adjust and assess how you are doing. Although I mention self-assessment as one of the first steps of gaining leadership skills, it is also important to reflect on your progress and skills periodically throughout your learning process. The skill of self-reflection is a skill that is often taught to us as nurses. It is from our appraisal of clinical situations that we learn what works, what does not work, and how to anticipate for the future. So too with learning leadership skills, it is important to be able to take the time to look at how you have adopted your new skills. What aspects of your new leadership style do you like? What seems to be less effective? What areas would you like to have more practice in? How well do you communicate your vision? How are you at collaborating with others? Are you able to lead others? Are you able to critically evaluate information and use it to create change? If the answers to these questions are "yes," then keep doing what you are doing. If the answer to some or all of these questions is "no," then redirect your focus, identify your assets and ways to overcome your challenges, and then try out your new strategy. From this ongoing self-reflection, you will eventually find the right mix of skills and expertise to be the leader you envision yourself being.

## ■ JUST THE BEGINNING

Once you have gained some practical experience in leadership and using your advanced practice skills, you will be well on your way to fulfilling the role and competencies of the DNP. It is important to remember that the process of being a leader takes time, and it is an evolutionary process that will be both challenging and rewarding. Leadership is both a skill and an art form. Just like any other skill, the more you do "it," the easier "it" becomes. As you transition into the role of DNP, you will cross many milestones, and being a leader and gaining the skills to be a successful leader are included in those milestones. Now more than ever, the field of nursing and the health care environment, in general, is changing at speeds that far exceed the changes we have seen historically. It is truly a time of limitless boundaries, and as clinicians, visionaries, and systems-level experts, the DNP graduate of today has the opportunity to change the landscape of health care for generations to come.

## ■ REFERENCES

American Association of Colleges of Nursing (AACN). (2006). *The essentials of doctoral education for advanced nursing practice* [Pdf]. Retrieved from http://www.aacn.nche.edu/dnp/pdf/essentials.pdf

Archer, D., & Cameron A. (2008). *Collaborative leadership: How to succeed in an interconnected world*. Butterworth-Heinemann: Burlington, MA. ISBN: 0750687053.

Clawson, J. G. (2006). *Level three leadership: Getting below the surface* (3rd ed.). Upper Saddle River, NJ: Pearson Prentice Hall.

French, J. P., & Raven, B. (1959). The bases of social power. In D. Cartwright (Ed.), *Studies in social power*. Ann Arbor, MI: University of Michigan Press.

Goleman, D. (1998). *What makes a leader?* Harvard Business Review (pp. 82–91) [Pdf]. Retrieved from http://www.lesaffaires.com/uploads/references/743_what-makes-leader_Goleman.pdf

Institute of Medicine (IOM). (2010). *The future of nursing: Leading change, advancing health*. Retrieved from http://www.nap.edu/catalog.php?record_id=12956#toc

Leader. (n.d.). In *Merriam-Webster Dictionary*. Retrieved from http://www.merriam-webster.com/dictionary/leader

CHAPTER 10

# Developing the Leadership Skill Set for the Executive Nurse Leader

Jeanette Ives Erickson, Marianne Ditomassi, and Jeffrey M. Adams

Opportunities and strategies for leadership improvement in the health care system have been well-documented. Yet, direct funding and support of nursing administration research has traditionally not been a high priority for federal or private grant making institutions. The increasing acuity of patients, the demand for reducing cost of providing health services, and the need for establishing structures that lead to a more efficient, effective, timely, equitable, safe, and patient-centered (Institute of Medicine [IOM], 2001) delivery system all require expert nurse leadership. Thus, focus and development of expert executive nurse leaders are more important than ever. This chapter will explore the efforts, experiences, and framing of executive nurse leadership through an organization's commitment to development and utilization of a program of research within this population.

## ■ EBP AND KBP—EVIDENCE- AND KNOWLEDGE-BASED MANAGEMENT PRACTICE

An important distinction in setting an organizational executive nurse leadership agenda is the commitment to evidence-based practice (EBP) and, perhaps more importantly, knowledge-based practice (KBP) within the context of nursing administration and executive nurse leadership roles. EBP can be defined as the integration of best-research evidence with clinical expertise and patient values (Sackett, Straus, Richardson, Rosenberg, & Haynes, 2000). KBP can be best described as the interactive linkage between theory, research, and practice (Roy, 2007). While evidence and data have been widely adopted as drivers of clinical practice decisions, they have not been completely integrated in administrative or leadership practice. KBP provides a framework for both a basis and justification of executive nurse leadership practice. It places value on critical thinking and decision making, providing some latitude for managing social and political structures that are a daily part of executive leadership practice.

Parallel to the need for the adopting of EBP/KBP strategies, Magnet recognition validates executive nurse leadership and highlights the presence of a strong and collaborative professional practice environment (PPE). Grounded in research, Magnet recognition is the highest honor awarded to health care institutions by the American Nurses Credentialing Center (ANCC) for excellence in nursing services. The current Magnet recognition model heightens the importance of demonstrating the outcomes and effects of nurses' work (ANCC, 2008). This framework challenges executive nurse leaders to utilize KBP/EBP as part of a continuous critical review toward improving the structures and processes that support care delivery.

## ■ ADVANCING KNOWLEDGE/FRAMING THE EFFORTS

An important part of KBP is not only the utilization of evidence, but the participation and development of new knowledge to inform and advance the discipline and improve patient care, practice environments, and outcomes. The Agency for Healthcare Research & Quality (AHRQ), American Nurses Association (ANA), American Organization for Nurse Executives (AONE), and the National Institute for Nursing Research (NINR) have all identified nursing work environments, organizational structure, and patient outcomes research as funding priorities. Additionally, it can be surmised that these research initiatives will also lead toward the refinement of nursing administration educational curricula and continuing education strategies for the executive nurse leader.

Shortell, Gillies, and Devers (1995) first sounded the alarm for a need to understand and manage the complexities of health care institutions, with the recognition that new management and leadership skills are required. They proposed that health care leaders must generate the development of a new culture with an emphasis on managing horizontally, which calls for greater negotiation and conflict management skills, systems thinking, and team building. While this call, nearly two decades old, has not gone unheeded, adapting to manage the complexities of health care is a forever project, and success is closely tied to those with vision and focus. Within this context, tying or framing executive nurse leadership research to PPEs and/or patient outcomes serves as both a visionary approach and a focus that can be shared/ supported by the funding organizations; it also further defines and improves success for those in nursing executive leadership practice.

## ■ LEADERSHIP DEVELOPMENT TRAJECTORY—THE PROFESSIONAL PRACTICE MODEL

While a knowledge-based nursing leadership practice inclusive of research and theory has long been a part of efforts at the Massachusetts General Hospital (MGH), the coordinated efforts toward a focused executive nurse leadership strategy integrating and emphasizing the PPE began in 1996. At this time, the MGH nursing and patient care leadership first developed the MGH professional practice model (PPM) as represented in Figure 10.1 (Ives Erickson, 1996). A PPM is a conceptual, theoretical, and practical framework that provides nurses with an articulate, knowledge-based justification for practice of the profession. Developed and disseminated in 1996 and revised in 2007, the MGH PPM is grounded in values and beliefs that embrace patient-centered care in partnership with the nurse and other providers of care within the patient care environment.

With a well-designed PPM framework, nurses feel connected within the context of their relationships to the patient, to their own practice, to the roles of other providers in contributing to the plan, to other nurses, and to the institution. A framework

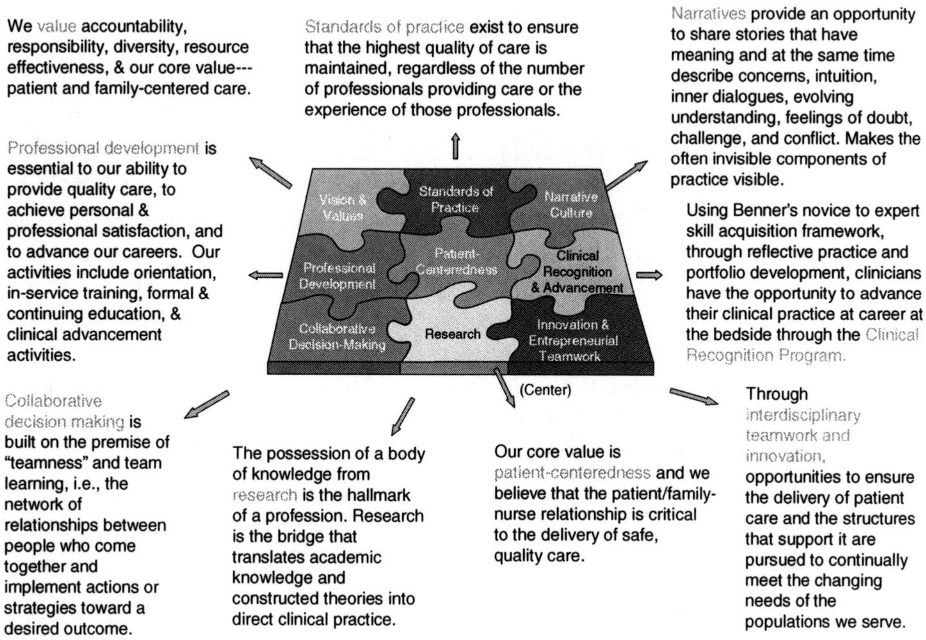
We value accountability, responsibility, diversity, resource effectiveness, & our core value--- patient and family-centered care.
Standards of practice exist to ensure that the highest quality of care is maintained, regardless of the number of professionals providing care or the experience of those professionals.
Narratives provide an opportunity to share stories that have meaning and at the same time describe concerns, intuition, inner dialogues, evolving understanding, feelings of doubt, challenge, and conflict. Makes the often invisible components of practice visible.
Professional development is essential to our ability to provide quality care, to achieve personal & professional satisfaction, and to advance our careers. Our activities include orientation, in-service training, formal & continuing education, & clinical advancement activities.
Vision & Values
Standards of Practice
Narrative Culture
Professional Development
Patient-Centeredness
Clinical Recognition & Advancement
Collaborative Decision-Making
Research
Innovation & Entrepreneurial Teamwork
Using Benner's novice to expert skill acquisition framework, through reflective practice and portfolio development, clinicians have the opportunity to advance their clinical practice at career at the bedside through the Clinical Recognition Program.
(Center)
Collaborative decision making is built on the premise of "teamness" and team learning, i.e., the network of relationships between people who come together and implement actions or strategies toward a desired outcome.
The possession of a body of knowledge from research is the hallmark of a profession. Research is the bridge that translates academic knowledge and constructed theories into direct clinical practice.
Our core value is patient-centeredness and we believe that the patient/family-nurse relationship is critical to the delivery of safe, quality care.
Through interdisciplinary teamwork and innovation, opportunities to ensure the delivery of patient care and the structures that support it are pursued to continually meet the changing needs of the populations we serve.

**FIGURE 10.1** Massachusetts General Hospital—Professional Practice Model (MGH PPM).

and structure supports the nurse in planning, managing, and adapting to change, and facilitates the identification of goals and strategies to improve outcomes. Articulation of a model for the nursing professionals within an organization provides a critical mass of energy to support resources, strength, and visibility within an often-complex structure. Routinely evaluating clinicians' perceptions of that practice model provides invaluable information toward the betterment of both the organization and patient care (Ives Erickson & Ditomassi, 2011).

## ■ EVALUATING THE PPE

Furthering this agenda, the Staff Perceptions of Professional Practice Environment (SPPPE) survey instrument comprised of the Revised Professional Practice Environment (RPPE) scale (Ives Erickson, Duffy, Ditomassi, & Jones, 2009), a derivative of the Professional Practice Environment (PPE) scale (Ives Erickson et al., 2004), was developed as a mechanism for evaluating and informing leaders as to opportunities to improve the care delivery practice environment. This instrument was based on the work of the initial Magnet study (McClure, Poulin, Sovie, & Wandelt, 1983), which began the research associating positive practice environments to better patient outcomes. The RPPE scale provides an assessment of eight organizational characteristics determined to be important to clinician satisfaction. These consist of autonomy, clinician–physician relations, control over practice, communication, teamwork, conflict management, internal work motivation, and cultural sensitivity.

## ■ DEVELOPING A CLIMATE OF INCLUSION

Adding to the knowledge development thread surrounding the PPE is the ongoing research focused on understanding the diversity of an organization's workforce and fostering a climate in which culturally competent and culturally sensitive care is delivered. The delivery of culturally competent care, and the nurses' abilities as leaders to create an environment to meet the individual needs of our patients in a sensitive, healing, and respectful way, must be a commitment of nurse leaders. If cultural diversity is to be viewed with an eye to the future, a shift in personal perspectives and values is necessary, whereby cultural competence cannot simply be about tolerance, as tolerance is a position of neutrality (Washington, Ives Erickson & Ditomassi, 2004). To meet this commitment, executive nurse leaders must strengthen their awareness, knowledge, and skills surrounding cultural concepts and ensure that these are shared and integrated into clinical practice as a mechanism to improve both the care of patients and the PPE in which clinicians work.

## ■ EXECUTIVE NURSE LEADERSHIP AND THE PRACTICE ENVIRONMENT

Parallel to the practice environment enhancement research, MGH also began to stress looking at the "source" of organizational executive nurse leadership. In doing so, researchers conducted a national survey of chief nurses to identify the skills needed to position nurse executives for success in an integrated delivery system (IDS) environment structure (Ives Erickson, 2002). Survey respondents included chief nurses of single-hospital facilities and leaders of multifacility IDSs. The 182 respondents identified critical skills needed to perform effectively at the IDS level, which are identified in Figure 10.2 and included the following: communication; strategic planning; financial management; creating vision, mission, and values; operations

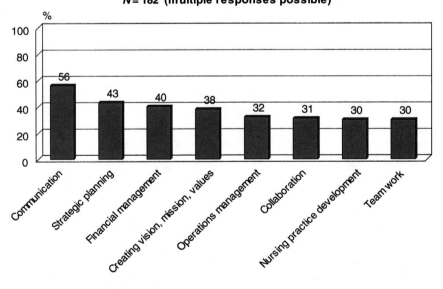

**FIGURE 10.2** Top skills necessary for success as CNO in IDS.

management; collaboration; nursing practice development; and teamwork (Ives Erickson, 2002). Analysis of qualitative responses revealed that different skills specific to the IDS were emphasized, yet, interestingly, all were closely related to other independently identified standards, such as PPE/RPPE scales mentioned previously (Ives Erickson et al., 2004, 2009) and to the core competencies of nurse executive practice (Business skills, Knowledge of the health care environment, Leadership skills, Professionalism, and Relationship building) as defined by American Organization of Nurse Executives (AONE, 2011).

## ■ EXECUTIVE NURSE LEADERSHIP INFLUENCE

Building on Ives Erickson's work, Adams, Duffy, and Clifford (2006) suggested that the approximately 5,000 chief nurses in the United States (Health Forum, 2006) serve as the gatekeepers for the advancement of the majority of the 3.1 million nurses practicing in the United States (Health Resources and Services Administration, 2008), yet were not maximizing influence in comparison with their C-suite counterparts (Adams et al., 2006, 2007), leaving us with the question, "Having gotten to that table, now what?"

Thus, from 2005 to present, in collaboration with Joyce C. Clifford, CEO of the Institute for Nursing Healthcare Leadership (INHL), MGH nurse researchers have conducted surveys at the annual INHL invitational seminars. This research thread aims at understanding the influence of the executive nurse leader and identifying how to maximize this influence. The findings from the series of INHL surveys (Adams et al., 2006, 2007, 2008) helped to identify and understand the factors, attributes, and process of influence within the executive nurse leadership population. The surveys have also played a significant role in understanding the knowledge, influence, and perceived success of the executive nurse leader. This work also informed and validated the influence factors, influence attributes, and process of influence as represented in the Adams Influence Model (AIM), and the Model of the Interrelationship of Leadership Environments and Outcomes for Nurse Executives (MILE ONE) as represented in Figure 10.3 (Adams, 2009).

## ■ THE ADAMS INFLUENCE MODEL

The AIM was developed as a framework for chief nurses to better understand the factors, attributes, and process of influence (Adams, 2009), as nursing influence has long been an identified shortcoming for the profession (Godden, 1995; Robert Wood Johnson Foundation, 2010). It guides executive nurse leaders in their practice through the recognition of five primary influence factors (authority, communication traits, knowledge-based competence, status, and use of time and timing) (Adams & Ives Erickson, 2011) and the associated attributes of each factor (Adams, 2009). Additionally, while the personal, interpersonal, and social systems interrelate, as represented within the outer circles of the AIM in Figure 10.3, it is important to note that interpersonal influence occurs within a two-person dyad for any single issue. As an example, a single issue may be the selection of a clinical information system. A dyad could include the agent (chief nurse) and a target of influence (superior, peer, or subordinate). As human beings, the agent (chief nurse) and the target of influence each possess qualities, characteristics, and skills that can be used in the influence process. It is the understanding and titration of these factors, attributes, and tactics that lead to achieved or missed influence efforts.

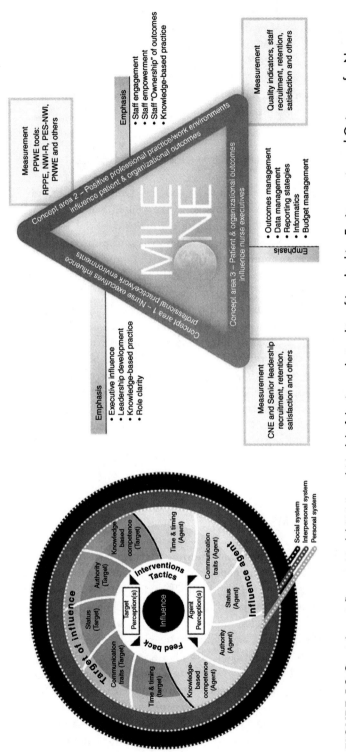
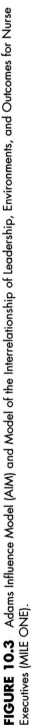

**FIGURE 10.3**  Adams Influence Model (AIM) and Model of the Interrelationship of Leadership, Environments, and Outcomes for Nurse Executives (MILE ONE).

Nursing leadership studies aimed at influence are extremely important. It has been identified that the application and understanding of influence begins with those tasked with motivating and securing support and resources (Yukl & Falbe, 1990). In no population is this more pertinent than within executive nursing leadership, with the complexities of sustained improvement of the PPE through the workforce development, changes to organizational budgets, and the continued evolution of our health care system. The AIM is an emerging nursing theory and provides a guide for executive nurse leaders to focus efforts, advance the discipline, and more broadly influence appropriate changes to nursing education, policy, practice, research, and theory.

## ■ THE MILE ONE

As suggested previously, the chief nurse's emphasis of practice is the PPE. Paying keen attention to articulating a shared PPM to guide practice is the key. The MILE ONE presented as a triangle in Figure 10.3 highlights the PPE as the focus of nurse executive practice (Adams, Ives Erickson, Jones, & Paulo, 2009). It provides suggested areas of emphasis, including leadership development, KBP, and clarification of role within the first leg of the model. With the emphasis on the development of a PPE, the nurse executive leader fosters an environment that leads to an engaged, empowered staff that "own" outcomes as depicted in the second leg of the triangle. The third leg highlights the impact of positive patient and organizational outcomes on the increased influence and power of the nurse executive leader in his/her role. Together, this framework encompasses most, if not all, EBP/KBP projects that occur in care delivery settings. The MILE ONE provides a literature-based structure toward understanding and guiding nurse executive, management, and staff nurse efforts toward maximizing patient outcomes and was developed as part of the review for this general program of research.

## ■ ADVANCING AN AGENDA FOR EXECUTIVE NURSE LEADERS

This chapter highlights the importance and value of an executive nurse leader perspective and provides a description of what many identify as a program of research. Admittedly, there are many additional nursing research endeavors and for KBP/EBP projects underway within one organization, most if not all ongoing improvement efforts can be linked to this general administrative-focused thread in one way or another. The specific work highlighted here continues to be utilized in research and practice and has expanded significantly in the literature. Our work around the PPE as an emphasis for the nurse executive leader has served as a basis for a twinning relationship between Shanghai Haushan Hospital in China and MGH as a mechanism to advance learning across organizations and cultures (Ives Erickson, Hong, & Ditomassi, in press). The work emphasizing the adoption of the core components of a PPE fosters autonomous and successful nursing care, even during disaster situations as identified through our staff deployed to Haiti during the 2010 earthquake (Ives Erickson, 2010). The RPPE has been translated into multiple languages (Chang, 2009) with use in a variety of settings across more than 70 sites internationally. The AIM has been applied to several nursing administration scenarios including chief nurse application during a sentinel event (Adams & Ives Erickson, 2011), influencing policy (Adams, Chisari, Ditomassi, & Ives, 2011), and as a guide for aspiring nurse leaders (Keys, 2011), and the MILE ONE has been applied to integration of standardized nursing language into electronic documentation (Adams, Denham, & Neumeister, 2010).

## ■ SUMMARY

Sally Reel (in Dahnke & Dreher, 2011, p. xiii) states that the challenge ahead for nursing is to take the path of most resistance rather than the easier road of least resistance. Although this was stated in the context of what educational preparation is required for nurses to "conduct research versus utilize research," her words of wisdom apply to how to navigate the care delivery redesign journey ahead. Executive nurse leaders having "successfully" managed and led in traditional hospital settings cannot rely on their past skill set to meet the demands of the future system of health care. Executive nurse leaders must critically reflect on their skill sets to identify any gaps. New skills are needed for leadership effectiveness during this time of continuous care delivery redesign. Health care, in particular, is an industry in the midst of radical change, requiring innovative, adaptive, and visionary leaders for the future. The KBP nurse executive, director, and manager are essential for the discipline. They will define the future of nursing and the direction of research and assimilate theory into their practice environment.

## ■ REFERENCES

Adams, J. M. (2009). *The Adams Influence Model (AIM): Understanding the factors, attributes and process of achieving influence.* Saarbrücken, Germany: VDM Verlag.

Adams, J. M., Chisari, R. G., Ditomassi, M., & Ives, E. J. (2011, July). Understanding and influencing policy: An imperative to the contemporary nurse leader. *Voice of Nursing Leadership.*

Adams, J. M., Denham, D., Neumeister, I. (2010). Applying the model of the interrelationship of leadership, environments & outcomes for nurse executives (MILE ONE): A community hospital's exemplar in developing staff nurse engagement through documentation improvement initiatives. *Nursing Administration Quarterly, 24*(3), 201–207.

Adams, J. M., Duffy, M. E., & Clifford, J. C. (2006). *Knowledge and influence of the nurse leader: A survey of participants from the 2005 conference.* Boston, MA: Institute for Nursing Healthcare Leadership.

Adams, J. M., & Ives Erickson, J. (2011). Applying the Adams influence model (aim) in nurse executive practice. *Journal of Nursing Administration, 41*(4), 186–192.

Adams, J. M., Ives Erickson, J., Duffy, M. E., Jones, D. A., Aspell Adams, A., & Clifford, J. C. (2007). *Knowledge and influence of the nurse leader: A survey of participants from the 2006 conference.* Boston, MA: Institute for Nursing Healthcare Leadership.

Adams, J. M., Ives Erickson, J., Jones, D. A., & Paulo, L. (2009). An evidence based structure for transformative nurse executive practice: The model of the interrelationship of leadership, environments & outcomes for nurse executives (MILE ONE). *Nursing Administration Quarterly, 33*(4), 280–287.

Adams, J. M., Paulo, L., Meraz-Gottfried, L., Aspell Adams, A., Ives Erickson, J., Jones, D. A., & Clifford, J. C. (2008). *Success measures for the nurse leader: A survey of participants from the 2007 INHL conference.* Boston, MA: The Institute for nursing healthcare leadership.

American Nurses Credentialing Center (ANCC). (2008). *A new model for ANCC's Magnet recognition program.* Retrieved from www.nursecredentialing.org

American Organization of Nurse Executives (AONE). (2011). *The AONE nurse executive competencies.* AONE. Retrieved from http://www.aone.org/resources/leadership%20tools/nursecomp.shtml

Chang, C. C. (2009). *Development and evaluation of psychometric properties of the Chinese version of the Professional Practice Environment Scale in Taiwan.* Unpublished doctoral dissertation, Boston College, Boston, MA.

Dahnke, M. D., & Dreher, H. M. (2011). *Philosophy of science for nursing practice: Concepts and application* (p. xiii). New York: Springer Publishing Company.

Godden, J. (1995). Victorian influences on the development of nursing. In G. Gray & R. Pratt (Eds.), *Scholarship in the discipline of nursing* (pp. 243–258). Melbourne, Australia: Churchill Livingstone.

Health Forum. (2006). *AHA guide to the health care field.* Chicago, IL: Health Forum LLC.

Health Resources and Services Administration. (2008). *National sample of registered nurses.* Retrieved August 20, 2011, from http://datawarehouse.hrsa.gov/nursingsurvey.aspx

Institute of Medicine (IOM). (2001). *Crossing the quality chasm: A new health system for the 21st century.* Washington, DC: National Academy Press.

Ives Erickson, J. (1996). MGH Professional Practice Model, *Caring Headlines.* Boston, MA: Massachusetts General Hospital.

Ives Erickson, J. (2002). Chief nurse executive role in integrated delivery systems: Initial impressions from a national survey of chief nursing officers, *The Robert Wood Johnson Foundation Executive Nurse Fellows Program.*

Ives Erickson, J. (2010, May). A nurse leader's perspective on disaster preparedness and response: Experiences from Haiti. *Voice of Nursing Leadership.*

Ives Erickson, J., & Ditomassi, M. (2011). Professional practice model: Strategies for translating models into practice. *Nursing Clinics of North America, 46*(1), 35–44 .

Ives Erickson, J., Duffy, M. E., Ditomassi, M., & Jones, D. (2009). Psychometric evaluation of the revised professional practice environment (RPPE) scale. *Journal of Nursing Administration, 39*(5), 236–243.

Ives Erickson, J., Duffy, M. E., Gibbons, M. P., Fitzmaurice, J., Ditomassi, M., & Jones, D. A. (2004). Development and psychometric evaluation of the professional practice environment (PPE) scale. *Journal of Nursing Scholarship, 36*(3), 279–285.

Ives Erickson, J. Hong, J., & Ditomassi, M. (2012). Promoting a culture of professional practice through a twinning relationship. *Journal of Nursing Administration, 42*(2), 117–122.

Keys, Y. (2011). Perspectives on executive relationships—Influence. *Journal of Nursing Administration, 41*(9), 347–349.

McClure, M. L., Poulin, M. A., Sovie, M. D., & Wandelt, M. (1983). *Magnet hospitals: Attraction and retention of professional nurses.* Washington, DC: American Nurses Publishing.

Robert Wood Johnson Foundation. (2010). *Nursing leadership from bedside to boardroom: Opinion leaders' perceptions.* Retrieved July 3, 2011, from http://www.rwjf.org/pr/product.jsp?id=55091

Roy, C. (2007). Nursing knowledge development and clinical practice. In S. C. Roy & D. A. Jones (Eds.), *Advances in nursing knowledge and the challenge for transforming practice* (pp. 3–38). New York, NY: Springer Publishing Company.

Sackett, D. L., Straus, S. E., Richardson, W. S., Rosenberg, W., & Haynes, R. B. (2000). *Evidence-based medicine. How to practice and teach EBM* (2nd ed.). New York, NY: Churchill Livingstone.

Shortell, S. M., Gillies, R. R., & Devers, K. J. (1995). Reinventing the American hospital. *The Milbank Quarterly, 73*(2), 131–60.

Washington, D., Ives Erickson, J., & Ditomassi, M. (2004). Mentoring the minority nurse leader of tomorrow. *Nursing Administration Quarterly, 28*(3), 165–169.

Yukl, G., & Falbe, C. M. (1990). Influence tactics and objectives in upward, downward, and lateral influence attempts. *Journal of Applied Psychology, 75*, 132–140.

# PART IV

# *The Scholarship of Practice*

*All health professionals should be educated to deliver patient-centered care as
members of an interdisciplinary team, emphasizing evidence-based practice,
quality improvement approaches, and informatics.*
—(Institute of Medicine, Crossing the Quality Chasm, 2001)

Doctor of nursing practice (DNP) graduates are expected to function as leaders within increasingly complex health care systems. Inherent to this role will be the ability to critically appraise and translate best evidence for patients, systems, and organizations; integrate and implement health information technology; and measure outcomes to improve patient care.

Part IV of this book reviews the core essentials of outcomes measurement, health information technology, and evidence-based practice. These inter-related concepts are woven throughout the DNP essentials and serve as the foundation for DNP practice. Additionally, this section serves as an example of DNP- and PhD-prepared nurses working together to generate new knowledge in the pursuit of best practice.

# CHAPTER 11

# Evidence-Based Practice: The Scholarship Behind the Practice

Valerie J. Fuller, Debra Kramlich, and Debra Palmer

*Knowledge is of no value unless you put it into practice.*

—Anton Chekhov

Evidence-based practice (EBP) is the cornerstone of the DNP role. It represents the practitioners' commitment to use all means possible to locate the best (most effective) evidence for any given problem and at all points of planning and contact with clients (Fischer, 2009). In Chapter 3 of this book, Dr. Crabtree aptly defines the role of nursing scholars in generating scientific evidence for practice and the translation of this evidence into practice to achieve optimal health outcomes. In Chapter 4, Dr. Andrist and Dr. Miller review the steps of an EBP capstone project, starting with the formulation of a burning question through to its development, implementation, evaluation, and dissemination. We continue to build on this concept in Chapter 11 by providing a general overview of EBP, including a nursing framework for EBP, challenges to its use, and implementation of EBP in the clinical setting. Exemplars of EBP capstone projects from recent graduates of Doctor of Nursing Practice can be found in Chapter 6.

## ■ EBP AND THE DOCTOR OF NURSING PRACTICE

It's become a well-known and troubling statistic that it takes one or two decades for original research to be put into routine clinical practice (Agency for Healthcare Research and Quality, 2001). Thus, the translation of research findings into sustainable improvements for clinical practice and patient outcomes remains a substantial obstacle to improving the quality of health care (AHRQ, 2001). This separation or knowledge "gap" between research and clinical practice has been well documented and cited in two landmark reports from the Institute of Medicine: *Crossing the Quality Chasm: A New Health System for the 21st Century* (2001) and *Health Professions Education: A Bridge to Quality* (2003). Both reports emphasized the need for additional education in EBP for all health care professionals.

In 2004, the American Association of Colleges of Nursing (AACN) released their position statement on the doctor of nursing practice and recommended that the content of such programs include analytic methodologies related to the evaluation of practice and the application of evidence for practice (AACN, 2004). This was later incorporated in the AACN's *Essentials of Doctoral Education for Advanced Nursing Practice* as Essential III, "Clinical Scholarship and Analytical Methods for Evidence-Based Practice" (AACN, 2006). This essential stresses the need for DNP graduates to translate research into practice in order to improve practice and outcomes of care. Specifically, the AACN recommends that DNP programs prepare graduates to

1. Use analytic methods to critically appraise existing literature and other evidence to determine and implement the best evidence for practice
2. Design and implement processes to evaluate outcomes of practice, practice patterns, and systems of care within a practice setting, health care organization, or community against national benchmarks to determine variances in practice outcomes and population trends
3. Design, direct, and evaluate quality improvement (QI) methodologies to promote safe, timely, effective, efficient, equitable, and patient-centered care
4. Apply relevant findings to develop practice guidelines and improve practice and the practice environment
5. Use information technology and research methods appropriately to

   • Collect appropriate and accurate dates to generate evidence for nursing
   • Inform and guide the design of databases that generate meaningful evidence for nursing practice
   • Analyze data from practice
   • Design evidence-based interventions
   • Predict and analyze outcomes
   • Examine patterns of behavior and outcomes
   • Identify gaps in evidence for practice

6. Function as practice specialist or consultant in collaborative knowledge-generating research
7. Disseminate findings from EBP and research to improve health care outcomes

(AACN, 2006, p. 12)

## ■ EBP, QUALITY IMPROVEMENT (QI), AND NURSING RESEARCH

Numerous synonyms exist for EBP—evidence-based medicine, evidence-based nursing, evidence-based health care, and others. Likewise, there exists an abundance of EBP definitions. Broadly defined, EBP is the integration of best research evidence with clinical expertise and patient values (Sackett, Rosenberg, Gray, Haynes, & Richardson, 1996). Defining what EBP is, and is not, is an important first step in understanding the concept of evidence. EBP is not nursing research, research utilization, or Quality Improvement (QI), and while these terms are inextricably linked, there are distinct differences. For example, an EBP project can lead to a research study or a QI project (Beyea & Slattery, 2006). One of the most important distinctions between QI and research lies within the intent. QI intends to improve systems and processes with the goal of improving outcomes. The intention of research is to generate new knowledge, with the results being generalizable to a larger population (Newhouse,

Pettit, Poe, & Rocco, 2006). We have defined these terms in the next section in order to provide additional understanding and context for their use in the literature.

### Definitions of Research Utilization, Nursing Research, and Quality Improvement (QI)

*Research utilization* is the process of using research findings to improve patient care. According to Titler (2002), it involves dissemination of scientific knowledge, study critique, synthesis of research findings, determination of the applicability of findings, developing a research-based practice standard, implementation of the standard, and evaluation. This term is most closely linked to EBP and is often considered a subset of EBP (Cullen, Titler, & Belding-Schmitt, 2009).

Polit and Beck (2008) define *nursing research* as systematic inquiry designed to develop trustworthy evidence about issues of importance to the nursing profession. Nursing research involves the application of a methodology (quantitative or qualitative) to investigate a phenomenon of interest in order to develop, refine, or extend nursing knowledge (Bond, n.d.; Polit & Beck, 2008; Titler, 2002).

QI utilizes a system to monitor and evaluate the quality and appropriateness of care (outcomes) based on EBP and research (Bond, n.d.). Often, QI projects involve solving a problem in a particular setting as opposed to attempting to generalize across all settings and populations (Beyea & Slattery, 2006).

In summary, EBP may encompass the above terms, but its process is more rigorous and systematic. In EBP, scientific evidence is analyzed, synthesized, and placed in an integrative review. The results are then integrated into the context of clinical expertise and patients values from which best practices are developed (Spector, n.d.).

### ■ DEFINITION AND HISTORY OF EBP

*Evidence-based medicine* (EBM) has been defined as "the conscientious and judicious use of current best evidence in making decisions about the care of individual patients" (Sackett et al., 1996). Historically, EBM was developed as an educational strategy in the medical curriculum as a means of promoting clinical learning (Jennings & Loan, 2001). This process shifted decision making from an intuitive, authoritative approach to an objective, scientific, and outcome-based approach. With EBM, interventions and clinical outcomes drive problem solving rather than a process approach as used in nursing since the late 1970s (Dale, 2006). EBM has been criticized that it has an experimental perspective on research and a strong "clinical trials" orientation, and therefore defines evidence in quantitative terms and largely ignores qualitative and hermeneutic forms of evidence (French, 1999). In this view, the evidence answers the question, "Can it work?" without being concerned with, "How it works" or, "Is it worth it?" (Lomas, Culyer, McCutcheon, McAuley, & Law, 2005). This approach devalues evidence obtained from other sources such as expert knowledge, clinical experience, patient preferences, stakeholder consultations, and nonexperimental research. To add to the growing difficulties of evidence translation, today's focus is on patient-centered health care, creating philosophical tensions between health care as an objective scientific endeavor and health care as intimate encounters with individuals captured in an exceptional time and circumstance.

As the use of evidence became more popular, the phraseology changed and such terms as evidence-based nursing (EBN) and EBP emerged from evidence-based medicine (French, 2002). Evidence-based nursing is defined as "integration of the best evidence available, nursing expertise, and the values and preferences of the individuals, families, and communities who are served" (Sigma Theta Tau International, 2005). Regardless of terminology, the premises of EBP include actual scientific-based clinical practices rather than practices based upon tradition, a focus on individualized care, valuing the contribution of clinical expertise, and incorporating patients' expectations into the plan of care (Hudson, Duke, Haas, & Varnell, 2008). In a study by Banning (2005), focus-group interviews were conducted to explore the understanding of nurses on evidence, EBP, and EBM, and to identify the uptake of research evidence in the workplace (Banning, 2005). The authors concluded that nurses had a variety of differing views and understanding of EBP and could not differentiate EBP from EBM nor identify different levels of evidence. This study supports the belief that there is confusion among nurses regarding EBP.

In 2005, the Canadian Health Services Research Foundation conducted a systematic review to examine the concept of evidence by those who produce evidence and those who make decisions based on evidence. The foundation determined that evidence defined as a science is valued by methodological tests and information gained through rigorous processes and procedures defined as scientific. When evidence is defined colloquially, it becomes valued as it relates to context-sensitive applications specific to the circumstances in which it is applied. Therefore, evidence is uncertain, complex, dynamic, and rarely complete, which adds to the challenges to negotiate and adopt a common definition for translation into practice (Lomas et al., 2005).

Following the definition of evidence, the scientific evidence must be integrated with the patient and family preferences along with nurses' explicit and tacit knowledge. The actual role the patients play in their decision making has not yet been formalized, but it is essential that health care practitioners acknowledge patients' choices (Chummun & Tiran, 2008).

Knowledge-translation strategies and interprofessional education and collaboration aim to improve health care processes and outcomes (Zwarenstein & Reeves, 2006). Governmental agencies are becoming more involved in actively promoting change in health care organizations, where mandatory public reporting of health care quality initiatives are increasingly transparent to the public. The translation of knowledge and evidence needs to be relayed in messages that are clearly heard by potential target audiences and beneficiaries, including clinicians, administrators, patients, and families (Gordon & Brown, 2005).

Research by Benner (1996) demonstrated that nurses come to clinical situations and decision making inherently with a sense of what is good and right. These values are often unspoken and unrecognized but profoundly influence a nurse's decision making. In addition, clinical judgments are extremely complex, often made under very stressful situations, in fractions of a minute and with other staff who may have competing interests (Tanner, 2006). Nurses may be reluctant to embrace the EBP or research paradigm, not understanding the research language and EBP concepts; however, they do collectively seek to provide the best care to their patients.

The paradigm of knowledge translation has seen remarkable uptake in a short period of time, with national organizations around the world endorsing knowledge translation as a means for applying scientific evidence into practice. Although specific terminology may differ slightly, the broad concept of knowledge translation refers to the implementation of research-derived evidence within a complex system of exchange among stakeholders (Reimer-Kirkham, Varcoe, Browne, Khan, & McDonald, 2009).

### ■ RESEARCH UTILIZATION AND EBP MODELS

There are growing numbers of EBP models to assist practitioners in moving evidence into practice. While it is beyond the scope of this chapter to discuss each model in detail, a table of the most commonly cited models is listed below. In addition, the following section provides

### TABLE 11.1 Research Utilization and EBP Models

| Research Utilization and EBP Models | Authors | Year |
| --- | --- | --- |
| CURN (Conduct and Utilization of Research in Nursing) | Horsley, J., Crane, J., Crabtree, M., & Wood, D. | 1983 |
| Ottawa Model | Logan, J., & Graham, I. | 1998 |
| Rosswurm & Larrabee Model | Rosswurm, M., & Larrabee, J. | 1999 |
| Stetler Model | Stetler, C. | 2001 |
| Iowa Model | Titler, M., Kleiber, C., Steelman, V., Rakel, B., Budreau, G., Everett, L., Buckwalter, K., Tripp-Reimer, T., & Goode, C. | 2001 |
| ACE Star Model of Knowledge Transformation | Stevens, K. | 2004 |
| PARIHS Model (Promoting Action on Research Implementation in Health Services) | Rycroft-Malone, J. | 2004 |
| Johns Hopkins Model | Newhouse, R., Dearhold, S., Poe, S., Pugh, L., & White, K. | 2005 |
| Multisystem Model of Knowledge Integration & Translation (MKIT) | Palmer, D., & Kramlich, D. | 2011 |

a detailed overview of the Multisystem Model of Knowledge Integration and Translation (MKIT) as an example (Table 11.1).

### ■ USE OF THE MKIT TO EMPLOY EBP

A model is a schematic description that takes essential components of a process and attempts to explain the relationships between them (Wolf & Greenhouse, 2007). Models serve as a map illustrating to the user how to get from one point to another. With the acceleration of the EBP paradigm has come the development of many research utilization and EBP models to assist practitioners.

Each of these models has strengths and limitations. A model may be linear or unidirectional, designed for individual or organizational use, difficult for novice evidence users to understand, lacking an algorithm that is easy to follow, focused on empirical knowledge alone, or ignoring the importance of practitioners' tacit knowledge.

The process for innovation is often quite complex and cannot be reduced to a simple, linear model (Van De Ven, Polley, Garud, & Venkataraman, 1999). Quality and safety processes in literature, such as *plan, do, study, act* have implicit ongoing interconnections (Thor et al., 2004). Action research incorporates spirals of learning, doing, and reflection that are well recognized with embedded ongoing cyclical processes (Titchen & Manley, 2006). Cyclical process patterns are not new to innovations.

Traditional models of research have separated research and practice into distinct domains, thereby expanding the already significant divide between theorists and practitioners.

Rycroft-Malone and Bucknall (2010) suggest that the application of frameworks and models to research can make a difference in our understanding of the processes involved and the outcomes that result. The MKIT (Palmer & Kramlich, 2011) addresses the limitations of linear systems thinking and is supported with a well-established conceptual framework. The cyclical process of the MKIT is ongoing reflection, action, monitoring of outcomes, and reflection. Tacit knowledge integrated with the research literature and patients' values can be catapulted by the formation of communities of practice (CoP), allowing for the sharing of knowledge and expertise for better patient care. This fundamental component of true knowledge translation begins with creating opportunities for interaction between both the evidence creators and users.

It is becoming more apparent that advances in health care are limited by the failure to translate research findings into practice. EBP programs have emerged, while the science for health care practitioners to implement the new knowledge to consumers has lagged behind. There is also emerging literature recognizing that the practitioner's tacit knowledge is grossly undervalued. The MKIT model, supported by CoP, integrates explicit and tacit knowledge and scientific evidence to practice. The application of the MKIT for the integration of knowledge management and clinical process improvements allow for a higher performing organization.

Operating within the theoretical framework of CoP (Wenger, McDermott, & Snyder, 2002), the MKIT is circular rather than unidirectional with reflective inquiry, knowledge seeking or generation, integration, implementation, evaluation, mentoring, and reflective inquiry. CoP was originated in learning theory when anthropologists Jean Lave and Etienne Wenger popularized the term while studying apprenticeship as a learning model. CoP are defined as "groups of people who share a concern, a set of problems, or a passion about a topic, and who deepen their knowledge and expertise in this area by interacting on an ongoing basis" (Wenger et al., 2002; p. 4). CoP are formed when a group of people come together to share a common domain of interest to share knowledge and other resources to advance practice and improve patient care.

The steps of the MKIT are straightforward for the knowledge seeker evaluating practice through searching, creating, integrating, and translating new evidence into practice by forming strategic partnerships. These strategic partnerships employ a microsystem or "bottom up" approach to identifying and resolving problems with an interdisciplinary group of frontline workers to sustain the solution. The advanced practice registered nurse (APRN) will engage in reflective practice upon challenging clinical situations that lead to forming a clinical question. This will guide the literature search and development of a researchable question. Based upon the results of the literature search, the APRN will then decide to develop policies and protocols to move the evidence into practice or develop a research study to generate evidence if little is found. After implementing the changes in practice, it is imperative to monitor the patient outcomes. The MKIT encourage pilot testing with a small group of clinicians and patients to demonstrate the feasibility of the change in practice (Palmer & Kramlich, 2011). If the outcomes are favorable from a pilot test, change could then be made in practice in other units, with other like populations and monitored over time to determine its impact on the environment, staff, costs, and the patient and family. The APRN should disseminate the results of the changes in practice by presentations and/or publications for others to elicit the knowledge for their organizations and to advance the state of the science. All of the steps occur within the micro, meso, and macro organizational levels, and it is imperative that the APRN engage key stakeholders, change agents, and early adopters in the process in order to successfully implement change.

A multitude of issues and factors come together to identify the complexity and scope of patient safety and quality care, as well as the necessity for intricate strategies to create change within health care systems and processes of care. Advanced practice nurses typically take care of several patients, each with conflicting, yet simultaneous, needs. Increasing patient acuity, decreasing length of hospital stay, and increasing mandated governmental regulations have all contributed to the complexity of clinical practice challenging APRNs today. In using EBP by employing the easy-to-use MKIT, the APRN is in the forefront of engaging in initiatives to continually improve quality by striving for excellence (Hughs, 2008).

## ■ WHAT IS EVIDENCE?

EBP has been defined in various ways, with most definitions including elements of explicit (research-based, external) knowledge, clinician expertise (tacit knowledge), and patient preferences (Melnyk & Fineout-Overholt, 2010; Sackett et al., 1996; Samara, 2007). In the past, double-blind randomized controlled trials (RCT), meta-analyses, and systematic integrative reviews have been held as gold standards for applying evidence to practice. We now understand that clinicians' tacit knowledge has been undervalued and can be a powerful source of evidence to inform practice. Terms such as research utilization, knowledge translation, and research or knowledge integration have been used interchangeably to describe EBP, often creating confusion. With the Institute of Medicine's goal that 90% of health care decisions be evidence based by 2020, it is imperative that the DNP be able to identify the source, level, quality, and strength of the evidence to inform practice.

Evidence can arise from a variety of sources. Instant access to electronic databases and journals, global knowledge sharing, and even social networking make information readily accessible to clinicians and consumers. Conversely, time taken to publish study results continues to be delayed by 4 to 8 years depending on results, with longer lag times found for studies that produce less favorable results (known as time-lag bias) (Hopewell, Clarke, Stewart, & Tierney, 2007). Publication bias, poor quality studies, inadequate sample sizes, and direct health care marketing to consumers compromise the quality of the evidence available for informing practice, so the DNP must be able to apply methods for grading the level, quality, and strength of the best available evidence.

There are over 100 systems for *grading the level of evidence,* which refers to the design of a study or source of evidence; the most widely used are the Agency for Healthcare Research and Quality (AHRQ); the Cochrane Collaboration; nursing models such as Stetler, Melnyk, Titler, and the Registered Nurses Association of Ontario; other professional health care organizations; and collaborative models such as Strength of Recommendation Taxonomy, Grade of Recommendations Assessment, Development and Evaluation, Consolidated Standards of Reporting Trials, and Appraisal of Guidelines for Research and Education. Most models utilize a similar level of evidence hierarchy, with systematic reviews at the top and expert opinion at the bottom (Figure 11.1).

Practice decisions should not be based solely on the level of evidence; it is important to consider the quality and strength of the evidence. *Quality* refers to how well a study was conducted and determined by individuals appraising the evidence. *Strength* is a combination of the design and quality of the study and the consistency of the results when more than one study measures the same variables. It indicates the extent to which one can be confident that adherence to the recommendation will do more good than harm. Evidence from a well-designed nonexperimental study or opinion from a respected expert may be more beneficial than that from a poorly designed RCT.

The best available external evidence must be combined with clinical expertise, proficiency, and judgment acquired through experience and practice. Results from a well-designed RCT may be inappropriate for an individual patient. Also, some situations may not require an RCT or cannot wait for such evidence to be produced. Application of evidence to inform

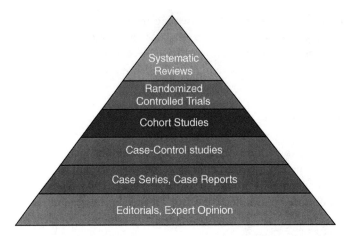

**FIGURE 11.1** Evidence hierarchy. Retrieved from http://gollum.lib.uic.edu/nursing/node/12

practice should consider all factors related to patient preference including quality and quantity of life, risk-benefit analysis, and cost.

## ■ CHALLENGES TO ENGAGEMENT IN EBP

Numerous challenges to health care professionals' engagement in EBP, including acceptance, adoption, and implementation, have been cited in the literature. Barriers occur at both the individual and the institutional level. It is important for the DNP to be aware of potential challenges and to recognize the importance of the role the DNP plays in the promotion of EBP.

While most health care professionals generally possess a positive attitude toward EBP and consider it important for patient outcomes, the challenges often delay or prevent implementation. Individual challenges to EBP include difficulty finding time to search for and appraise the evidence; the enormous amount of literature; lack of skills necessary to implement EBP (understanding terminology and statistics, identification of gaps in knowledge and practice, literature searching strategies, ability to determine validity of studies, application of findings to patient problems, and incorporation of patient preferences); lack of organizational support; negative attitudes from peers and other members of the health care team; lack of autonomy and confidence in the ability to effect change; insufficient resources, such as library support, computers, journals, and databases; and patient demands (Hannes et al., 2007; Hutchinson & Johnston, 2004; Majid et al., 2011; Melnyk & Fineout-Overholt, 2010; Nagy, Lumby, McKinley, & MacFarlane, 2001; Sams et al., 2004; Solomons & Spross, 2011).

Pravikoff, Tanner, and Pierce (2005) studied the readiness of nurses for EBP by conducting a nationwide study of registered nurses across the United States to ascertain their perceptions of access to tools to obtain evidence and whether or not they have the skills to do so (Pravikoff et al., 2005). The authors found that nurses acknowledged that they needed information for effective practice, but were not prepared to use the information resources. They had little or no education in searching databases to find evidence, nor did they have the critiquing skills to evaluate the evidence (Pravikoff et al., 2005). When nurses were not able to answer clinical questions, they most frequently turned to a colleague rather than searching for empirical evidence. This may not always provide the best evidence or knowledge.

Organizational barriers are closely related to the obstacles described by health care professionals. Infrastructures, such as library services and computers, may be inadequate to support EBP. With increasing constraints and demands on health care organizations, there may be insufficient resources in terms of administrative support and financial incentives to allow practitioners to engage in EBP projects. Organizational leaders may themselves lack the knowledge, attitudes, and skills to promote EBP (Solomons & Spross, 2011).

Practitioner misperceptions concerning EBP continue to impede the implementation of proven-effective practices. Some practitioners continue to believe that the double-blind RCT is the only valid evidence to inform practice. They often disregard evidence from well-designed QI projects and quasi-experimental and descriptive studies as insignificant. Other practices are so steeped in tradition that the best evidence cannot influence them. This can be quite intimidating to frontline practitioners (Hannes et al., 2007; Hutchinson & Johnson, 2004).

The number of resources available to assist practitioners in engaging in EBP is growing and becoming more accessible. Use of a model, such as MKIT, to assist individuals through the EBP process within the larger organization will address potential barriers before they arise. Educational programs to teach EBP skills are available online, reducing the need to attend workshops and conferences. Databases such as the National Guidelines Clearinghouse and the Cochrane Library provide evidence-based guidelines and systematic reviews that have already been appraised and graded.

As EBP becomes a standard practice for health care professionals, DNPs need to be able to successfully integrate the results of published research into practice, as well as to expand the knowledge base by conducting research as a regular part of clinical practice. These two challenges constitute a major cultural shift for clinicians, one that is complex to implement but far reaching in its implications for better patient care (Czerwinski, Cesaria, & Ashley, 2004)

DNPs are in an excellent position to promote EBP and help eliminate obstacles (Gerrish, Nolan, Guillaume, Kirshbaum, & Tod, 2011). They possess the educational preparation (knowledge and skills) and credential that bedside practitioners often lack. The role, responsibilities, and workload of the DNP are more conducive to engagement in EBP activities. They have developed relationships with various levels of the health care team, as well as formed professional networks, that promote collaborative practice. It is important for the DNP to cultivate those skills for successful implementation of EBP.

## ■ EBP PROJECTS

If you are still feeling uncertain of your ability to engage in EBP, you are not alone. Novice EBP users often wonder how to get started, where to find the evidence, how to implement the evidence, and whether such implementation will yield the expected outcome. The following are several examples of EBP projects conducted by frontline staff that may inspire confidence and emphasize the myriad ways the DNPs can promote EBP.

### Pediatric Pain Assessment

A staff nurse working in a pediatric intensive care unit (PICU) felt dissatisfied with the scales used for assessment of pain in children. There were four scales and several were complicated and difficult to use, and none were appropriate or validated for the PICU population. Concurrently, patient satisfaction scores regarding pain management in children were below benchmark, and chart audits showed poor compliance with pain assessment documentation. This nurse had recently been introduced to the FLACC (Face, Legs, Activity, Cry, Consolability) scale (Merkel et al., 1997), which seemed like a more appropriate scale for the patient population and was consistent with other 0-to-10 scales. A thorough critical analysis of the literature revealed that pain management did not improve following staff education. Implementation of a valid, objective pain assessment and documentation tool appropriate for the patient population did seem to improve pain management, as did improved documentation. Staff surveys regarding knowledge of pain assessment, documentation policies, best practices, and chart audits were conducted. Education about the FLACC scale, pediatric pain assessment, and the pain documentation policy was then provided to all staff in the form of a paper packet, a computer-based program, resource binders, and staff mentors. Charts were again audited 1 month and 4 months post education to assess for change in documentation. Postimplementation surveys were also administered to assess for change in knowledge. Documentation of pain using objective criteria, patient satisfaction with pain management, and staff satisfaction with the pain scales available all improved following implementation of the FLACC scale. Institutional policy was changed to replace several of the previously used pain scales with the FLACC scale.

## Family Presence During Resuscitation

Nurses and physicians in the intensive care units were experiencing more requests for family presence during resuscitation. With no policy, guidelines, or additional support staff, the experiences of staff and families were not always positive. One staff nurse with personal experience of being denied family presence during the resuscitation of a loved one pursued the implementation of a guideline to support families and staff during such events. The literature was rich with evidence to support the practice, numerous professional nursing and medical associations endorsed the practice, and a published guideline to assist in presenting the option for family presence existed. There were still many obstacles to simply implement such a guideline, including firmly entrenched beliefs, fears, and misperceptions. Using the MKIT, the staff nurse performed a critical analysis of the literature, formed a multidisciplinary team, and methodically worked to gain consensus for development of a guideline to support families during resuscitation of their loved one, whether or not bedside presence was requested or allowed. The guideline has been successfully implemented for over 3 years with improved family and staff satisfaction as a result.

## Detecting Deterioration in Children

It has been well documented that signs of clinical deterioration may be apparent hours before cardiac arrest in acutely ill patients, and early detection may prevent adverse outcomes (Monaghan, 2005; Parshuram, Hutchison, & Middaugh, 2009). One of the attending pediatric intensivists expressed concern about anecdotal cases of missed early signs of deterioration and suggested implementation of the pediatric early warning score (Monaghan, 2005). This idea was met with little interest, and it seemed that the proposal had hit a dead end. A staff nurse then conducted a chart audit of children who had been transferred from the pediatric inpatient unit to the PICU over the previous 18 months and found that of 161 unexpected transfers, there were 33 missed opportunities for early detection and intervention, including several cardiorespiratory arrests. This evidence was brought forward to nursing and physician leadership, which renewed interest in implementation of an early detection of deterioration scoring system. Concurrently, the institution was approached by developers of the Bedside Paediatric Early Warning System (Parsharum et al., 2009) to collaborate on validation of this scale. This partnership has resulted in a significant reduction in adverse outcomes: >80% reduction in cardiorespiratory arrest events; 2.5-fold increase in the number of rapid response team evaluations per patient day; 3.5-fold increase in the number of rapid response team evaluations that resulted in avoidance of an unplanned transfer to the PICU; and a 60% reduction in the deterioration events per patient day.

## Fall and Injury Risk Assessment in Children

As part of the Joint Commission's 2005 National Safety Goals, acute care facilities are required to implement a fall-prevention program and evaluate its effectiveness. Fall-prevention programs have proven to be an effective intervention for the adult and geriatric populations; screening tools have been developed, tested, and deemed reliable and valid. Conversely, development of a fall-prevention instrument for pediatrics has proven to be challenging. Recognizing the need to choose a pediatric fall risk assessment instrument that would be appropriate for the patient population and acceptable to staff, a team that included several staff nurses and an experienced staff nurse research mentor conducted a study investigating the reliability, specificity, and sensitivity of five pediatric fall scale instruments (Harvey, Kramlich, Chapman, Parker, & Blades, 2010). Findings indicated that while almost all of the instruments showed acceptable reliability and sensitivity, specificity for all five scales was lacking. Furthermore, the study demonstrated that none of the five instruments adequately assessed risk of injury from falls. Pediatric nurses involved in this study expressed great concern regarding a patient's risk of injury from a fall and indicated that it should be a priority when assessing a child. Much of the published pediatric fall–related literature focused on the development and testing of screening instruments and the implementation of fall-prevention programs. There were no studies that investigated nursing perceptions of pediatric falls. Bedside pediatric nurses play a significant role in protecting their patients against falls and are frequently the individuals responsible for reporting a fall occurrence. Because of those concerns, staff felt it would be important to clearly and accurately define a reportable fall before implementation of a pediatric fall and injury risk assessment tool and prevention program. Therefore, an exploratory study of pediatric health care practitioners' perception of a reportable fall occurrence is underway to help provide the basis for a definition, with the intent of development of a fall prevention program and screening tool with better reliability, sensitivity, and specificity. Results are currently pending.

## ■ ADDITIONAL RESOURCES FOR EBP

Table 11.2 provides a list of additional resources for EBP.

### TABLE 11.2 EBP Websites and Addresses

| | |
|---|---|
| Agency for Healthcare Research & Quality | www.ahrq.gov/clinic/epcix.htm |
| Agree Collaboration | www.agreecollaboration.org |
| Center for Evidence-Based Medicine | www.cebm.net/ |
| Cochrane Collaboration | www.cochrane.org |
| Evidence-Based Nursing Online | ebn.bmjjournals.com/ |
| GRADE Workgroup | www.gradeworkinggroup.org |
| Institute of Medicine (IOM) | www.iom.edu |
| Joanna Briggs Institute | www.joannabriggs.edu.au/about/home |
| National Guideline Clearinghouse | www/guideline.gov |
| National Institute for Nursing Research | www.nih.gov/ninr/ |
| Registered Nurses Association of Ontario | www.rnao.org |
| Sigma Theta Tau International | www.nursingsociety.org |

*(continued)*

**TABLE 11.2   EBP Websites and Addresses (Continued)**

| | |
|---|---|
| TRIP Database | www.tripdatabase.com |
| University of Iowa | www.uihealthcare.org/otherservices |
| University of Minnesota | evidence.ahc.umn.edu/ebn.htm |
| University of Texas School of Nursing | www.acestar.uthscsa.edu/ |
| U.S. National Library of Medicine/NIH | www.nlm.nih.gov/hsrinfo/evidence_based_practice.html |
| Virginia Henderson Intl Nursing Library | www.nursinglibrary.org/vhl/ |
| Zebra Consulting, LLC | www.zebraconsult.com |

■ **SUMMARY**

EBP is a process that enables clinicians to seek out best practices and determine if and how these practices can be incorporated into patient care (Poe & White, 2010). The DNP is uniquely prepared to synthesize clinical expertise with EBP to improve patient outcomes, provide clinical leadership, and transform health care.

■ **REFERENCES**

Agency for Healthcare Research and Quality. (2001). *Translating research into practice (TRIP)-II fact sheet.* Retrieved July 3, 2011, from http://www.ahrq.gov/research/trip2fac.htm

American Association of Colleges of Nursing. (2004). *AACN position statement on the practice doctorate in nursing.* Washington, DC: Author.

American Association of Colleges of Nursing. (2006). *The essentials of doctoral education for advanced practice nursing.* Retrieved from www.aacn.nche.edu/publications/position/dnpes sentials.pdf

Banning, M. (2005). Conceptions of evidence, evidence-based medicine, evidence-based practice and their use in nursing: Independent nurse prescribers' views. *Journal of Clinical Nursing, 14*(4), 411–417.

Benner, P., Tanner, C., & Chesla, C. (1996). *Expertise in nursing practice: A possible role for the consultant nurse.* New York, NY: Springer Publishing Company.

Beyea, S. C., & Slattery, M. J. (2006). *Evidence-based practice in nursing: A guide to successful implementation.* Retrieved July 5, 2011, from http://www.hcmarketplace.com/supplemental/3737_browse.pdf

Bond, S. (n.d.). *Evidence-based practice: What's in it for you* [PowerPoint slides].

Chummun, H., & Tiran, D. (2008). Increasing research evidence in practice: A possible role for the consultant nurse. *Journal of Nursing Management, 16*(3), 327–333.

Cullen, L., Titler, M. G., & Belding-Schmitt, M. (2009). *Online webcourse: Evidence-based practice.* Retrieved July 13, 2011, from www.uihealthcare.org/otherservices.aspx?id=225170

Czerwinski, B. S., Cesaria, S. K., & Ashley, M. H. (2004). Integrating research: Into daily nursing practice. *Journal of Nursing Administration, 34*(3), 117–119.

Dale, A. (2006). Determining guiding principles for evidence-based practice. *Nursing Standard, 20*(25), 41–46.

Fischer, J. (2009). Evidence-based practice. In J. Fischer, *Toward evidence-based practice: Variations on a theme* (pp. 451–468). Chicago, IL: Lyceum Books, Inc.

French, P. (1999). The development of evidence-based nursing. *Journal of Advanced Nursing, 29*(1), 72–78.

French, P. (2002). What is the evidence on evidence-based nursing? An epistemological concern. *Journal of Advanced Nursing, 37*(3), 250–257.

Gerrish, K., Nolan, M., Guillaume, L., Kirshbaum, M., & Tod, A. (2011). The role of advanced practice nurses in knowledge brokering as a means of promoting evidence-based practice among clinical nurses. *Journal of Advanced Nursing, 67*(9), 2004–2014.

Gordon, W., & Brown, M. (2005). Building research capacity: The role of partnerships. *American Journal of Physical Medicine & Rehabilitation, 84*(12), 999–1004.

Hannes, K., Vandersmissen, J., De Blaeser, L., Peeters, G., Goedhuys, J., & Aertgeerts, B. (2007). Barriers to evidence-based nursing: a focus group study. *Journal of Advanced Nursing, 60*(2), 162–171.

Harvey, K., Kramlich, D., Chapman, J., Parker, J., & Blades, E. (2010). Exploring and evaluating five pediatric falls assessment instruments and injury risk indicators: An ambispective study in a tertiary care setting. *Journal of Nursing Management, 18*(5), 531–541.

Horsley, J., Crane, J., Crabtree, M., Wood, O. (1983). *Using research to improve nursing practice: A guide.* New York, NY: W. B. Saunders.

Hopewell, S., Clarke, M. J., Stewart, L., & Tierney, J. (2007). Time to publication for results of clinical trials. *Cochrane Database of Systematic Reviews, (2).*

Hudson, K., Duke, G., Haas, B., & Varnell, G. (2008). Navigating the evidence-based practice maze. *Journal of Nursing Management, 16*(4), 409–416.

Hughes, R. G. (Ed.). (2008). *Patient safety and quality: An evidence-based handbook for nurses.* Rockville, MD: Agency for Healthcare Research and Quality.

Hutchinson, A. M., & Johnston, L. (2004). Bridging the divide: A survey of nurses' opinions regarding barriers to, and facilitators of, research utilization in the practice setting. *Journal of Clinical Nursing, 13*(3), 304–315.

Institute of Medicine. (2001). *Crossing the quality chasm: A new health system for the 21st century.* Washington, DC: The National Academies Press.

Institute of Medicine (2003). *Health professions education: A bridge to quality.* Washington, DC: National Academies Press.

Jennings, B. M., & Loan, L. A. (2001). Misconceptions among nurses about evidence-based practice. *Journal of Nursing Scholarship, 33*(2), 121–127.

Logan, J., Graham, I. (1998). Toward a comprehensive interdisciplinary model of health care research use. Scientific Community, *20*(2), 227–246.

Lomas, J., Culyer, T., McCutcheon, C., McAuley, L., & Law, S. (2005). *Conceptualizing and combining evidence for health system guidance.* Retrieved September 24, 2010, from http://www.chsrf.ca/migrated/pdf/insightAction/evidence_e.pdf

Majid, S., Foo, S., Luyt, B., Zhang, X., Theng, Y., Chang, Y., & Mokhtar, I. A. (2011). Adopting evidence-based practice in clinical decision making: Nurses' perceptions, knowledge, and barriers. *Journal of the Medical Library Association, 99*(3), 229–236.

Melnyk, B. M., & Fineout-Overholt, E. (Eds.). (2010). *Evidence-based practice in nursing & healthcare* (2nd ed.). Philadelphia, PA: Wolters Kluwer Health/Lippincott Williams & Wilkins.

Merkel, S. I., Voepel-Lewis, T., Shayevitz, J. R., & Malviya, S. (1997). The FLACC: A behavioral scale for scoring postoperative pain in young children. *Pediatric Nursing, 23*(3), 293–297.

Monaghan, A. (2005). Detecting and managing deterioration in children. *Paediatric Nursing, 17*(1), 32–35.

Nagy, S., Lumby, J., McKinley, S., & MacFarlane, C. (2001). Nurses' beliefs about the conditions that hinder or support evidence-based nursing. *International Journal of Nursing Practice, 7*(5), 314–321.

Newhouse, R., Dearholt, S., Poe, S., Pugh, L., & White, K. (2005). Evidence-based practice, a practical approach to implementation. *JONA, 35*(1):35–40.

Newhouse, R. P., Pettit, J. C., Poe, S., & Rocco, L. (2006). The slippery slope: Differentiating between quality improvement and research. *Journal of Nursing Administration, 36*(4), 211–219.

Palmer, D., & Kramlich, D. (2011). An introduction to the multisystem model of knowledge integration and translation. *Advances in Nursing Science, 34*(1), 29–38.

Palmer, D. (2010). *Utilizing an evidence-based practice model at the bedside* [PowerPoint slides].

Parshuram, C. S., Hutchison, J., & Middaugh, K. (2009). Development and initial validation of the bedside paediatric early warning system score. *Critical Care, 13*(4), R135.

Poe, S. S., & White, K. M. (2010). *Johns Hopkins nursing evidence-based practice: Implementation and translation.* Indianapolis, IN: Sigma Theta Tau International.

Polit, D. F., & Beck, C. T. (2008). *Nursing research: Generating and assessing evidence for nursing practice* (8th ed.). Philadelphia, PA: Wolters Kluwer/Lippincott Williams & Wilkins.

Pravikoff, D. S., Tanner, A. B., & Pierce, S. T. (2005). Readiness of U.S. nurses for evidence-based practice. *American Journal of Nursing, 105*(9), 40–51.

Reimer-Kirkham, S., Varcoe, C., Browne, A. J., Khan, K. B., & McDonald, H. (2009). Critical inquiry and knowledge translation: Exploring compatibilities and tensions. *Nursing Philosophy, 10*(3), 152–166.

Rosswurm, M., & Larrabee, J. (1999). A model for change to evidence-based practice. *Image—The Journal of Nursing Scholarship, 31*, 317–322.

Rycroft-Malone, J. (2004). The PARISH framework: A framework for guiding the implementation of evidence-based practice. *Journal of Nursing Care Quality, 19*(4), 297–304.

Rycroft-Malone, J., & Bucknall, T. (2010). Using theory and frameworks to facilitate the implementation of evidence into practice. *Worldviews on Evidence-Based Nursing, 7*(2), 57–58.

Sackett, D. L., Rosenberg, W. M., Gray, J. A., Haynes, R. B., & Richardson, W. S. (1996). Evidence based medicine: What it is and what it isn't. *British Medical Journal, 312*, 71–72.

Samara, K. (2007). A framework for discovering KM forces: The fifth element. *Journal of Knowledge Management Practice, 8*(1).

Sams, L., Penn, B. K., & Facteau, L. (2004). The challenge of using evidence-based practice. *Journal of Nursing Administration, 34*(9), 407–414.

Sigma Theta Tau International Honor Society Of Nursing. (2005). *Evidence-based nursing position statement.* Retrieved July 26, 2011, from http://www.nursingsociety.org/aboutus/PositionPapers/Pages/EBN_positionpaper.aspx

Solomons, N. M., & Spross, J. A. (2011). Evidence-based practice barriers and facilitators from a continuous quality improvement perspective: An integrative review. *Journal of Nursing Management, 19*(1), 109–120.

Spector, N. (n.d.). *Evidence-based healthcare in nursing regulation.* Retrieved July 5, 2011, from http://www.ncsbn.org/Evidence_based_HC_Nsg_Regulation_updated507withname.pdf

Stetler, C. (2001). Updating the Stetler model of research utilization to facilitate evidence-based practice. *Nursing Outlook, 49*, 272–278.

Stevens, K. (2004). *Academic Center for Evidence Based Practice.* Retrieved November 20, 2010, from www.acestar.uthscsa.edu/Learn-Illodel.htm

Tanner, C. A. (2006). Thinking like a nurse: A research based-model of clinical judgment in nursing. *Journal of Nursing Education, 45*(6), 204–211.

Thor, J. L., Wittlov, K., Herrlin, B., Brommels, M., Svensson, O., Skar, J., & Ovretveit, J. (2004). Learning helpers: How they facilitated improvement and improved facilitation-lessons from a hospital-wide quality improvement initiative. *Quality Management in Health Care, 13*(1), 60–74.

Titchen, A., & Manley, K. (2006). Spiraling towards transformational action research: Philosophical and practical journeys. *Educational Action Research, 14*(3), 333–356.

Titler, M. G. (2002). *Toolkit for promoting evidence-based practice.* Iowa City, IA: The University of Iowa Hospital and Clinics, Dept. of Nursing Services and Patient Care.

Titler, M., Kleiber, C., Steelman, V., Rakel, B. A., Budreau, G., Everett, L. Q., ... Goode, C. J. (2001). The Iowa Model of Evidence-Based practice to promote quality care. *Critical Care Nursing Clinics of North America, 13*(4), 497–509.

Van De Ven, A. H., Polley, D. E., Garud, R., & Venkataraman, S. (1999). *The innovation journey.* New York, NY: Oxford University Press.

Wenger, E., McDermott, R., & Snyder, W. M. (2002). *Cultivating communities of practice: A guide to managing knowledge.* Boston, MA: Harvard Business School Press.

Wolf, G. A., & Greenhouse, P. K. (2007). Blueprint for design: Creating models that direct change. *Journal of Nursing Administration, 37*(9), 381–387.

Zwarenstein, M., & Reeves, S. (2006). Knowledge translation and interprofessional collaboration: Where the rubber of evidence-based care hits the road of teamwork. *Journal of Continuing Education in the Health Professions, 26*(1), 46–54.

CHAPTER 12

# The Scholarship Supporting Leadership, Organizations, and Systems as They Adopt Evidence-Based Practice

Marjorie Splaine Wiggins and Kristiina Hyrkäs

Over the course of the last few decades, a theme of evidence-based approaches to practice, management, and education has become increasingly dominant in published literature (see e.g., Rycroft-Malone et al., 2004). However, scholars have largely focused on trying to understand individual-level barriers/facilitators and individual characteristics related to research utilization (Fink, Thompson, & Bonnes, 2005; Melnyk et al., 2004; Squires, Estabrooks, Gustavsson, & Wallin, 2011). As the importance of evidence-based practice (EBP) is becoming increasingly recognized, the scholarship behind organizations, systems, and identification of different media to bridge the research–practice divide are gaining more attention and popularity. However, the knowledge to practice gap remains wide in the 21st century; the transfer and uptake of research findings in health care settings has been surprisingly slow despite considerable efforts by the scientific community and investment of funds into health care research (Straus, Graham, & Mazmanian, 2006). This includes research and development of theoretical approaches on how knowledge transfer could be supported (Estabrooks, 2007; Estabrooks, Thompson, Lovely, & Hofmeyer, 2006). An interesting, recent systematic review by Squires and colleagues (Squires et al., 2011) has found that nurses' use of research is moderate to high and has remained relatively consistent over time until the early 2000s. The authors admit that this finding may be overly optimistic given the methodological problems inherent in the majority of the studies. However, this systematic review raises two important and timely issues: (1) there is clearly a need for the use of standard measures, and (2) there is a need for well-designed studies that examine nurses' use of research and assess the effects of varying levels of research use on patient outcomes.

It is natural today for bedside clinicians to change assumptions and long-standing practices based on evidence supporting something better (Ahrens, 2005). However, it may be more difficult to move an entire organization and, in turn, an entire health care system toward the same evidence-based way of thinking and behaving. In the same way that nursing practice needs to constantly change, the organizations and systems within health care need to evolve to meet the changing needs of the populations and the communities which they serve by actively bringing research-based knowledge into practice and promoting its utilization to improve the quality, cost effectiveness, and safety of health care delivery and service outcomes (Agency for Healthcare Research and Quality, 2008).

Today there is a great deal of scholarship behind the practice of nursing (Mohide & Coker, 2005). In much the same way, there are evidence-based practices (EBPs) and a body of scholarship that support the ability of organizations and systems to remain viable and flexible while promoting evidence-based/informed practice that optimizes the quality of care.

According to the literature, the most successful implementation of EBP seems to occur when: (1) evidence is scientifically robust and matches professional consensus and patients' preferences; (2) the context is receptive to change with sympathetic cultures, strong leadership, and appropriate monitoring and feedback systems; and (3) there is appropriate facilitation of change with input from skilled external and internal facilitators (Rycroft-Malone, 2004).

This chapter focuses on EBP from the organizational and systems perspective and evidence-based management and administration from the decision makers' perspective. It includes information about the assessment of environmental readiness and the examination of elements that can enhance the change process. Finally, it explores the future of EBP.

## ■ MAJOR PROFESSIONAL ORGANIZATIONS' AND POLICY-MAKING BODIES' EMPHASIS ON EBP

Today, at least three major professional and health organizations as well as policy-making bodies are emphasizing the importance of EBP: (1) The Institute of Medicine (Greiner & Knebel, 2003), (2) The Joint Commission (Joint Commission, 2003), and (3) the American Nurses Credentialing Center (Greiner & Knebel, 2003). According to the Institute of Medicine, EBP is a necessary and valuable tool for future progress, and as a project goal, by the year 2020, 90% of all clinical decisions should be supported by accurate, timely, and up-to-date clinical information that is supported by the best available evidence (Olsen, Aisner, & McGinnis, 2007). The Joint Commission has recognized the benefits of EBP and requires, for example, that disease-specific certifications be based on national standards, effective use of evidence-based clinical practice guidelines, and performance measurement and improvement. The Joint Commission has provided resources for implementation of EBP, including *Putting Evidence to Work* (2003) that focuses on concepts, principles, and techniques of EBP and provides tools for appraising evidence. It also provides examples of starting or improving EBP programs, and supplies tools and templates for incorporating patients' values in shared decision making (The Joint Commission, 2003).

In nursing, one of the most influential organizations is the American Nurses Credentialing Center, a subsidiary of the American Nurses Association. The American Nurses Credentialing Center Magnet Recognition Program® recognizes health care organizations that provide the very best in patient care and is the gold standard for nursing practice. A significant component of the program emphasizes the expectation that the nurses in an organization use EBP in their nursing care. Organizations that achieve Magnet status possess established and evolving programs related to EBP and resources are in place to support the advancement of EBPs and research in all clinical settings (American Nurses Credentialing Center, 2008). The Magnet Recognition Program® relies heavily on current evidence and the use of best practices and has been able to demonstrate strong outcomes.

Over the years, the literature, as outlined below, has provided a significant body of knowledge cataloging those outcomes. One of the earliest outcome studies looked at 39 of the original Magnet hospitals with 195 control hospitals selected from non-Magnet U.S. hospitals with over 100 Medicare discharges adjusted for severity. The study found that the Magnet hospitals had a 4.6% lower mortality rate (Aiken, Smith, & Lake, 1994). In 2008, Aiken and colleagues published a study that collected data from 10,184 nurses and 232,342 surgical patients in 168 hospitals in Pennsylvania, which found that the surgical mortality rates were more than 60% in poorly staffed hospitals with the poorest patient care environments than in hospitals with the better care environments. In the publication, the authors of the study suggest that one point for improvement would be to implement the blueprint for the American Nurses Credentialing Center Magnet designation (Aiken, Clarke, Sloane, & Cheney, 2008). Another study of Magnet environments demonstrated that hospitals with higher levels of Magnet characteristics and nurses who have increased access to empowering structures were significantly related to higher perceived patient safety climate (Armstrong, Laschinger, & Wong, 2009).

## ■ CONTEXT AND CULTURE—A SHIFT TO EXPLORING ORGANIZATIONAL FACTORS

There is a growing consensus in the literature that the challenges of EBP and transferring research into clinical practice are more due to organizational factors than to attributes of individual clinicians or the methods/models by which the evidence/research findings are disseminated (Cummings, Estabrooks, Midodzi, & Hayduk, 2007; Pettengill, Gillies, & Clark, 1994). Given that the majority of health care organizations are very complex today, it is important to focus the discussion first on the organizational context. It is possible to claim, based on the literature (Scott-Findlay & Golden-Biddle, 2005), that organizational context shapes the utilization of research in practice through its individuals, group behavioral norms, and innovations.

Interest in organizational features on EBP and research use started in the late 1990s. Over the years, Kitson and colleagues (Kitson, Harvey, & McCormack, 1998; McCormack et al., 2002; Rycroft-Malone et al., 2002; Rycroft-Malone et al., 2004) conducted pioneering studies that demonstrated that factors such as culture and leadership influence research use. Scott and colleagues (Scott, Estabrooks, Allen, & Pollock, 2008) found that uncertainty within an organizational context (e.g., inconsistent management) significantly hindered nurses' use of research in practice. Recent studies have illuminated how the organizational and contextual features influencing research utilization work and interact. For example, Cummings and colleagues (Cummings et al., 2007) report that there are relationships among features of organizational context (e.g., responsive administration, relational capital, and hospital size), nurses' research utilization, and adverse patient events. They found that the organizational characteristics mentioned above correlated with better leadership, culture, and evaluation and led to greater research use by nurses and ultimately fewer adverse events. The findings and strong evidence described above suggest very clearly that strategies (e.g., built-in, established organizational structure and support for clinical enquiry, functional and effective processes for EBP activities, including resources and mechanisms to sustain momentum and interest over time) to develop the organizational context are the first step to research utilization and a starting point to strengthen the EBP in an organization (Schulman, 2008). Today the literature is rich with descriptions of different strategies, approaches, and educational programs that promote EBP in the clinical setting. The reader can learn more valuable information from, for example, the following articles: Mohide and Coker (2005); Fineout-Overholt, Melnyk, and Schultz (2005); Larkin et al. (2007); Newhouse, Dearholt, Poe, Pugh, and White (2007); Barnsteiner, Reeder, Palma, Preston, and Walton (2010).

## ■ MODELS OF EBP AND RESEARCH UTILIZATION

The models of EBP, research dissemination, and utilization started to emerge in the late 1970s.[1] The first models developed by Stetler and Marram (1976) and Funk and colleagues (Funk, Tornquist, & Champagne, 1989) were important milestones historically because these models started a "new era" in nursing by de-emphasizing rituals and traditions, as well as raising awareness about the importance of applying research findings in nursing practice.

Today, there are EBP models available both for individual practitioners and organizations. For example, Melnyk and Fineout-Overholt (2005) introduce models developed by DiCenso and colleagues (DiCenso, Cullum, Ciliska, & Guyatt, 2005) for individual practitioners and four models for organizations: the Iowa Model (Titler, 2002), Rosswurm and Larrabee's model (Rosswurm & Larrabee, 1999), the Advancing Research and Clinical Practice Through Close Collaboration model (Melnyk & Fineout-Overholt, 2002), and Kitson's model (Kitson, 1999). These models have been developed to help nurses move evidence into practice. It is assumed that the use of a model leads to a systematic approach to EBP, prevents incomplete implementation, promotes timely evaluation, and maximizes use of time and resources (Gawlinski & Rutledge, 2008). Review of every available model is beyond the scope of this chapter. Instead, the discussion will be focused on processes that help organizations choose models of EBP.

Because there are several EBP models available, the selection and adoption process of a model for an organization is an important decision. An example of this process utilizing a systematic approach has been described by Gawlinski and Rutledge (2008) and Mohide and Coker (2005). The first step for selecting a model is to establish a structure or forum (e.g., use of an existing nursing research committee, formation of an EBP council, or appointment of a task force) in which discussions can occur about various EBP models, their advantages and disadvantages, and their applicability to organizational needs. The second step is to review and systematically evaluate a selection of the models. Gawlinski and Rutledge (2008) suggest focusing on (1) the history and development of the EBP model; (2) any revisions of the model over time; (3) overall concepts in the EBP model, process, and flow of the model; and (4) publications describing how the model has guided EBP changes in other facilities. Mohide and Coker (2005) emphasize that there seem to be, in fact, three important core criteria for evaluation: clarity and conciseness, comprehensiveness, and ease of use by direct care nurses. The final selection of a model should be based on an evaluation of (1) how easy the EBP model is to understand and whether it guides the user in the EBP process, (2) direction of the model for conducting research, (3) the flow of steps in the model and whether this is similar to the flow of practice algorithms, and (4) decision points in the EBP model regarding opportunities for thoughtful reflection and decision making (Gawlinski & Rutledge, 2008). Once the model is chosen, the third and final step is its dissemination and use. Several strategies, including strong leadership support, can be used for the dissemination/education and integration of the selected model, such as incorporating a class about EBP and the selected

[1] Estabrooks, Thompson, Lovely, and Hofmeyer (2006) published *A Guide to Knowledge Translation Theory*. This guide includes helpful definitions regarding EBP concepts, models, and theories of knowledge translation.

model into orientation, adding content about the EBP model in preceptor development programs and/or nursing grand rounds, and incorporating education into the annual skills and competency forums (Gawlinski & Rutledge, 2008).

Nurse leaders are instrumental in supporting nurses with resources to apply and utilize research/evidence to their practice. Research utilization means the use of research in clinical practice, and is one of the many components underpinning EBP. Estabrooks (1999) has provided helpful clarification regarding this concept by identifying three forms of research utilization: (1) direct research utilization, (2) indirect research utilization, and (3) persuasive research utilization. *Direct research utilization* means the application of research findings and (instrumental) use of findings when giving patient care. *Indirect research utilization* means the use of research findings to change thinking or opinions (but not necessarily behavior) in response to how to, for example, approach certain patient care situations. *Persuasive research utilization* means the use of research findings to persuade others, for example, decision makers to make changes in conditions, policies, or practices relevant to nurses, or the health of individuals or groups (Estabrooks, 1999, 2007).

Although there are models of research utilization available, a resourceful leader will find it important to identify factors that affect research utilization prior to developing strategies to promote research use in practice. The literature shows (Godin, Bélanger-Gravel, Eccles, & Grimshaw, 2008) that nurses' attitudes seem to be predictors of behavior and ultimately successful implementation of EBP. Today, there are several instruments available to measure research utilization in general, but it is important to note that the concepts that comprise nurses' attitudes toward using research are based on different definitions, because there is no specific theory to guide research utilization (Estabrooks, 2007). It is thus crucial to identify and review a variety of instruments and their theoretical and psychometric properties before selecting how to measure, implement, and test strategies to increase the adoption of research utilization in practice. Frasure (2008) recently conducted a systematic review describing and evaluating the instruments used to measure nurses' attitudes toward research utilization that were developed and published from 1982 to 2007 in nursing journals. The paper reports an in-depth analysis of 14 instruments. Four instruments were developed using constructs from Roger's diffusions of innovations theory. One instrument was influenced by not only Roger's theory but also multiple theories; eight instruments did not designate a specific theory, and one remains unclassified. The author also used Estabrooks' framework/definition of research utilization and found that indirect and overall research utilization were measured in all of the 14 instruments, 10 measured direct research utilization, and 9 measured persuasive research utilization. The methodological process to find the strongest instrument and weighting the evidence were also described in this article.

## ■ LEADERSHIP PERSPECTIVE ON EBP

Transformational leadership is an approach that has been shown to have a high impact on both practice changes in nursing and on the development of an organizational culture that is more receptive to progression and change (Shaw, 2005). One model of transformational leadership that is evidence-based and has stood the test of time was developed by Kouzes and Posner in the early 1980s when they conducted a research project that looked at what people did when they felt they were at their personal best when leading others (Kouzes & Posner, 2007). Kouzes and Posner's leadership model is described in the best-selling book, *The Leadership Challenge* (4th ed.); it is grounded in extensive research and found to be applicable in the United States, Europe, Asia, Australia, and elsewhere around the world. The conceptual framework is based on interviews of leaders at all levels and written case studies from personal best leadership practices in both public and private organizations. When empirical research was repeated 20 years after the model was developed, the concepts and principles of the model remained unchanged (Kouzes & Posner, 2002). Supported by hundreds of external research studies and utilized by academics (Yukl, 2001) and organizational leaders, the model has been analyzed, tested, critiqued, and applied with repeated success and validation (Kouzes & Posner, 2000–2011). The conceptual framework of the model is comprised of five practices of exemplary leadership: (1) model the way, (2) inspire a shared vision, (3) challenge the process, (4) enable others to act, and (5) encourage the heart. Kouzes and Posner postulate that when leaders understand that leadership is a relationship and the five practices are used, they are better able to perform at their personal best and success is sure to follow (Kouzes & Posner, 2002). The Leadership Practices Inventory used to measure the five practices was developed through a triangulation of qualitative and quantitative research methods and studies (Kouzes & Posner, 2000). Both a self-report and observer form of the Leadership Practices Inventory have been developed. The instruments measure the five key practices: modeling the way, inspiring a shared vision, challenging the process, enabling others to act, and encouraging the heart (Kouzes & Posner, 2007). Under the key practices, the authors have identified 10 commitments of leadership that should be followed to be successful in using the model (Table 12.1).

**TABLE 12.1  Five Practices of Exemplary Leadership and Ten Commitments of Leadership**

| Practice | Commitments |
| --- | --- |
| **Model the way** | 1. Clarify values by finding your voice and affirming shared ideals |
| | 2. Set an example by aligning actions with shared values |
| **Inspire a shared vision** | 3. Envision the future by imagining exciting and ennobling possibilities |
| | 4. Enlist others in a common vision by appealing to shared aspirations |
| **Challenge the process** | 5. Search for opportunities by seizing the initiative and by looking outward for innovative ways to improve |
| | 6. Experiment and take risks by constantly generating small wins and learning from experience |
| **Enable others to act** | 7. Foster collaboration by building trust and facilitating relationships |
| | 8. Strengthen others by increasing self-determination and developing competence |
| **Encourage the heart** | 9. Recognize contributions by showing appreciation for individual excellence |
| | 10. Celebrate the values and victories by creating a spirit of community |

*Source:* Adapted from Kouzes & Posner, 2007.

Relationship is a key word in understanding this model. In fact, two of the most powerful statements in *The Leadership Challenge* are the last sentences of the book. "Leadership is not an affair of the head. Leadership is an affair of the heart" (Kouzes & Posner, 2002, p. 351). Kouzes and Posner are not the only contemporaries who feel leadership is about the heart. Others speak of love when they reference leadership.

> Exercising leadership is a way of giving meaning to your life by contributing to the lives of others. At best, leadership is a labor of love. Opportunities for these labors cross your path every day, though we appreciate through the scar tissue of our own experiences that seizing these opportunities takes heart. (Heifetz & Linsky, 2002, p. 211)

Effective leadership and relationships/emotional intelligence are key in developing an environment that supports the effort and institutional energy required for evidence-based culture.

## ■ EMOTIONAL INTELLIGENCE

In a 1998 article entitled "What Makes a Leader" published in the *Harvard Business Review*, Daniel Goleman articulated the five components of emotional intelligence (EI) in the business workplace with a particular emphasis on management and leadership skill.

*(1) Self-awareness* refers to "the ability to recognize and understand (your) moods, emotions, and the effects on others."

*(2) Self-regulation* is the second component and refers to "the ability to control or redirect disruptive impulses and moods" and "to think before acting."

*(3) Motivation*, the third component, refers to "a passion to work for reasons that go beyond money or status" and "a propensity to pursue goals with energy and persistence."

*(4) Empathy* is reflected in "the ability to understand the emotional makeup of other people" and to treat "people according to their emotional reactions."

*(5) Social skill* is a "proficiency in managing relationships and building networks" and an "ability to find common ground and build rapport." (Goleman, 1998)

Goleman's five components of EI yielded a valuable insight on how managers can develop leadership skills in the (business) workplace by having insight on their own behavior. This work in the late 1990s demonstrated that by focusing on the relationships with colleagues and listening rather than reacting on impulse will assist managers to function with leadership and increase motivation in the business workplace.

EI has also been a focus of interest in nursing for a while. For example, Akerjordet and Severinsson (2008) have conducted a systematic review (literature from 1997 to 2007) focusing on EI and how this is linked to nursing leadership. The findings of the review report, among other things, that nurses leaders with high EI

• Demonstrate a caring attitude
• Nurture a greater sense of safety
• Act out of commitment (i.e., desire) as opposed to obligation or guilt, reflecting one's own values
• Manage their emotions in functional ways and make a greater number of rational decisions

- Are more likely to use supportive behaviors and provide rewards in the form of psychological benefits, as they are more sensitive to their own and their followers' feelings and emotions
- Have self-awareness and authentic empathy that facilitates real understanding and builds relationships of trust by appealing to the heart
- Contribute positive empowering processes in the organization by having authentic empathy, wisdom, and respect for others' experiences.

According to Akerjordet and Severinsson (2008), EI seems to have several implications for organizational development processes by creating highly energized and synchronized teams. In other words, EI nurse leaders may bring awareness about what the team collectively is able to create by direct encouragement, positive expectations, and tangible opportunities to learn new skills, valuing personal responsibility, initiative, and innovation. EI nurse leaders stimulate the creativity of their team using self-control against criticism and feeling less threatened by the changes that creative ideas may imply to the team. EI nurse leaders are also able to respond constructively to changes in others' emotional stages, seeking out new opportunities. EI nurse leaders nurture a supportive work climate in which people feel energized to do their best and encourage high performance based on mutual trust. In the literature, Akerjordet and Severinsson (2008) conclude that emotionally intelligent nurse leadership is characterized by self-awareness and supervisory skills that highlight positive empowerment processes and thus create a favorable work climate exemplified by resilience, innovation, and change. It is possible to argue that EI included in a set of leadership skills offers new ways of thinking for nurse leaders, especially how this can be utilized to strengthen the EBPs in an organization.

## ■ ORGANIZATIONAL CHANGE THEORIES

Change can be planned or unplanned but in either case it is rarely easy. There are several theories about the nature of change and assumptions related to how successful change can be encouraged and facilitated. Many of these explain the phenomena of change process, define the leader's role, and explain why change participants are so often resistant to change (Stichler, 2011).

An early model of change developed by Lewin described change as a three-stage process. The first stage he called "unfreezing." It involves overcoming inertia and dismantling the existing "mind set." At this juncture, leaders need to bypass defense mechanisms to effectively manage resistance. In the second stage, change or movement occurs. Three actions can facilitate movement at this stage, which include persuading employees to agree that the status quo is not beneficial to them and encouraging them to view the problem from a fresh perspective; working together on a quest for new, relevant information; and connecting the views of the group to well-respected, powerful leaders that also support the change (Kritsonis, 2004–2005). This can be a period of confusion and transition. The third and final stage he called "freezing." This is a critical step without which change may not be sustained over time. It is the process of integrating the new values into that of the community. This includes reinforcing new patterns through both formal and informal mechanisms such as policies and procedures.

While Lewin's theory of change is popular, it is but one of several that can be used to successfully manage and sustain change. It is useful to consider various theories/models and how they resonate with the values and beliefs of the organization. For example, the three theories listed below also explain the phenomenon of change process, describe the leader's role, and explain why change participants are often resistant to change: (1) Lippitt's and colleagues theory of change that extends Lewin's three stages to seven with more emphasis on the role and responsibility of the leader as the change agent in planning, integrating, and sustaining the change over time, as contrasted to the evolution of the change. (2) Ajzen's theory of reasoned action and planned behavior that emphasizes, among other things, individual's social environment, subjective norms, and (positive) attitudes regarding the change to actually occur. (3) Prochaska and DiClement's theory describes change as a cyclical, not linear process composed of stages such as precontemplation, contemplation, preparation, action, maintenance (Kritsonis 2004–2005; Stichler 2011). Careful consideration and selection of the appropriate model can help to ensure success. For example, Grant, Colello, Riehle, and Dende (2010) demonstrated the utility and effectiveness of Lewin's theory as they undertook the significant practice change of moving the shift-to-shift report to the patient's bedside. They also note the importance of key characteristics of a Magnet organization to their success. Conversely, one can imagine that without critical thinking, mechanically applying a theory with no consideration of organizational context or its structures and processes would not likely produce the desired outcomes.

## ■ IMPLEMENTATION OF EBP AND ACTION RESEARCH

Many authors in the nursing literature (Gerrish et al., 2007; Kitson et al., 1998; Rycroft-Malone et al., 2002; Thompson, Estabrooks, Scott-Findlay, Moore, & Wallin, 2007) have analyzed the question of why it is so difficult to use or adopt research findings. The categories that have been utilized and that found helpful to better understand the obstacles have often been based on barriers identified by Funk and colleagues (Funk, Champagne, Wiese, & Tornquist, 1991). The four major categories that have many times been considered as the obstacles to research utilization in practice are (1) characteristics of the adopter (i.e., values, skills, and awareness); (2) characteristics of the organization (i.e., setting) (3) characteristics of the innovation (i.e., qualities of the research), and (4) characteristics of the communication (i.e., presentation and accessibility of the research). Several authors (Denis, Hébert, Langley, Lozeau, & Trottier, 2002; Dopson, FitzGerald, Ferlie, Gabbay & Locock, 2002; Meijers et al., 2006) have recommended that characteristics of the context, the (new) knowledge, people/actors involved, and their possible interactions (roles) should be taken into account when implementing (EBP) changes in practice. It has also been acknowledged that the factors influencing the use/implementation and adoption of research findings and new knowledge are diverse and complex processes.

The challenges around the implementation of EBP and the research–practice gap have led researchers like Munten and colleagues (Munten, van den Bogaard, Cox, Garretsen, & Bongers, 2010) to explore different methodologies, more specifically, action research, as an answer and a suitable strategy for EBP because this directly addresses the problem of the division between practice and research/knowledge, and participation of those involved in the context (Dick, 2004; Noffke & Somekh, 2005; Sharp, 2005).

### What Is Action Research?

The origins of action research lie in the beginning of the 20th century, and Lewin is often cited in the literature as the person who first used this term (Waterman, Tillen, Dickson & de Koning, 2001). His interest was a social science that could help to resolve social conflicts and problems combining research and change (action). According to this methodology, an action researcher not only intends to collect data/knowledge about a particular situation but also to (help) improve the situation while investigating it. Two criteria are fundamental to action research. First, an intervention is carried out as a part of cyclic process that is composed of problem identification/diagnosis, planning, action (implementation of change and monitoring), and evaluation/reflection before starting a new cycle/situation analysis. The second criterion of action research concerns the partnership between the researcher and those being involved/investigated in the research process. In fact, partnership is seen as an essential feature of this methodology for implementing change in practice and for developing practical knowledge. This partnership also enhances the accessibility of the knowledge/evidence created to a wider public than the researcher, and thus helps to achieve the emancipatory and empowering intent of action research.

## What Is Known About Implementing EBP in Nursing Using Action Research?

It is possible to claim that action research has been widely utilized in nursing and health care research since the early 1980s (Hyrkäs, 1997; Munn-Giddings, McVicar, & Smith, 2008). The literature contains indication that action research is suitable methodology for bridging the gap between practice and research, and for implementing new knowledge. However, the potentials of action research methodology from EBP perspective have just started to become a focus of interest in the literature. In a very recent paper, Munten et al. (2010) reviewed 21 action research studies published from 1999 to 2007. The findings showed that very few interventions were aimed specifically at changing leadership and culture, even though these factors seem to be the biggest obstacles to the implementation of EBP (e.g., McCormack et al. 2002). However, there were other frequently occurring interventions, such as changes to communication and personal contacts, which could also have contributed (indirectly) to altering culture, which is reflected and supported through other outcomes measures. It was not possible to draw conclusions based on the findings of this study whether action research is more or less successful in implementing EBP compared to designs that are less cyclic and not based on partnership between the researcher and those being investigated. However, the findings of this review demonstrated that a participatory approach led to results that were less expected than with a nonparticipatory approach to implementation (e.g., nurses were feeling personally responsible for a developed guideline, teams were feeling responsible for the changes of care and development of expertise because of knowledge sharing). The authors (Munten et al., 2010) conclude, with an element of caution, that implementation of EBP using action research is a promising approach. Several authors (Carey, Buchan, & Sanson-Fisher, 2009; MacDavitt, Cieplinski & Walker, 2011) have proposed small tests of change as a cyclical process for implementing best evidence into clinical practice. Like action research, this is an alternative approach to a randomized clinical trial in which clinicians pilot test a change and measure its effectiveness in producing desired clinical changes. These tests of change are generally limited in scope and duration. The caution, as argued by Scott-Findlay and Golden-Biddle (2005), is that evaluating outcomes in the very short term may fail to recognize the benefits of using evidence from research. In fact, rapid cycles of small changes may be counter-productive and create frustration rather than build momentum toward the adoption of evidence-based practices (Carey et al., 2009).

## ■ READINESS FOR CHANGE

Although a great emphasis has been placed on EBP implementation, organizations and individuals within the organizations need to systematically assess whether or not their institution is ready for the EBP. *Environmental readiness* refers to the ability of the health care environment to respond to change and implement process that can improve care. In other words, organizational readiness is a stage of preparedness, psychologically and behaviorally, for change. This requires having necessary knowledge, skills, resources, and support (Weiner, 2009). Organizational readiness is a critical precursor to successful implementation of (complex) changes in practice and sustaining change as a part of the culture. It has been speculated in the literature (Smith & Donze, 2010) that 50% of efforts for organizational change fail because organizational leaders have not established sufficient readiness for change. It is thus possible to argue that the best time to assess organizational readiness for change is before its implementation; therefore, the organizational leader's role is crucial. Furthermore, to successfully implement EBP, it is important not only to recognize the interactions between the organizational, interdisciplinary team, and individual levels but also to understand the effects of organizational culture, infrastructure, and available resources (Smith & Donze, 2010).

One of the most important steps and the first step from an organizational perspective is to assess the organizational context and readiness for EBP. This allows, for example, leaders to plan and pave the path for the right direction to promote adoption. French and colleagues (French et al., 2009) have conducted a review on the current literature and instruments in an attempt to answer the question: What can management theories offer evidence-based practice? The authors conducted a structured search in major health care and management databases and focused on four major domains: research utilization, research activity, knowledge management, and organizational learning. As a result, 30 measurement tools were identified and appraised. Eighteen instruments from the four domains were selected for a closer analysis. The instruments measure three major organizational attributes (i.e., vision, leadership, and a learning culture) and four different types of knowledge stages (i.e., need, acquisition of new knowledge, knowledge sharing, and knowledge use). The authors conclude that these concepts measure the absorptive and receptive capacity of organizations. Weiner and colleagues (Weiner, Amick, & Lee, 2008) have also conducted an extensive review of the literature in health services research focusing on the conceptualization and measurement of organizational readiness for change. The authors found 106 peer-reviewed articles and 43 instruments measuring the concept. The review revealed, among other things, that there were different perspectives to operationalize the concept and limited evidence of reliability and validity for many instruments.

Newhouse (2010) has presented an overview of the most recent instruments to assess organizations' readiness for EBP in nursing. An interesting observation is that the Promoting Action on Research Implementation in Health Services (PARIHS) framework and its major concepts of evidence, facilitation, and context have been used as a foundation for all three instruments: the Context Assessment Instrument (CAI), Alberta Context Tool (ACT), and Organizational Readiness to Change Assessment (ORCA). Each instrument measures the readiness of the work context for EBP specifically. The CAI contains 37 items and it measures five domains: collaborative practice, evidence-informed practice, respect for persons, practice boundaries, and evaluation (McCormack, McCarthy, Wright, Slater & Coffey, 2009). The second instrument, ACT, is composed of 56 items and the core dimensions include leadership, culture, evaluation, social capital, structural and electronic resources, formal and informal interactions, and organizational slack (Estabrooks, Squires, Cummings, Birdsell & Norton, 2009). The third instrument, ORCA, contains 77 items and these measure three domains: evidence (i.e., research, clinical experience, and patient preference), context (i.e., leadership culture, staff culture, leadership behavior, measurement/leadership feedback, opinion leaders, and general resources), and facilitation (i.e., leadership practices, clinical champions, leadership implementation roles, implementation team roles, implementation plan, project communication, project progress tracking, project resources and context, and project evaluation) (Helfrich, Li, Sharp, & Sales, 2009). The validity and reliability of these instruments have been tested and they have been widely used in the United States, Canada, and Europe.

## ■ NURSING READINESS FOR EBP

It is possible to claim that the barriers and facilitators for EBP are well known today (Kajermo et al., 2010). Several studies looking at why nurses do not use EBP have shown that lack of time is the most common barrier. The other very commonly reported barriers are workload and resource constraints, lack of access to resources and equipment, and resistance to change (Ploeg, Davies, Edwards, Gifford, & Miller, 2007). The facilitators include, for example, provision of protected time to find, read, appraise, and implement research; participatory management; colleague support; champions; and mentorship. Responding to the perceived barriers and assessing nurses' readiness for the EBP implementation include factors not only at the individual but also at organizational level (context): leaders, administrators, and different groups of stakeholders (Ploeg et al., 2007).

It has been commonly suggested in the literature (Bosch, van der Weijden, Wensing, & Grol, 2007; Shaw et al., 2005) that the best strategy to bridge the gap between research and practice is to identify the barriers first and then implement tailored strategies that account for these typically context-dependent barriers. Some evidence supports this approach (Kajermo et al. 2010); however, it is important to revisit and reassess the strategies because little is known about how the barriers should be identified and by whom and what interventions are effective for overcoming specific barriers. Kajermo and colleagues (2010) have just recently conducted a systematic review on this topic. The authors' recommendation is that various contextual and human factors enhancing research use in a given organizational context should be studied and interventions should be tailored and carefully evaluated.

Recently, an EBP Belief Scale and an EBP Implementation Scale have been developed to assess the nursing/nurses readiness for utilizing EBP and to identify perceived barriers within organization (Melnyk, Fineout-Overholt, & Mays, 2008). Other instruments are also available today, for example, the EBP Confidence Scale (Salbach & Jaglal, 2011) and EBP Self-Efficacy Scale (Tucker, Olson, & Frusti, 2009). The EBP Confidence Scale provides an opportunity to evaluate health care professionals' beliefs in their ability (i.e., self-efficacy) to undertake EBP activities, and this measurement can increase our understanding of health care professionals' readiness to engage in EBP activities. The EBP Self-Efficacy Scale has been developed to assess self-rating regarding one's ability to carry out EBP. This instrument could also be used to predict changes in EBP practices over time and ultimately patient outcomes.

## ■ DIFFUSION OF INNOVATIONS

New evidence is coming into the profession on a daily basis but it is well known that adoption of this evidence takes time. It has been speculated in the literature that, on an average, it may take about 17 years to move from research trials to clinical practice (Tucker et al., 2009). The diffusion and adoption of innovations is a sociopolitical process in which the benefits and risks of technologies are distributed unevenly and locally defined, and thus have differentiated influences on individual decision makers. In this context, decision making that supposes a unified evaluation based on evidence is unlikely to fully explain diffusion patterns (Denis et al., 2002). Changing practice to reflect the latest evidence needs to be valued by the practitioner and not create additional, time-consuming work.

The work of Everett Rogers gives valuable insight into what enhances diffusion of innovations, which can readily be applied to EBP. Diffusion scholars have long recognized that an individual's decision about adoption of an innovation requires a process that occurs over time as opposed to an instantaneous decision (Rogers, 2003). Rogers also identified attributes that impact the rate of adoption and postulates that the variances in the rate of adoption are due to five attributes: (1) relative advantage, (2) compatibility, (3) complexity, (4) trialability, and (5) observability. Relative advantage or the degree to which this innovation is better than the idea it supersedes is most likely the strongest attribute in the speed of adoption (Rogers, 2003). However, that may not be enough to adopt a new best practice if it is more costly or time consuming. Compatibility is the degree to which an innovation is perceived as consistent with existing values, past experiences, and needs of potential adopters (Rogers, 2003). Complexity is another attribute. If an innovation is seen as difficult to understand or implement, it will be set aside by busy clinical practitioners who already have too many demands on their time. Trialability, the fourth attribute, offers the opportunity to experiment with an innovation on a limited basis to see its advantages and see how it fits into the context of the organization. Finally, observability provides the opportunity for others to see the application of the innovation before they devote time and resources to adopting the innovation. All these attributes have impact on the adoptions of innovations or new evidence and should be carefully considered and addressed to facilitate adoption of evidence.

The majority of statements from policy makers and in policy documents on evidence-based practice implementation draw on classic diffusion of innovation models, the most influential of which remains Rogers. However, it is critically important to realize that individuals and groups involved in setting clinical policy are part of highly complex networks of social relationships that affect their practice. This complexity and variability of local contexts ensure that there are no magic bullets for introducing evidence-based improvements in care (Dopson et al., 2002).

One key criticism of Rogers is that his theory of diffusion of innovation is linear. Given the complexity of the health care environment, it is highly possible and often probable that adoption of innovations, even those with a very strong scientific basis, does not occur in readily defined stages. In fact, Denis et al. (2002) have discussed four propositions that appear to have specific practice implications on the topic of effective and efficient adoption of innovations. The authors introduce a two-by-two grid design in which the two axes of the grid reflect variations in time (i.e., rapid adoption vs. slow adoption) and emergence of evidence (i.e., leading vs. lagging evidence). The four "cells" (i.e., "success," "overadoption," "prudence," and "underadoption") were found to be helpful with understanding the events leading to different overall outcomes. Denis et al. (2002) suggest that those interested in promoting wisdom in the adoption of innovations must become deeply aware of the specific ways in which they are likely to interact with their social contexts.

## ■ WHAT IS NEXT FOR EBP?

This question is answered from two different perspectives: (1) translation/implementation science and (2) the increasing needs for interdisciplinary collaboration.

Implementing EBPs is challenging and, as discussed, the difficulties may be largely explained by contextual factors. Thus, it is possible to claim that, in order to promote EBP, (new) strategies are needed that address the complexity and systems of care, leadership, and ultimately change the prevailing health care cultures. According to Titler (2010), if we want to upgrade knowledge about promoting and sustaining adoption of EBPs in health care, *translation science* needs more studies that test implementation/translation interventions into practice. The author defines *translation/implementation science* as: "the investigation of methods, interventions, and variables that influence adoption of EBPs by individuals and organizations to improve clinical and operational decision-making in health care." In other words, examples of translation studies could focus on

- Facilitators and barriers to knowledge uptake and use—what works, for whom in what circumstances, in what type of settings
- Organizational predictors of adherence to EBP guidelines
- Attitudes toward EBP
- Factors that explain the underlying mechanisms of effective interventions

*Translation science* is still young, and although there is a growing body of knowledge in this area, there are many unanswered questions. Titler (2010) has pointed out that, for example, the "knowledge transfer framework" introduced by the Agency for Healthcare Research and Quality (Nieva et al., 2005), provides a helpful guiding framework for testing and/or selecting strategies to promote adoption of EBP. The model encompasses the core processes, actors and activities, and also three major strategies: (1) knowledge creation and distillation, (2) diffusion and dissemination, (3) adoption, implementation, and institutionalization. Titler (2007) has also developed a translation research model based on Roger's diffusion of innovation framework. In this model, translation/diffusion of innovation/EBP is influenced by its characteristics and the manner in which it is communicated to users in a social system (see Figure 12.1).

It is possible to assume that these two models described above would not only serve as very useful and helpful frameworks for an overview of scientific findings about implementation

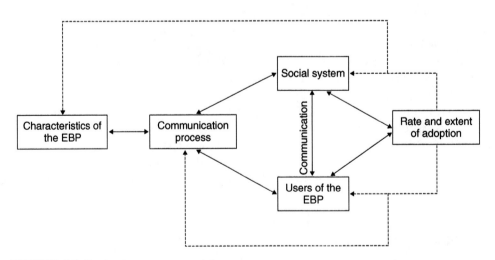

**FIGURE 12.1** Implementation model.

*Source:* Redrawn from Rogers (2003) and Titler and Everett (2001a). (Copyright by Marita Titler.)

strategies (for DNPs) but also useful tools for clinical investigators developing research initiatives and programs.

The literature shows developments of evidence-based practices for medicine (EBM), nursing (EBN), psychology (EBPP), social work (EBSWP), and public health (EBPH) and it is possible to claim that evidence-based practices are becoming increasingly important for interdisciplinary teams in patient care (Satterfield et al., 2009). However, because the training of practitioners in the health professions stand apart, their vocabulary, conceptual frameworks, and research methods (evidence) often differ as well, thereby impeding cross-disciplinary translation and research utilization. It is thus not a surprise that there are common challenges across disciplines focusing on "shared" EBPs. According to Satterfield and colleagues (2009), these include (1) how "evidence" should be defined and weighted, (2) how and when patients' preferences and other contextual factors should be entered into the clinical decision-making process, (3) definition of the "expert," and (4) what other variables should be considered when selecting an EBP (e.g., age, social class, community resources, and local expertise). The commonly known EBM model, also called "three circle model," emphasizes research evidence, clinical expertise, and patients' preferences. Compared with EBM, EBN utilizes the same concepts but it usually relies also on evidence from nonrandomized studies, qualitative research, and even quality improvement and patient satisfaction studies. In contrast, EBPP relies exclusively on research evidence, singling out treatments that do not have the best empirical support. Furthermore, the clinical expertise (in psychology) has been defined as composed of such competencies as assessment, diagnostic judgment, systematic case formulation, and treatment planning. There is also an official description how the competencies are acquired and the role of the expert in the clinical decision-making process. In the evidence-based social work (EBSWP) model, the key concepts are research evidence, client's preferences and actions, and client's state and circumstances. However, professional expertise replaces clinical expertise in this model, reflecting social workers' roles in management and policy in addition to clinical practice. Furthermore, the political, professional, economic, and sociohistorical perspectives of the context are taken into consideration. Like other disciplines, social work has debated the criteria and relevant weight for evidence. Today, social workers consider evidence from different types of qualitative studies because of its insight into clients' experiences and context, and quantitative studies because of its objectivity and precision in addressing the efficacy and cost-effectiveness of alternative intervention options. In the EBPH model, the perspective has been extended to communities' input and preferences in decision making. The key concepts in the public health model are evidence, population needs and values, and resources. Although fewer RCTs are available, the evidence relies on public health surveillance and the policies rely on cross-sectional studies, quasi-experimental designs, and time-series analyses. The "experts" in public health are drawn from many disciplines and, thus, there is no single credential that certifies a public health practitioner.

The literature demonstrates (Cohen & Hersh, 2004) that the critique on EBM has focused on (1) evidence that is defined too narrowly, (2) the unclear role and value of practitioners and their expertise, (3) ignored resources and/or contextual factors, and (4) low attention to clients' preferences. As described above, these perspectives are, in fact, addressed in the behavioral and social sciences of health and their emphasis on EBPs. It is particularly helpful to see how each discipline (nursing, psychology, social work, and public health) has utilized the original EBM model as a starting point and expanded the scope of what is considered as evidence. These disciplines have also demonstrated that many different practice questions are important from EBP perspectives and that the best study design depends on the question asked. Psychology has illuminated how to specify criteria for evidence-based treatments and also introduced these to training programs. Both psychology and social work have emphasized the importance of client characteristics as potential moderators of the outcomes. Social work has also drawn attention to institutional and environmental contexts. Public health addresses the issue of how resource availability influences decision making. Finally, both nursing and psychology have recognized the importance of patient characteristics and preferences to decisions regarding clinical care.

In the future, the transdisciplinary perspective could/should incorporate each discipline's most profound contributions and attempt to address remaining deficiencies. From the transdisciplinary perspective, the environment and organizational factors would create a cultural context that could not only moderate but also strengthen the EBP. It is possible to assume that environment/context and organization are becoming increasingly important to evidence-based decisions for all disciplines. One of the core concepts from the transdisciplinary perspective is thus "best available evidence," and "expertise" is possible to see as one of the resources needed to implement health services, including competence at performing the EBP process, assessment, communication/collaboration, and engagement/intervention. Because clinical expertise is a resource, it could be evaluated as a part of the decision-making process. Decision making would be a core concept, and in the center of the EBP model this would mean a cognitive action that turns evidence into contextualized EBP. The collaborative EBP model would assume that health decisions are not solely the practitioner's but are shared among practitioner(s), clients, and other affected stakeholders. The collaborative model would not only just support practice but also research endeavors across traditional disciplinary silos.

■ SUMMARY

EBP for the way we provide and manage patient care has grown in the literature over the past few decades. More recent literature is focused on transferring evidence into practice so patients and leaders can reap the benefit of new evidence that supports better practice, which leads to more positive patient outcomes. Organizations that accredit and support health care endorse the use of EBP. One organization, the American Nurses Credentialing Center, even goes so far as to require proof of its use in the organization to recognize the organization for Magnet status. Still, adopting EBP is difficult in complex environments such as health care. However, organizational context and leadership can influence the scholarship behind organizations and systems. The role of leaders is key in creating an environment that facilitates the adoption and sustainability of the use of EBP. Creating structures and providing resources that support clinical scholarship is the first critical step in the process. The second is to utilize models that help facilitate dissemination and the utilization of EBP. Evidence-based leadership models, like Kouzes and Posner's model for transformational leadership, provide support and guidance for individuals to take organizations to a new level. Supported by numerous research studies, their model has stood the test of time and has all the elements to create the transformation required in complex environments. Organizational change theories and methods to evaluate readiness for change are important to understand and help prepare for change. The future success of applying evidence to practice may lie in the current work of translational research. The science of translational research is embryonic but holds great promise in closing the evidence-to-practice gap. The scientific and leadership knowledge embedded in the doctor of nursing practice (DNP) curriculum helps ready DNPs to take a leading role in uniting disciplines to research new ways of improving care to increase health and well-being and improve the lives of those who are served by the health care system. Now, more than ever, this leadership is needed. The emerging presence of DNPs throughout the health care system can facilitate this important work that, to date, has been challenging for so many years.

# ■ REFERENCES

Agency for Healthcare Research and Quality (2008). National healthcare quality report 2007. *2007 National Healthcare Quality & Disparties Reports.* Retrieved from http://www.ahrq.gov/qual/nhqr07/nhqr07.pdf

Ahrens, T. (2005). Evidenced-based practice: priorities and implementation strategies. *AACN Clinical Issues, 16*(1), 36–42.

Aiken, L. H., Clarke, S. P., Sloane, D. M., & Cheney, T. (2008). Effects of hospital care environment on patient mortality and nurse outcomes. *Journal of Nursing Administration, 38*(5), 223–229.

Aiken, L. H., Smith, H. L., & Lake, E. T. (1994). Lower medicare mortality among a set of hospitals known for good nursing care. *Medical Care, 32*(8), 771–787.

Akerjordet, K., & Severinsson, E. (2008). Emotionally intelligent nurse leadership: A literature review study. *Journal of Nursing Management, 16*(5), 565–577.

American Nurses Credentialing Center. (2008). *Application manual: Magnet recognition program* [Brochure]. Washington, DC: Author.

Armstrong, K., Laschinger, H., & Wong, C. (2009). Workplace empowerment and Magnet hospital characteristics as predictors of patient safety climate. *Journal of Nursing Care Quality, 24*(1), 55–62.

Barnsteiner, J. H., Reeder, V. C., Palma, W. H., Preston, A. M., & Walton, M. K. (2010). Promoting evidence-based practice and translational research. *Nursing Administration Quarterly, 34*(3), 217–225.

Bosch, M., van der Weijden, T., Wensing, M., & Grol, R. (2007). Tailoring quality improvement interventions to identified barriers: A multiple case analysis. *Journal of Evaluation in Clinical Practice, 13*(2), 161–168.

Carey, M., Buchan, H., & Sanson-Fisher, R. (2009). The cycle of change: Implementing best-evidence clinical practice. *International Journal for Quality in Health Care, 21*(1), 37–43.

Cohen, A. M., & Hersh, W. R. (2004). Guest editorial: Criticisms of evidence-based medicine. *Evidence-Based Cardiovascular Medicine, 8,* 197–198. doi:10.1016/j.ebcm.2004.06.036

Cummings, G. G., Estabrooks, C. A., Midodzi, W. K., & Hayduk, L. (2007). Influence of organizational characteristics and context on research utilization. *Nursing Research, 56*(4), S24–S39.

Denis, J. L., Hébert, Y., Langley, A., Lozeau, D., & Trottier, L. H. (2002). Explaining diffusion patterns for complex health care innovations. *Health Care Management Review, 27*(3), 60–73.

DiCenso, A., Cullum, N., Ciliska, D., & Guyatt, G. (2005). Introduction to evidence-based nursing. In A. DiCenso, G. Guyatt, & D. Ciliska (Eds.), *Evidence based nursing: A guide to clinical practice* (pp. 3–19). St. Louis, MO: Elsevier Mosby.

Dick, B. (2004). Action research literature: Themes and trends. *Action Research, 2*(4), 425–444. doi:10.1177/1476750304047985

Dopson, S., FitzGerald, L., Ferlie, E., Gabbay, J., & Locock, L. (2002). No magic targets! Changing clinical practice to become more evidence based. *Health Care Management Review, 27*(3), 35–47.

Estabrooks, C. A., Squires, J. E., Cummings, G. G., Birdsell, J. M., & Norton, P. G. (2009). Development and assessment of the Alberta Context Tool. *BMC Health Services Research, 9*(234). doi:10.1186/1472–6963–9–234

Estabrooks, C. A. (1999). The conceptual structure of research utilization. *Research in Nursing & Health, 22*(3), 203–216.

Estabrooks, C. A. (2007). Prologue: A program of research in knowledge translation. *Nursing Research, 56*(4), S4–S6.

Estabrooks, C., Thompson, D., Lovely, J., & Hofmeyer, A. (2006). A guide to knowledge translation theory. *Journal of Continuing Education in the Health Professions, 26*(1), 25–36.

Fineout-Overholt, E., Melnyk, B. M., & Schultz, A. (2005). Transforming health care from the inside out: Advancing evidence-based practice in the 21st century. *Journal of Professional Nursing, 21*(6), 335–344.

Fink, R., Thompson, C. J., & Bonnes, D. (2005). Overcoming barriers and promoting the use of research in practice. *Journal of Nursing Administration, 35*(3), 121–129.

Frasure, J. (2008). Analysis of instruments measuring nurses' attitudes towards research utilization: A systematic review. *Journal of Advanced Nursing, 61*(1), 5–18.

French, B., Thomas, L. H., Baker, P., Burton, C. R., Pennington, L., & Roddam, H. (2009). What can management theories offer evidence-based practice? A comparative analysis of measurement tools for organisational context. *Implementation Science, 4*(28). doi:10.1186/1748–5908–4-28

Funk, S. G., Champagne, M. T., Wiese, R. A., & Tornquist, E. M. (1991). Barriers to using research findings in practice: The clinician's perspective. *Applied Nursing Research, 4*(2), 90–95.

Funk, S. G., Tornquist, E. M., & Champagne, M. T. (1989). A model for improving the dissemination of nursing research. *Western Journal of Nursing Research, 11*(3), 361–367.

Gawlinski, A., & Rutledge, D. (2008). Selecting a model for evidence-based practice changes: A practical approach. *AACN Advance Critical Care, 19*(3), 291–300.

Gerrish, K., Ashworth, P., Lacey, A., Bailey, J., Cooke, J., Kendall, S., & McNeilly, E. (2007). Factors influencing the development of evidence-based practice: A research tool. *Journal of Advanced Nursing, 57*(3), 328–338.

Godin, G., Bélanger-Gravel, A., Eccles, M., & Grimshaw, J. (2008). Healthcare professionals' intentions and behaviours: A systematic review of studies based on social cognitive theories. *Implementation Science, 3*(36). doi:10.1186/1748–5908–3-36

Goleman, D. (1998). What makes a leader? *Harvard Business Review, 76*(6), 93–102.

Grant, B., Colello, S., Riehle, M., & Dende, D. (2010). An evaluation of the nursing practice environment and successful change management using the new generation Magnet Model. *Journal of Nursing Management, 18*(3), 326–331.

Greiner, A. C., & Knebel, E. (Eds.). (2003). *Health professions education: A bridge to quality.* Washington, DC: The National Academies Press.

Heifetz, R. A., & Linsky, M. (2002). *Leadership on the line: Staying alive through the dangers of leading.* Boston: Harvard Business Press.

Helfrich, C. D., Li, Y. F., Sharp, N. D., & Sales, A. E. (2009). Organizational readiness to change assessment (ORCA): Development of an instrument based on the Promoting Action on Research in Health Services (PARIHS) framework. *Implementation Science, 4*(38). doi:10.1186/1748–5908–4-38

Hyrkäs, K. (1997). Can action research be applied in developing clinical teaching?. *Journal of Advanced Nursing, 25*(4), 801–808.

Kajermo, K. N., Boström, A. M., Thompson, D. S., Hutchinson, A. M., Estabrooks, C. A., & Wallin, L. (2010). The BARRIERS scale—the barriers to research utilization scale: A systematic review. *Implementation Science, 5*(32). doi:10.1186/1748–5908–5-32

Kitson, A., Harvey, G., & McCormack, B. (1998). Enabling the implementation of evidence based practice: A conceptual framework. *Quality in Health Care, 7*(3), 149–158.

Kitson, A. (1999). Research utilization: Current issues, questions, and debates. *Canadian Journal of Nursing Research, 31*(1), 13–22.

Kouzes, J. M., & Posner, B. Z. (2000, June). *Leadership practices inventory: Psychometric properties.* Retrieved from http://media.wiley.com/assets/56/95/lc_jb_psychometric_properti.pdf

Kouzes, J. M., & Posner, B. Z. (2000–2011). *The leadership challenge website.* Retrieved from http://www.leadershipchallenge.com/WileyCDA/Section/id-131011.html

Kouzes, J. M., & Posner, B. Z. (2002). *The leadership practices inventory: Theory and evidence behind the five practices of exemplary leaders.* San Francisco: John Wiley & Sons Inc.

Kouzes, J. M., & Posner, B. Z. (2007). *The leadership challenge* (4th ed.). San Francisco: Jossey-Bass.

Kritsonis, A. (2004–2005). Comparison of change theories. *International Journal of Scholarly Academic Intellectual Diversity, 8*(1). Retrieved from http://www.nationalforum.com/ Electronic%20Journal%20Volumes/Kritsonis,%20Alicia%20Comparison%20of%20 Change%20Theories.pdf

Larkin, M. E., Griffith, C. A., Capasso, V. A., Cierpial, C., Gettings, E., Walsh, K., & O'Malley, C. (2007). Promoting research utilization using a conceptual framework. *Journal of Nursing Administration, 37*(11), 510–516.

MacDavitt, K., Cieplinski, J. & Walker, V. (2011) Implementing small tests of change to improve patient satisfaction. *Journal of Nursing Administration, 41*(1), 5–9.

McCormack, B., Kitson, A., Harvey, G., Rycroft-Malone, J., Titchen, A., & Seers, K. (2002). Getting evidence into practice: The meaning of 'context'. *Journal of Advanced Nursing, 38*(1), 94–104.

McCormack, B., McCarthy, G., Wright, J., Slater, P., & Coffey, A. (2009). Development and testing of the Context Assessment Index (CAI). *Worldviews on Evidence-Based Nursing, 6*(1), 27–35.

Meijers, J. M., Janssen, M. A., Cummings, G. G., Wallin, L., Estabrooks, C. A., & Halfens, R. Y. (2006). Assessing the relationships between contextual factors and research utilization in nursing: Systematic literature review. *Journal of Advanced Nursing, 55*(5), 622–635.

Melnyk, B. M., Fineout-Overholt, E., Feinstein, N. F., Li, H., Small, L., Wilcox, L., & Kraus, R. (2004). Nurses' perceived knowledge, beliefs, skills, and needs regarding evidence-based practice: Implications for accelerating the paradigm shift. *Worldviews on Evidence-Based Nursing, 1*(3), 185–193.

Melnyk, B. M., Fineout-Overholt, E., & Mays, M. Z. (2008). The evidence-based practice beliefs and implementation scales: Psychometric properties of two new instruments. *Worldviews on Evidence-Based Nursing, 5*(4), 208–216.

Melnyk, B. M., & Fineout-Overholt, E. (2002). Putting research into practice, Rochester ARCC. *Reflections on Nursing Leadership, 28*(2), 22–25.

Melnyk, B. M., & Fineout-Overholt, E. (2005). *Evidence-based practice in nursing and healthcare: A guide to best practice.* Philadelphia: Lippincott Williams & Wilkins.

Mohide, E. A., & Coker, E. (2005). Toward clinical scholarship: Promoting evidence-based practice in the clinical setting. *Journal of Professional Nursing, 21*(6), 372–379.

Munn-Giddings, C., McVicar, A., & Smith, L. (2008). Systematic review of the uptake and design of action research in published nursing research, 200–2005. *Journal of Research in Nursing, 13*(6), 465–477. doi:10.1177/1744987108090297

Munten, G., Van Den Bogaard, J., Cox, K., Garretsen, H., & Bongers, I. (2010). Implementation of evidence-based practice in nursing using action research: A review. *Worldviews on Evidence-Based Nursing, 7*(3), 135–157.

Newhouse, R. P., Dearholt, S., Poe, S., Pugh, L. C., & White, K. M. (2007). Organizational change strategies for evidence-based practice. *Journal of Nursing Administration, 37*(12), 552–557.

Newhouse, R. (2010). Instruments to assess organizational readiness for evidence-based practice. *Journal of Nursing Administration, 40*(10), 404–407.

Nieva, V. F., Murphy, R., Ridley, N., Donaldson, N., Combes, J., Mitchell, P., . . . Carpenter, D. (2005). From science to service: A framework for the transfer of patient safety research into practice. In K. Henriksen, J. Battles, E. Marks, & D. Lewin (Eds.), *Advances in patient safety: From research to implementation* (Vol. 2). Rockville, MD: Agency for Healthcare Research and Quality. Retrieved from www.ncbi.nlm.nih.gov/books/NBK20499

Noffke, S., & Somekh, B. (2005). Action research. In B. Somekh & C. Lewin (Eds.), *Research methods in the social sciences* (pp. 89–96). London, UK: Sage Publications Ltd.

Olsen, L., Aisner, D. & McGinnis, J. M. (Eds.). (2007) *Roundtable on evidence-based medicine: The learning environment*. Washington, DC: National Academies Press.

Pettengill, M. M., Gillies, D. A., & Clark, C. C. (1994). Factors encouraging and discouraging the use of nursing research findings. *Image. Journal of Nursing Scholarship, 26*(2), 143–147.

Ploeg, J., Davies, B., Edwards, N., Gifford, W., & Miller, P. E. (2007). Factors influencing best-practice guideline implementation: Lessons learned from administrators, nursing staff, and project leaders. *Worldviews on Evidence-Based Nursing, 4*(4), 210–219.

Rogers, E. M. (2003). *Diffusions of innovations* (5th ed.). New York: Free Press.

Rosswurm, M. A., & Larrabee, J. H. (1999). A model for change to evidence-based practice. *Image. Journal of Nursing Scholarship, 31*(4), 317–322.

Rycroft-Malone, J., Kitson, A., Harvey, G., Seers, K., Titchen, A., & Estabrooks, C. (2002). Ingredients for change: Revisiting a conceptual framework. *Quality and Safety in Health Care, 11*(2), 174–180.

Rycroft-Malone, J., Seers, K., Titchen, A., Harvey, G., Kitson, A., & McCormack, B. (2004). What counts as evidence in evidence-based practice? *Journal of Advanced Nursing, 47*(1), 81–90.

Rycroft-Malone, J. (2004). The PARIHS framework—a framework for guiding the implementation of evidence-based practice. *Journal of Nursing Care Quality, 19*(4), 297–304.

Salbach, N. M., & Jaglal, S. B. (2011). Creation and validation of the evidence-based practice confidence scale for health care professionals. *Journal of Evaluation in Clinical Practice, 17*(4), 794–800. doi:10.1111/j.1365–2753.2010.01478.x

Satterfield, J., Spring B., Brownson, R., Mullen, E., Newhouse, R., Wakler B. & Whitlock, E. (2009). Towards a transdisciplinary model of evidence-based practice. *The Milbank Quarterly, 87*(2), 368–390.

Schulman, C. S. (2008). Strategies for starting a successful evidence-based practice program. *AACN Advance Critical Care, 19*(3), 301–311.

Scott, S. D., Estabrooks, C. A., Allen, M., & Pollock, C. (2008). A context of uncertainty: How context shapes nurses' research utilization behaviors. *Qualitative Health Research, 18*(3), 347–357.

Scott-Findlay, S., & Golden-Biddle, K. (2005). Understanding how organizational culture shapes research use. *Journal of Nursing Administration, 35*(7–8), 359–356.

Sharp, C. (2005, September 30). *The improvement of public sector delivery: Supporting evidence based practice through action research*. Retrieved from http://www.scotland.gov.uk/Publications/2005/09/2890219/02201

Shaw, B., Cheater, F., Baker, R., Gilles, C., Hearnshaw, H., Flottorp, S., & Robertson, N. (2005). Tailored interventions to overcome identified barriers to change: Effects on professional practice and health care outcomes. *Cochrane Database of Systematic Reviews, 20*(3).

Shaw, T. (2005). Leadership in practice development. In M. Jasper & M. Jumaa (Eds.), *Effective healthcare leadership* (1st ed., pp. 207–221). Oxford, UK: Blackwell Publishing Ltd.

Smith, J. R., & Donze, A. (2010). Assessing enviromental readiness: First steps in developing an evidence-based practice implementation culture. *Journal of Perinatal and Neonatal Nursing, 24*(1), 61–71.

Squires, J. E., Estabrooks, C. A., Gustavsson, P., & Wallin, L. (2011). Individual determinants of research utilization by nurses: A systematic review update. *Implementation Science, 6*(1). doi:10.1186/1748–5908-6–1

Squires, J. E., Hutchinson, A. M., Boström, A. M., O'Rourke, H. M., Cobban, S. J., & Estabrooks, C. A. (2011). To what extent do nurses use research in clinical practice? A systematic review. *Implementation Science, 6*(21). doi:10.1186/1748–5908–6-21

Stetler, C. B., & Marram, G. (1976). Evaluating research findings for applicability in practice. *Nursing Outlook, 24*(9), 559–563.

Stichler, J. F. (2011). Leading change: One of leader's most important roles. *Nursing for Women's Health, 15*(2), 166–170.

Straus, S. E., Graham, I. D., & Mazmanian, P. E. (2006). Knowledge translation: Resolving the confusion. *The Journal of Continuing Education in the Health Professions, 26*(1), 3–4.

The Joint Commission (2003). *Putting evidence to work: Tools and resources.* Washington, DC: The Joint Commission Resources.

Thompson, D. S., Estabrooks, C. A., Scott-Findlay, S., Moore, K., & Wallin, L. (2007). Interventions aimed at increasing research use in nursing: A systematic review. *Implementation Science, 2*(15). doi:10.1186/1748–5908-2-15

Titler, M. G. (2002). Use of research in practice. In G. LoBiondo-Wood & J. Haber (Eds.), *Nursing research: Methods, critical appraisal and utilization* (5th ed.). St. Louis, MO: Mosby.

Titler, M. G. (2010). Translation science and context. *Research & Theory for Nursing Practice, 24*(1), 35–55.

Titler, M. (2007). Translating research into practice. *American Journal of Nursing, 107*(6), 26–33.

Tucker, S. J., Olson, M. E., & Frusti, D. K. (2009). Evidence-based practice self-efficacy scale: Preliminary reliability and validity. *Clinical Nurse Specialist: The Journal for Advanced Nursing Practice, 23*(4), 207–215.

Waterman, H., Tillen, D., Dickson, R., & De Koning, K. (2001). Action research: A systematic review and guidance for assessment. *Health Technology Assessment, 5*(23), iii–157.

Weiner, B. J., Amick, H., & Lee, S. D. (2008). Review: Conceptualization and measurement of organizational readiness for change. *Medical Care Research and Review, 65*(4), 379–436. doi:10.1177/1077558708317802

Weiner, B. J. (2009). A theory of organizational readiness for change. *Implementation Science, 4*(67), 1–9. doi:10.1186/1748–5908-4-67

Yukl, G. A. (2001). *Leadership in organizations* (5th ed.). Upper Saddle River, NJ: Prentice Hall.

CHAPTER 13

# Health Information Technology and the Transformation of Health Care in the 21st Century

Lena Sorensen

We must teach for the future. This means teaching to *find* rather than to know; *question* rather than answer; *achieve* rather than accomplish; *inspire* rather than inform.
—Patricia Flatley Brennan[1]

With today's major advancement in information and communication technology (ICT) in health care, there is both a critical need for change in the way that health care is delivered and for an opportunity to look to the future to ensure that these developments result in improvements in quality, access, and efficiencies of all health care systems. With this call for a transformation of the current health care system, there is also a need to develop new practice models that better integrate the patient into all aspects of their health and disease management (IOM, 1999, 2001). Initially, software tools were developed to support institutional functions (i.e., management and financial) and data collection for providers. Now, new technologies are being designed to interface across the spectrum of the health care system, with all participants focusing on the development of both software and hardware innovations (i.e., wireless, hand-held, mobile devices, smart phones, tablets, Web-based interactive sites, etc.) to enhance full communication and information exchange among all users. Where once the electronic health record (EHR) was the only tool central to hospital care, now there is a call to extend that record and all health information and communication beyond these boundaries to the patient (through Patient Portals and personal health records [PHR]) and community (Brennan, Norcross, Grindrod, & Sopher, 2004; Curran & Curran, 2005; Dickerson & Sensmeier, 2010; Dorr et al., 2007). The 21st century is a "whole new world"; new technologies have become ubiquitous in all areas of society and they are becoming essential tools to ensuring quality and safety in the delivery and management of health care (Buntin, Burke, Hoaglin, & Blumenthal, 2011). Along with these enhancements come significant challenges:

---

[1] Cited in The TIGER Initiative 2007 *Evidence and Informatics Transforming Nursing: 3-Year Action Steps Toward a 10-Year Vision*, p. 3.

ensure all clinical information systems are secure and confidential, interoperable with diverse systems, and designed with the user in mind. Many refer to today's health care as "ehealth" (Bates & Wright, 2009; Eysenbach, 2001; Oh, Rizo, Enkin, & Jadad, 2005), emphasizing the integral role of electronic technologies in all aspects of health care.

## ■ WHAT IS BIOMEDICAL INFORMATICS?

Informatics is a term that first appeared in the 1970s, *informatique*, as referring to the computer milieu. As computers become more integrated into health care, the study of informatics became more developed. The American Medical Informatics Association defines biomedical informatics (BMI) as "the interdisciplinary field that studies and pursues the effective uses of biomedical data, information, and knowledge for scientific inquiry, problem solving, and decision making, motivated by efforts to improve human health" (AMIA, 2011 at www.amia. org/about-amia/science-informatics). BMI is an umbrella term that includes the research and application of all aspects of informatics in a diverse group of disciplines (medical, nursing, pharmacology, medical imaging, dental, and consumer informatics) (Figure 13.1). BMI integrates computer, communication, cognitive, and information sciences with clinical knowledge.

## ■ WHAT IS NURSING INFORMATICS?

The definition of nursing informatics has gone through many changes since Graves and Corcoran (1989) first defined it as "Computer science, information science, and nursing science combined to assist in the management and processing of nursing data, information and knowledge to support the practice of nursing and the delivery of nursing care" (pg. 227). In this original definition, the emphasis was on technology. As the definition evolved, it changed to include the central focus on the concepts of data, information, and knowledge incorporating the critical roles and elements of nursing practice (Staggers & Thompson, 2002). The newest definition expands the definition to recognize the role of "wisdom," a fundamental form of knowledge that goes into designing new processes that improve the quality of health care (ANA, 2008). Thus, the 2008 ANA definition of nursing informatics has become increasingly complex:

> a specialty that integrates nursing science, computer science and information science to manage and communicate data, information, knowledge and wisdom in nursing practice. Nursing informatics facilitates the integration of data, information and knowledge to support patients, nurses and other providers in their decision-making in all roles and settings. This support is accomplished through the use of information technology and information structures, which organize data, information and knowledge for processing by computers.

Nursing informatics is recognized in all aspects of nursing across the globe. The International Medical Informatics Association-Nursing Informatics Group (IMIA-NI) states "Nursing informatics science and practice integrates nursing, its information and knowledge and their management with information and communication technologies to promote the health of people, families, and communities world wide."

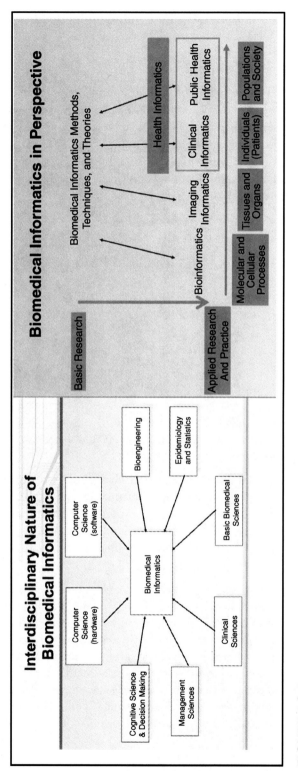

**FIGURE 13.1**  Interdisciplinary biomedical informatics.

*Source:* www.amia.org/about-amia/science-informatics

### ■ WHAT IS EHEALTH? SHIFTING HEALTH CARE LANDSCAPE: GLOBAL AND NATIONAL PERSPECTIVES

The word *ehealth* can be described as follows:

> an emerging field in the intersection of medical informatics, public health and business, referring to health services and information delivered or enhanced through the Internet and related technologies. In a broader sense, the term characterizes not only a technical development, but also a state-of-mind, a way of thinking, an attitude, and a commitment for networked, global thinking, to improve health care locally, regionally, and worldwide by using information and communication technology. (Eysenbach, 2001)

Eysenbach (2001) identifies the 10 "e's" of ehealth:

1. *Efficiency*
2. *Enhancing quality of care*
3. *Evidence based*
4. *Empowerment of consumers and patients*
5. *Encouragement of a new relationship between the patient and health professional*
6. *Education*
7. *Enabling*
8. *Extending*
9. *Ethics*
10. *Equity*

In addition to these 10 essential e's, Eysenbach insists that ehealth should also be easy to use, entertaining, and exciting to ensure successful engagement of all users. Moreover, current definitions focus on access to eliminate health disparities:

> Many observers believe that the use of emerging interactive health information technologies...can help to improve the quality, capacity, and efficiency of the health care system. eHealth has the potential to improve access to the health care system for traditionally underserved populations and to increase the capacity to provide tailoring and customization for individual patients and consumers. (Ahern et al., 2006, cited in Hernandez, 2009)

Increasing use of innovative interactive health information systems does not in and of itself guarantee equity of access to health care for all people. Providers must understand the design and use of these interactive systems and the informational needs and search strategies of diverse populations to produce systems that are tailored to their communities of care. Competent leaders in health care practice who are both informatics literate and confident in their use of emerging interactive information technologies are better able to assess the needs of their patient populations, design systems that meet these needs, and identify resources to enable patients in the knowledge and use of these systems (Booth, 2006; Constantelou & Karounou, 2005; Maag, 2006; Skiba, 2007, 2008a, 2008b, 2009a; Turesco & Rhoads, 2008; Weiner, 2008).

As health care is changing, there is also an evolving shift away from a *provider-controlled system* to a *consumer driven system* that insists on patient-centered care, collaboration among all stakeholders, and care tailored to the needs of diverse communities. In 1999, the first IOM report entitled *To Err Is Human* appeared. This text reported on the thousands of deaths and injuries due to preventable medical errors in today's health care system, recognizing not only that decreasing these errors would require system-wide changes, but also that ICTs need to be a critical component to these solutions. Two subsequent IOM reports, *Crossing the Quality Chasm: The IOM Health Care Quality Initiative* (2001) and *Health Professions Education: A Bridge to Quality* (2003a) each recommended changes to ensure adequate preparation of health care providers to meet the demands of an increasingly diverse U.S. population. These recommendations can be summarized as follows: (1) redesign the way health professionals are trained to emphasize safety and quality improvement; (2) increase the teaching of evidence-based, patient-centered practice and provision of opportunities for interdisciplinary training; and (3) maximize the utilization of information technologies to better manage information and knowledge systems. These recommendations are not only recognized in the United States but also identified as essential for a 21st century global society (Hammond, Bailey, Boucher, Spohr, & Whitaker, 2010; Haux, 2006; Dentzer, 2010; WHO, 2011; ICN, 2011).

The recent 10-year agenda for improving national health, *Healthy People 2020*, set benchmarks for improvement to the current health care system, focused on improved communication strategies and health information technology to ensure access to health information (full description of objectives are accessible at: http://www.healthypeople.gov/2020/topicsobjectives2020/overview.aspx?topicid=18). It is well documented that access to quality health care and health information is a critical component for improving quality of life for all people. Only through meeting all of these charges will the United States and global health care systems be able to improve patient safety and quality care.

Currently, very few U.S. hospitals use even a basic EHR (also called electronic medical record [EMR] or electronic patient record, terms that are often used interchangeably) in a single unit, and the majority of U.S. physicians do not use any EHR in their own practices (HIMSS, 2011). The IOM (2003b) recommended that the EHR should include: (1) longitudinal collection of electronic health information for and about persons, where health information is defined as information pertaining to the health of an individual or health care provided to an individual; (2) immediate electronic access to person- and population-level information by only authorized users; (3) provision of knowledge and decision-support that enhance the quality, safety, and efficiency of patient care; and (4) support of efficient processes for health care delivery. Critical building blocks of a health information system are the EHRs maintained by providers (e.g., hospitals, nursing homes, and ambulatory settings) and by patients themselves (also called PHR). The Healthcare Information and Management Systems Society (HIMSS) has developed an EMR (EHR) adoption model to evaluate the status of implementation of EMR/EHRs and provides a scoring system for hospitals on an 8-step scale of EHR development (Figure 13.2).

Informed and coordinated national leadership is another essential component of necessary change. In 2004, President Bush created the National Health Information Technology Coordinator at the Department of Health and Human Services. In 2009, President Obama strengthened this goal for the national implementation of an effective EHR through the legislative order, *Health Information Technology for Economic and Clinical Health Act*, which provided incentives through the Centers for Medicare and Medicaid Services to ensure that EHRs are used in a meaningful way (Blumenthal & Tavenner, 2010). The *American Recovery and Reinvestment Act* of 2009 specifies three main components of what it calls *"Meaningful Use."*

1. The use of a certified EHR in a meaningful manner, such as eprescribing.
2. The use of certified EHR technology for electronic exchange of health information to improve quality of health care.
3. The use of certified EHR technology to submit clinical quality and other measures.

| US EMR Adoption Model<sup>SM</sup> | | | |
|---|---|---|---|
| Stage | Cumulative Capabilities | 2011 Q1 | 2011 Q2 |
| Stage 7 | Complete EMR; CCD transactions to share data; data warehousing; data continuity with ED, ambulatory, OP | 1.0% | 1.1% |
| Stage 6 | Physician documentation (structured templates), full CDSS (variance & compliance), full R-PACS | 3.5% | 4.0% |
| Stage 5 | Closed-loop medication administration | 5.9% | 6.1% |
| Stage 4 | CPOE, clinical decision support (clinical protocols) | 10.7% | 12.3% |
| Stage 3 | Nursing/clinical documentation (flow sheets), CDSS (error checking), PACS available outside radiology | 48.4% | 46.3% |
| Stage 2 | CDR, controlled medical vocabulary, CDS, may have document Imaging; HIE capable | 14.1% | 13.7% |
| Stage 1 | Ancillaries - lab, rad, pharmacy - all installed | 6.7% | 6.6% |
| Stage 0 | All three ancillaries not installed | 9.6% | 10.0% |

Data from HIMSS Analytics™ Database © 2011          N = 5,275  N = 5,310

**FIGURE 13.2**   HIMSS US EMR adoption model 2011.

*Source:* www.himssanalytics.org/home/index.aspx

Over a 5-year period, *"Meaningful Use"* will be implemented in three stages: Stage 1 (2011 and 2012) sets the baseline for building an infrastructure that promotes the use of electronic data capture and information sharing (Health Information Exchange), Stage 2 (expected to be implemented in 2013) expands these functions into advanced clinical practices that extends these functionalities to the patient, and Stage 3 (expected to be implemented in 2015) further extends the goal of *"Meaningful Use"* that demonstrates improved health outcomes (see http://healthit.hhs.gov/portal/server.pt/community/healthit_hhs_gov__incentive_programs_for_electronic_health_records_%28ehrs%29/3355). The goal of *"Meaningful Use"* is to ultimately stimulate the rapid adoption of effective EHR by hospitals and providers. These incentives have important implications for nurses (Barton, 2011; Jacobsen & Juste, 2010; Murphy, 2009; Westra et al., 2010). Nurses are central to these principles for improving the quality of health care for all "by promoting care coordination, improving continuity of care, reducing medical errors, improving population health, reducing health disparities, and reducing chronic disease (HIMSS, 2010, at http://www.himss.org/ASP/topics_FocusDynamic.asp?faid=395).

## ■ NURSING INFORMATICS COMPETENCIES FOR THE 21ST CENTURY

In this information age, nurses, as knowledge workers (Conrad & Sherrod, 2011), need new knowledge and skills to be able to use 21st century technologies (Barton, 2005; Garde, Harrison, & Hovenga, 2005; Gassert, 2008). Because much of health care depends on these ICTs to communicate and capture the delivery of health care, patients also must acquire specific competencies to be able to actively engage in their own health care. In order to ensure an ongoing improvement of health care delivery, it is essential that everyone has the knowledge and skills to use technological innovations (Gentles, Lokker, & McKibbon, 2010; Gordon, 2011; Volandes & Paasche-Orlow, 2007).

Recognizing this need, AHIMA and AMIA (2008) have produced a set of core foundational health information management and informatics competencies for any individual working with EHRs. The AHIMA/AMIA informatics domains include: basic computer literacy skills, health information literacy and skills, health informatics skills using EHRs and PHRs, privacy and confidentiality of health information skills, and health information and data technical security skills. It thus becomes critical that leaders in health care must have enhanced informatics competencies to be able to provide the vision and development of ongoing innovations in health care delivery (Skiba, 2008b; Zeng & Bell, 2008).

Nurses must be central to this movement to ensure the implementation of an EHR in all health care settings, and the goals of new technology directives are congruent with nursing aims for quality health care (Barton, 2011; Jacobsen & Juste, 2010; Murphy, 2009; Sensmeier, 2010a, 2010b). Nurses have always put the patient at the center of their practice and have identified effective communication across the continuum of care as essential to ensuring quality health care. But, the one area in which nursing has not yet fulfilled this promise is ensuring that all nurses have the knowledge and skills to use these new technologies within their practices. The nursing informatics community has taken this on as a critical agenda through their development of *Technology Initiative Guiding Educational Reform (TIGER)* in 2005, seeking to "identify information/knowledge management best practices and effective technology capabilities for nurses... to create and disseminate action plans that can be duplicated within nursing and other multidisciplinary health care training and workplace settings" (TIGER, 2009).

As the largest group of health providers (55% of all providers), nurses must be prepared to meet these challenges of the 21st century society and the ehealth revolution, which are transforming society through the diffusion of innovative information and communication technologies (Booth, 2006; Gassert, 2008; Greenhalgh, Robert, MacFarlane, Bate, & Kyriakidou, 2004; Hersh, 2006; TIGER, 2009). TIGER has identified four categories of competencies for all nurses:

1. Computer Competencies
2. Information Literacy Competencies
3. Information Management/Informatics Competencies
4. Attitudes and Awareness

In developing basic computer competencies that nurses need, they have recommended adopting the International Computer Driving License (ICDL), which is also called the *European Computer Driving License*, whose learning modules mirror basic computer competencies as gathered by the TIGER team.

- Module 1—Concepts of information technology
- Module 2—Using the computer and managing files
- Module 3—Word processing
- Module 4—Spreadsheets
- Module 5—Database
- Module 6—Presentation
- Module 7—Information and communication

The TIGER collaborative also found that many health care providers lack the ability to use informatics, a core competency in the 21st century.

- Majority of more than 2.8 million licensed nurses lack skills to use online evidence to support evidence-based practice
- Nurse executive leaders lack information technology competency and knowledge to lead EHR programs at their work
- Nursing education has not included informatics competencies that have been identified as needed in the curriculum
- Numbers of PhD-prepared nurse informaticists are inadequate to prepare for the additional 6,000 nurse informaticists needed by 2010
- Nursing faculty shortage is compounded by nurses' lack of information technology skills needed to teach required informatics competencies. (Gassert, 2008)

The National League for Nursing's *Nurse Educators 2006: A Report of the Faculty Census Survey of RN and Graduate Programs* reported these trends:

- Significant nursing faculty shortages
- Increasing use of part-time faculty
- An aging faculty
- Few incentives to recruit new, younger nursing faculty

It has been well documented that health information literacy plays a critical factor in the health outcomes and access to quality care of patients. Health literacy as defined by the Institute of Medicine and Healthy People 2010 states:

The degree to which individuals have the capacity to obtain, process, and understand basic health information and services needed to make appropriate health decisions. (HHS, 2000; Institute of Medicine, 2004)

As providers, we must be knowledgeable about how the design and availability of health information for our communities reflects the unique needs of those patient populations. Understanding the core building blocks of health care informatics, information, technology, and application of these resources provides clinicians the foundation to effectively infuse this knowledge to their practice. Designing clinical information systems that improve the efficiency and quality of the captured data and how this data is represented is not simply done by reproducing the ways that data is captured in current work processes. Nurses need to be able to critically analyze clinical processes to assess where in the workflow process improvements can be made in the way things are done by using technology to support bottlenecks. One method is to do a workflow analysis detailing every aspect of the process and then modeling it in a "process map" (California HealthCare Foundation, 2011; Tavakoli, 2008). Workflow analysis of a clinical process begins with an understanding of clinical practice.

A workflow refers to the interaction of processes (made up of tasks) through which a practice (clinic or hospital) provides health care to patients—for instance giving a medication, doing an intake or registering the patient. Process mapping, or flowcharting, involves diagramming all of the tasks required to carry out a process, and identifying the points at which one process intersects with another. Process analysis, or workflow analysis, helps to identify the inefficiencies and bottlenecks revealed by the process mapping. (California HealthCare Foundation, 2011)

Knowing how to do a mapping of a workflow analysis that allows us to identify inefficiencies within our practices and for the recipients of these processes will help nurses to be informed, active participants in the planning and design of these evolving health ICTs.

## ■ EHEALTH COMPETENCIES FOR THE CONSUMER/PATIENT

Just as health care has evolved into ehealth, patients are evolving into epatients (Internet users who have searched for health information) as they increasingly turn to the Internet as a source for health information (Goldberg et al., 2011). In a recent study of people living with a chronic disease or a disability, the Pew Internet and American Life Project (Fox, 2007) found:

- 51% used the Internet to find health information
- 75% of epatients with chronic conditions say the information they found in their last search *affected a decision about how to treat an illness or condition*
- 69% of epatients with chronic conditions say the information *led them to ask a doctor new questions or to get a second opinion from another doctor*
- 57% of epatients with chronic conditions say the information *changed the way they cope with a chronic condition or manage pain*
- 56% of e-patients with chronic conditions say the information *changed the way they think about diet, exercise, or stress management.* (Fox, 2007, p. ii)

This raises an additional challenge for nurses today. Just as nurses must increase their own ehealth literacy competencies, they must also be alert to these competencies for their patients. But additional challenges are faced by the nurses in this role when one considers the diverse characteristics of the patient populations being served, especially linguistic and literacy levels.

For the first time, the U.S. Department of Education's 2003 National Assessment of Adult Literacy contained a health literacy component. This survey found that 36% of the adult U.S. population—approximately 87 million people—has only basic or below-basic health literacy levels and that the cost of low health literacy to the U.S. economy is in the range of $106 billion to $236 billion annually (Kutner, Greenberg, Jin, & Paulsen, 2006).

As health educators and providers, we must tackle this problem from multiple perspectives. Effective use of tailored information and communication technologies to populations with low health literacy is an effective method for combating this problem (Gentles, Lokker, & McKibbon, 2010; USDHH, 2011).

One model widely respected, *Lily Model of eHealth Literacy* and assessment scale, (Norman & Skinner, 2006a, 2006b) identified six essential literacies, organized into two central types: *analytic* (traditional, media, and information) and *context-specific* (computer, scientific, and health). The *Lily model* is an effective tool in assessing and developing methods to ensure that all patients will be prepared to be active users of these ICTs that are now central to health care today and in the future (Figure 13.3).

ICTs are now being designed that enable patients to not only monitor their own health data through diverse telehealth systems, but also enable them to enter their health experiences and data (referred to as "observations of daily living") so that it interfaces with the EHR, ultimately enhancing a seamless communication and information exchange across the health delivery continuum. Over the past decade, Patient Portals

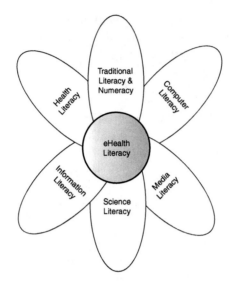

**FIGURE 13.3** Lily model of ehealth literacy.

*Source:* http://www.jmir.org/2006/2/e9

have become standard tools for many hospitals and practices that provide a secure Web platform that provides patients access to all or parts of their EHR and a way to communicate privately with their providers (Lin, Wittevrongel, Moore, Beaty, & Ross, 2005; Rodriguez, 2010; Sorensen, Shaw, & Casey, 2009). More recently, there is a call for a more consumer-driven system referred to as an electronic PHR, which is defined as "a private, secure application through which an individual may access, manage, and share his or her health information. The PHR can include information that is entered by the consumer and/or data from other sources such as pharmacies, labs, and health care providers" (Jones, Shipman, Plaut, & Selden, 2010, p. 244). In recent years, Robert Wood Johnson Foundation's *Project HealthDesign* has been supporting the design of ICTs that enhance a more comprehensive engagement of patients in this continuum of care. *Project HealthDesign* is "... working to demonstrate how to improve participants' health and well-being by helping them capture, understand, interpret and act on observations of daily living data" (see http://www.projecthealthdesign.org/projects/current_projects).

Another innovative example of the use of an emerging technology that allows the patient to control their observations of daily living is *PatientsLikeMe* (Frost & Massagli, 2008; Wicks et al., 2010), an online community-based information sharing system that exploits the functionalities of Web 2.0. *PatientsLikeMe* "is committed to putting patients first... by providing a better, more effective way for [patients] to share [their] real-world health experiences in order to help [them]self, other patients like [them] and organizations that focus on [their] conditions" (see http://www.patientslikeme.com). These are only two of a growing number of patient-centered or initiated strategies that are being developed today.

## ■ PREPARING THE NEW PROVIDERS

ICTs are ubiquitous in today's health care system. Nurses must be familiar and comfortable with a wide range of technologies, planning, designing, evaluating, and integrating these tools into all aspects of their practice. The nurse's role now also includes the responsibility to help patients and their families become competent technology users as well. Smith (2004) identified several categories of technologies that are needed for such a clinical transformation:

- Information systems—including financial, clinical, and hospital information systems
- Biomedical monitoring systems—including noninvasive blood pressure and home monitoring devices
- Connectivity or communications—through dial-in or satellite connections, Local Area Networks, and Wide Area Networks
- Patient safety—networked alarm systems, computerized provider order entry, smart IV pumps, barcode medication administration systems, and eprescribing
- Business and clinical decision support systems
- Education and reference—through patient bedside Internet access, networked patient education systems, and unit-based Internet access for nursing personnel

Yet, a systematic literature review of the state of informatics competency levels in the U.S. nursing workforce found evidence of inadequate competency in all nursing roles to meet these emerging job-related needs (Hart, 2008). Thus there remains an urgent need.

In Robert Wood Johnson Foundation's *Charting Nursing's Future* (2005 & 2009) report examining the impact of the nursing faculty shortage, four elements were identified that determine the demand for faculty to meet health care workforce needs: (1) critical increase in nursing workforce demand, (2) current inadequate supply of nurses and nursing faculty to meet these demands, (3) increasing standards and lengthy process of educational preparation of nursing faculty, and (4) increasing student/faculty ratios and stressful workloads, which contribute to low productivity of nursing faculty. Solutions to these barriers include increased time for faculty preparation, enhanced resources that relieve workload stressors, and enhanced image of faculty role.

In 2008, the National League for Nursing (NLN) published *Preparing the Next Generation of Nurses to Practice in a Technology-Rich Environment: An Informatics Agenda*, outlining essential content and competencies needed by 21st century practitioners because of their concern that only 50% to 60% of those surveyed had informatics content integrated into their school's curriculum. This report recommends that all nursing faculty

- Participate in faculty development programs to achieve competency in informatics
- Designate an informatics champion in every school of nursing to: (1) help faculty distinguish between using instructional technologies to teach versus using informatics to guide, document, analyze, and inform nursing practice; and (2) translate state-of-the-art practices in technology and informatics that need to be integrated into the curriculum
- Incorporate informatics into the curriculum
- Incorporate ANA-recognized standard nursing language and terminology into content. (NLN, 2008)

The American Association of Colleges of Nursing (AACN, 2006) has also connected the crisis in the nursing workforce shortage with nursing faculty shortages. AACN used the Price Waterhouse Coopers 2007 report, *What Works: Healing Healthcare Staffing Shortages*, which recommends two solutions: (1) developing public–private partnerships, and (2) using technology as a training tool.

## ■ CONCLUSION: LOOKING INTO THE FUTURE AND EMERGING TECHNOLOGIES

As health care increasingly shifts its focus toward patient-centered care, nurses are now seeing telehealth applications and a broad expansion of user-centered interactive tools (often through Web 2.0 platforms) intended to give patients a more meaningful role. Research is beginning to show that many of these innovations improve the quality of health for many users (Ahern et al., 2011; Detmer, Bloomrosen, Raymond, & Tang, 2008; Goldberg et al., 2011; Or & Karsh, 2009). As we look at these emerging trends in health information technologies, we also see increasing use of social networking tools (i.e., Facebook, Flickr, blogs, Wiki, Twitter) (Ciesielka, 2008; Wink, 2010) and virtual environments (like Second Life) (Ahern & Wink, 2010; Beard, Wilson, Morra, & Keelan, 2009; Skiba, 2009b; Wiecha, Heyden, Sternthal, & Merialdi, 2010) engage increasingly diverse and technology-literate patient populations in today's society (Kamel Boulos & Wheeler, 2007; Skiba, 2007, 2008a, 2008b). These are positive outcomes of the ehealth revolution.

As the largest group of health providers, nurses play a central role in the transformation to an innovative ehealth care system. Thus, as the United States faces a critical nursing shortage, compounded by a nursing faculty shortage, nursing leaders and educators must be prepared to ensure that all nurses are expert enough to meet 21st century demands. By ensuring both their knowledge of current and emerging technologies for ehealth and their ability to use these tools competently, nursing leaders and educators will pave the way for the use of these health care informatics into all aspects of our teaching and practice (Curran, 2008; Skiba, Connors, & Jeffries, 2008).

## ■ REFERENCES

Ahern, N., & Wink, D. M. (2010). Virtual learning environments: Second life. *Nurse Educator,* *35*(6), 225–227.

Ahern, D. K., Woods, S. S., Lightowler, M. C., Finley, S. W., & Houston, T. K. (2011). Promise of and potential for patient-facing technologies to enable meaningful use. *American Journal of Preventive Medicine, 40*(5 Suppl. 2), S162–172.

AHIMA & AMIA (2008). *Joint Work Force Task Force: Health information management and informatics core competencies for individuals working with electronic health records.* Retrieved from http://library.ahima.org/xpedio/groups/public/documents/ahima/bok1_040723.pdf

American Association of Colleges of Nursing. (AACN) (2006). *Essentials of doctoral education for advanced nursing practice.* Washington, DC: National Center for Health Education.

American Nurses Association. (2008). *Nursing informatics practice scope and standards of practice.* Washington, DC: Author.

Barton, A. J. (2005). Cultivating informatics competencies in a community of practice. *Nursing Administration Quarterly, 29*(4), 323–328.

Barton, A. J. (2011). The electronic health record and "meaningful use": Implications for the clinical nurse specialist. *Clinical Nurse Specialist, 25*(1), 8–10.

Bates, D. W. & Wright, A. (2009). Evaluating eHealth: Undertaking robust international cross-cultural eHealth research. *PLoS Med, 6*(9), e1000105.

Beard, L., Wilson, K., Morra, D., & Keelan, J. (2009). A survey of health-related activities on second life. *Journal of Medical Internet Research, 11*(2), e17.

Blumenthal, D., & Tavenner. M. (2010). The "meaningful use" regulation for electronic health records. *NEJM, 363*(6), 501–504.

Booth R.G. (2006). Educating the future eHealth professional nurse. *International Journal of Nursing Education Scholarship, 3*(1), Article 13.

Brennan, P. F., Norcross, N., Grindrod, D., & Sopher, M. (2004). "Community-wide Information Systems Design: Concepts and an Illustration," *Medinfo 2004, 11,* 192–196.

Buntin, M. B., Burke, M. F., Hoaglin, M. C., & Blumenthal, D. (2011). The benefits of health information technology: A review of the recent literature shows predominantly positive results. *Health Affairs, 30*(3), 464–471.

California HealthCare Foundation. (2011). *Workflow analysis for EHR deployment.* Retrieved from http://www.chcf.org/publications/2010/03/ehr-deployment-techniques

Ciesielka, D. (2008). Using a Wiki to meet graduate nursing education competencies in collaboration and community health. *Journal of Nursing Education, 47*(10), 473–476.

Conrad, S., & Sherrod, D. (2011). Nurse managers as knowledge workers. *Nursing Management, 42*(2), 47–48.

Constantelou, A., & Karounou, V. (2005). *Skills and competencies for the future of eHealth.* IPTS (Institute of Prospective Technological Studies) Report. Retrieved from www.ehealthstrategies.com/files/skills_ehealth.mht

Curran, C. R. (2008). Faculty development initiatives for the integration of informatics competencies and point-of-care technologies in undergraduate nursing education. *Nursing Clinics of North America, 43*(4), 523–533.

Curran, M. A., & Curran, K. E. (2005). The e-health revolution: Competitive options for nurse practitioners as local providers. *Journal of the American Academy of Nurse Practitioners, 17*(12), 495–498.

Dentzer, S. (2010). e-health's promise for the developing world. *Health Affairs, 29*(2), 229.

Detmer, D., Bloomrosen, M., Raymond, B., & Tang, P. (2008). Integrated personal health records: Transformative tools for consumer-centric care. *BMC Medical Informatics & Decision Making, 8,* 45.

Dickerson, A. E., & Sensmeier, J. (2010). Sharing data to ensure continuity of care. *Nursing Management, 41*(7), 19–22.

Dorr, D., Bonner, L. M., Cohen, A. N., Shoai, R. S., Perrin, R., Chaney, E., et al. (2007). Informatics systems to promote improved care for chronic illness: A literature review. *Journal of the American Medical Informatics Association, 14*(2), 156–163.

Eysenbach, G. (2001). What is eHealth? *Journal of Medical Internet Research, 3*(2), e20. Retrieved from http://www.jmir.org/2001/2/e20/

Fox, S. (2007). *E-patients with a disability or chronic disease.* Pew Internet and American Life Project. Retrieved from http://www.pewinternet.org/Reports/2007/Epatients-With-a-Disability-or-Chronic-Disease.aspx

Frost, J. H., & Massagli, M. P. (2008). Social uses of personal health information within PatientsLikeMe, an online patient community: What can happen when patients have access to one another's data. *Journal of Medical Internet Research, 10*(3), e15.

Garde, S., Harrison, D., & Hovenga, E. (2005). Skill needs for nurses in their role as health informatics professionals: A survey in the context of global health informatics education. *International Journal of Medical Informatics, 74*(11–12), 899–907.

Gassert, C. A. (2008). Technology and informatics competencies. *Nursing Clinics of North America, 43*(4), 507–21.

Gentles, S. J., Lokker, C., & McKibbon, K. A. (2010). Health information technology to facilitate communication involving health care providers, caregivers, and pediatric patients: A scoping review. *Journal of Medical Internet Research, 12*(2), e22.

Goldberg, L., Lide, B., Lowry, S., Massett, H. A., O'Connell, T., Preece, J., et al. (2011). Usability and accessibility in consumer health informatics current trends and future challenges. *American Journal of Preventive Medicine, 40*(5 Suppl. 2), S187–S197.

Gordon, J. (2011). Educating the patient: Challenges and opportunities with current technology. *Nursing Clinics of North America, 46*(3), 341–350.

Graves, J. R., & Corcoran, S. (1989). The study of nursing informatics. *Image, 21*(4), 227–231.

Greenhalgh, T., Robert, G., MacFarlane, F., Bate, P., & Kyriakidou, O. (2004). Diffusion of innovations in service organizations: Systematic review and recommendations. *The Millbank Quarterly, 82*(4), 581–629.

Hammond, W. E., Bailey, C., Boucher, P., Spohr, M., & Whitaker, P. (2010). Connecting information to improve health. *Health Affairs, 29*(2), 285–290.

Hart, M. D. (2008). Informatics competency and development within the US nursing population workforce: A systematic literature review. *CIN: Computers, Informatics, Nursing, 26*(6), 320–329; quiz 330–331.

Haux, R. (2006). Individualization, globalization and health—about sustainable information technologies and the aim of medical informatics. *International Journal of Medical Informatics, 75*(12), 795–808.

Hernandez, L. M. (2009). *Health literacy, eHealth, and communication: Putting the consumer first.* Washington, DC: The National Academies Press.

Hersh, W. (2006). Who are the informaticians? What we know and should know. *Journal of the American Medical Informatics Association, 13*(2), 166–170.

HIMSS. (2011). *2011 Nursing informatics workforce survey.* Retrieved from http://www.himss.org/ASP/topics_FocusDynamic.asp?faid=243

Institute of Medicine. (1999). *To err is human: Building a safer health system.* Washington, DC: National Academy of Sciences.

Institute of Medicine (IOM). (2001). *Crossing the quality chasm: The IOM health care quality initiative.* Washington, DC: National Academy of Sciences.

Institute of Medicine. (2003a). *Health professions education: A bridge to quality.* Washington, DC: National Academy of Sciences.

Institute of Medicine. (2003b). *Key capabilities of an electronic health record system letter report.* Committee on Data Standards for Patient Safety. Board on Health Care Services. Washington, DC: The National Academies Press.

International Council for Nurses (ICN). (2011). *eHealth.* Retrieved from http://www.icn.ch/pillarsprograms/ehealth/

Jacobsen, T., & Juste, F. (2010). Nursing in the era of "meaningful use". *Nursing Management, 41*(1), 11–13.

Jones, D. A., Shipman, J. P., Plaut, D. A., & Selden, C. R. (2010). Characteristics of personal health records: Findings of the Medical Library Association/National Library of Medicine Joint Electronic Personal Health Record Task Force. *Journal of the Medical Library Association, 98*(3), 243–249.

Kamel Boulos, M. N., & Wheeler, S. (2007). The emerging Web 2.0 social software: An enabling suite of sociable technologies in health and health care education. *Health Information and Libraries Journal, 24,* 2–23.

Kutner, M., Greenberg, E., Jin, Y., & Paulsen, C. (2006). *The health literacy of America's adults: Results from the 2003 National Assessment of Adult Literacy (NAAL).* U.S. Department of Education, Institute of Education Sciences. Retrieved from http://nces.ed.gov/pubsearch/pubsinfo.asp?pubid=2006483

Lin, C. T., Wittevrongel, L., Moore, L., Beaty, B. L., & Ross, S. E. (2005). An Internet-based patient-provider communication system: Randomized controlled trial. *Journal of Medical Internet Research, 7*(4), e47.

Maag, M. M. (2006). Nursing students' attitudes toward technology: A national study. *Nurse Educator, 31*(3), 112–118.

Murphy, J. (2009). Meaningful use for nursing: Six themes regarding the definition of meaningful use. *JHIM, 23*(4), 9–11.

National League for Nursing (NLN). (2006). *Nurse educators 2006: A report of the faculty census survey of RN and graduate programs.* Retrieved from http://www.nln.org/newsreleases/nurseeducators2006.htm

Norman, C. N., & Skinner, H. A. (2006a). eHealth literacy: Essential skills for consumer health in a networked world. *Journal of Medical Internet Research, 8*(2), e27. Retrieved from http://www.jmir.org/2006/2/e9

Norman, C. N., & Skinner, H. A. (2006b). eHEALS: The eHealth literacy scale. *Journal of Medical Internet Research, 8*(4), e27. Retrieved from http://www.jmir.org/2006/4/e27/

Oh, H., Rizo, C., Enkin, M., & Jadad, A. (2005). What is eHealth (3): A systematic review of published definitions. *Journal of Medical Internet Research, 7*(1), e1.

Or, C. K., & Karsh, B. T. (2009). A systematic review of patient acceptance of consumer health information technology. *Journal of the American Medical Informatics Association, 16*(4), 550–560.

Robert Wood Johnson Foundation (RWJF). (2004). The eHealth landscape.

RWJF. (2005). *Charting nursing's future.* Robert Wood Johnson Foundation. Retrieved from http://www.rwjf.org/pr/product.jsp?id=38074

RWJF. (2009). *Charting nursing's future, Part 2: How nurses are shaping, and being shaped by health information technologies.* Retrieved from www.hetinitiative.org/media/pdf/eHealth.pdf

Rodriguez, E. (2010). Using a patient portal for electronic communication with patients with cancer: Implications for nurses. *Oncology Nursing Forum, 37*(6), 667–671.

Sensmeier, J. (2010a). Alliance for nursing informatics statement to the Robert Wood Johnson Foundation Initiative on the future of nursing: Acute care, focusing on the area of technology, October 19, 2009. *CIN: Computers, Informatics, Nursing, 28*(1), 63–67.

Sensmeier, J. (2010b). Meaningful use: Making IT matter. *Nursing Management, 41*(9), 2–6.

Skiba, D. (2007). *The fourth wave: Collaboration, interactivity, & social networking.* ANIA Conference, Las Vegas, NV, April 2007.

Skiba, D. (2008a). Nursing education 2.0: Twitter and tweets: Can you post a nugget of knowledge in 140 characters or less. *Nursing Education Perspectives, 29*(2), 110–112.

Skiba, D. (2008b). Nursing education 2.0: Social networking for professions. *Nursing Education Perspectives, 29*(6), 370–371.

Skiba, D. (2009a). Nursing education 2.0: Should we as educators be crafting the next generation of nursing practice? *Nursing Education Perspectives, 30*(1), 48–49.

Skiba, D. (2009b). A second look at second life. *Nursing Education Perspectives, 30*(2), 12, 129–131.

Skiba, D., Connors, H. R., & Jeffries, P. R. (2008). Information technologies and the transformation of nursing education. *Nursing Outlook, 56*(5), 225–230.

Smith, C. (2004). New technology continues to invade healthcare: What are the strategic implications/outcomes? *Nursing Administration Quarterly, 28*(2), 92–98.

Sorensen, L., Shaw, R., & Casey, E. (2009). Patient portals: Survey of nursing informaticists. *Studies in Health Technology and Informatics, 146*, 160–165.

Staggers, N., & Thompson, C. B. (2002). The evolution of definitions for nursing informatics: A critical analysis and revised definition. *Journal of the American Medical Informatics Association, 9*(3), 255–261.

Tavakoli, F. (2008). Using work flow analysis and technology assessment to improve performance on quality measures. *The Joint Commission Journal on Quality and Patient Safety, 34*(5), 297–303.

Technology Initiative Guiding Educational Reform (TIGER). (2009). *Collaborating to integrate evidence and informatics into nursing practice and education: An executive summary.* Retrieved from www.tigersummit.com/uploads/TIGER_Collaborative_Exec_Summary_040509.pdf

Turesco, F., & Rhoads, J. (2008). *Equipped for efficiency: Improving nursing care through technology.* California Health Foundation. Retrieved from http://www.chcf.org/publications/2008/12/equipped-for-efficiency-improving-nursing-care-through-technology

US Department of Health and Human Services. (2011). *Healthy people 2020: National health promotion and disease prevention objectives.* Washington, DC: Author.

Volandes, A. E., & Paasche-Orlow, M. K. (2007). Health literacy, health inequality and a just healthcare system. *American Journal of Bioethics, 7*(11), 5–10.

Weiner, E. E. (2008). Technology: The interface to nursing educational informatics. *Nursing Clinics of North America, 43*(4), ix–x.

Westra, B. L., Subramanian, A., Hart, C. M., Matney, S. A., Wilson, P. S., Huff, S. M., . . . Delaney, C. W. (2010). Achieving "Meaningful Use" of Electronic Health Records through the integration of the Nursing Management Minimum Data Set. *JONA, 40*(7/8), 336–343.

World Health Organization (WHO). (2011). *Essential health technologies: eHealth for health care delivery.* Retrieved from http://www.who.int/eht/eHealthHCD/en/index.html

Wicks, P., Massagli, M., Frost, J., Brownstein, C., Okun, S., Vaughan, T., . . . Heywood, J. (2010). Sharing health data for better outcomes on PatientsLikeMe. *Journal of Medical Internet Research (JMIR), 12*(2), e19. Available online at: http://www.jmir.org/2010/2/e19

Wiecha, J., Heyden, R., Sternthal, E., & Merialdi, M. (2010). Learning in a virtual world: Experience with using second life for medical education. *Journal of Medical Internet Research, Jan-Mar; 12*(1), e1.

Wink, D. (2010). Social networking sites. *Nurse Educator, 35*(2), 49–51.

Zeng, X., & Bell, P. (2008). Web 2.0: What a health care manager needs to know. *Health Care Manager, 27*(1), 58–70.

# CHAPTER 14

# *Outcomes Measurement*

Lisa Colombo

Measurement of outcomes is a broad topic that has different meaning based on the context in which it is considered. Why something is being measured and what measures will inform the processes of care are important considerations in outcomes measurement. Measurement is done for various reasons in health care. The driving force for measurement in doctor of nursing practice (DNP) practice is for the improvement of quality of care. This chapter will review the purpose of outcomes measurement as it relates to DNP practice and discuss the use of measurement in improvement of quality of care for patients, safety for health care organizations, and to meet requirements from payors and regulators. The interrelationship between each of these perspectives will also be discussed.

## ■ OUTCOMES

Broadly, the term "outcomes" refers to the results of treatment or interventions or a change in health status as a result of care that is provided. They measure health care quality and efficacy (Kleinpell & Gawlinski 2005; Oermann & Floyd, 2002). As the emphasis on patient safety and quality has increased exponentially over the last several years, measurement of outcomes, or results, is essential to demonstrate effectiveness of care. The first step in managing outcomes for patients is measuring them. The measurement of outcomes provides useful information in the design and delivery of care and the continuous improvement in care processes (Hamric, Spross, & Hanson, 2009).

## ■ PURPOSE OF MEASUREMENT

The fundamental question to ask when reviewing outcomes measures is, "Why are we measuring?" The answer to this question will guide the journey to quality improvement. In general, measurement in health care is done for three specific purposes: research, improvement, and judgment. In research, measurement of outcomes is used to develop new knowledge. In practice, measurement of outcomes is used to drive improvement in processes, which will lead to improved patient outcomes (Solberg, Mosser, & McDonald,

1997). We also use outcomes measures to make judgments about evidence that results both from research and from improvement initiatives. For example, individuals (patients) *judge* the quality of their lives based on their perception of their health. In this example, health perception is an outcome of interest to an individual. In health care, measurements are often used for reporting aggregate results to regulators, legislators, and other parties that *judge* the data against specific standards or rules (Institute of Healthcare Improvement, 2011).

The Essentials of DNP Practice (American Association of Colleges of Nursing, 2006) describes the competencies required for DNP-prepared nurses. All of the essentials require skill at the doctoral level in outcomes measurement and the interpretation and use of outcomes measures to demonstrate competency. Essential II, *Organizational and Systems Leadership for Quality Improvement and Systems Thinking*, makes the case that outcomes measurement in practice is paramount to the improvement of quality of patient care and health outcomes.

In short, the overarching purpose for measurement in practice is to understand if improvements in practice lead to improvement in outcomes. Choosing the appropriate measures by which to judge process improvement is also important to the success of the effort.

## ■ DIFFERENCES BETWEEN MEASUREMENT FOR RESEARCH AND MEASUREMENT FOR IMPROVEMENT

Measurement for research is done to develop new knowledge and identify knowledge that will support improvement in quality of care. Measurement in practice is then used to bring that new knowledge into practice. Both are necessary to improve care; however, the methods of data collection and approaches to measurement vary according to the paradigm. See www.ihi.org/knowledge/Pages/HowtoImprove/ScienceofImprovement EstablishingMeasures.aspx for the comparison.

In research, there is a focus on rigor in research methods to control for biases and to ensure generalizability. In measurement for improvement, the goal is to perform rapid cycle tests of change, identify metrics to judge the effects of change, and incorporate learning from those interpretations into each consecutive improvement cycle to achieve the outcomes suggested by the research. In practice, measurement for improvement is the primary purpose for outcomes measurement.

## ■ TYPES OF MEASUREMENTS

It is important to understand that there are three types of measures, one of which is outcomes measures (Institute for Healthcare Improvement, 2011). These indicators give signals as to how a system is performing and what results are being achieved. Outcomes measures represent the voice of the customer (Lloyd, 2004). An example of an outcomes measure is the incidence of ventilator-associated pneumonia (VAP) in a population of critical care patients. VAP is the outcome of interest to the patient/customer/population.

Process measures represent the voice of the system (Institute for Healthcare Improvement, 2011). Evidence-based processes of care are processes which, when performed correctly, lead to improved patient outcomes (Chassin, Loeb, Schmaltz, & Wachter, 2010). Process measures help us to evaluate whether or not the system is performing as planned (Institute for

Healthcare Improvement, 2011). Using ventilator-associated pneumonia as the example again, measurement of the compliance with evidence-based VAP bundle (i.e., elevation of the head of the bed, daily "sedation vacations," peptic ulcer prophylaxis, deep vein thrombosis prophylaxis, and daily oral care with chlorhexidine) would constitute process measures which would identify if the established system was working properly.

In practice, it is important to measure both process and outcomes measures to evaluate the effectiveness of the processes intended to improve care. Measuring one without the other, such as measuring process without respect for outcomes, can lead to conclusions that may not support the improvement of quality of care.

The third type of measure is the balancing measure. This measure looks at a system from a different perspective and is intended to identify if changes made to improve outcomes have resulted in new problems in other parts of the system (Institute for Healthcare Improvement, 2011). For example, evaluation of processes that are put in place to reduce the length of stay for a population of patients should include the balancing measure of readmissions for that same population of patients. It would be important to know if reducing length of stay results in an increase in readmissions.

## ■ IMPORTANCE OF MEASUREMENT

The fundamental question is, "Why measure?" The answer is simple. Successful measurement is the cornerstone to successful improvement and, in practice, this is where the rubber meets the road. It helps us to determine if changes made lead to improvement.

Improvement in quality of care is not just a goal; it is a requirement in today's health care environment. In 1998, The Joint Commission (TJC) introduced the ORYX initiative, which was the first national program for hospital quality measurement (Chassin et al., 2010). This initiative required hospitals to collect and transmit data to TJC for a minimum of four core measure sets (TJC, 2011). Examples of core measure sets are acute myocardial infarction, heart failure, pneumonia, and the surgical care improvement project. The intent was to promote quality improvement efforts in TJC-accredited hospitals. The core measures, essentially, are evidence-based process of care measures, which, when executed correctly, lead to better patient outcomes. In 2004, the Centers for Medicare and Medicaid Services (CMS) aligned their efforts to collect quality data and began financially penalizing hospitals that did not report to CMS the same data that they collected and reported to TJC (Chassin et al., 2010).

Health care economics have also dictated that care should not only be effective but also be *cost effective*. Third party insurers are now linking quality metrics to payment. Beginning in October of 2012, Medicare will implement a system of value-based purchasing for hospitals. For the first time, hospitals will not only be paid based on the quantity but also the quality of services provided (Centers for Medicare & Medicaid Services, 2011).

The delivery and continuous improvement of high-quality, high-value health care requires attention to meaningful outcomes. Organizations that are high performers in the delivery of quality services are consistently asking whether or not specific processes of care add genuine value and if changes to those services represent improvement (Nelson, Batalden, Godfrey, & Lazar, 2011). Measurement both answers those questions and provides meaningful information to inform the improvement process.

## ■ RELATIONSHIP BETWEEN PROCESSES AND OUTCOMES

More than 30 years ago, a physician named Avedis Donabedian proposed a model for assessing health care quality based on structures, processes, and outcomes. He suggested that there was a relationship between structure, process, and outcome, and that each is influenced by the other. In effect, structure influences process and process influences outcome (Donebedian, 2005). See www.longwoods.com/articles/images/HQ82FEI-JardaliMLagaceF1.jpg for Donabedian's framework.

Important to note is that judgments on the appropriateness of processes to achieve desired outcomes are based on the premise that the processes are supported by a sound evidence base (Donabedian, 1988). Following Donabedian's model, compliance with processes known to improve quality will lead to desired outcomes. Therefore, measurement of processes or compliance with processes is a proxy for outcomes. Process measures can be used to assess the ability of a process to impact an outcome, and therefore should be used in conjunction with outcomes measures. The "goodness" of a process is only as good as the outcome that the process produces. Measurement of outcomes is essential to guide improvement. The goal is not measurement; the goal is improvement.

## ■ THE HEALTH CARE MEASUREMENT CONTINUUM

Measurement in health care can be broadly defined as a continuum that ranges from the subjective perceptions of the patient ("I feel good") to the highly objective data that is used to submit insurance claims. Along the continuum are various stakeholders: individuals/patients, providers, payors and regulators, accrediting bodies, and policy makers. Each stakeholder has a different perspective on what constitutes an outcome of interest to him or her. Perspectives and methods of measurement change as the stakeholder changes. Consider heart failure, diabetes mellitus, and nurse staffing as conditions that have outcomes associated with them. Table 14.1 demonstrates how perspectives change as stakeholders change.

As you move vertically down the table, you can see that the outcomes of interest change as the stakeholder changes. It is important to note that with the move toward value-based purchasing, alignment of outcomes of interest is beginning to occur. Take the example of nurse staffing. Both providers and payors are aligned in their concern for the outcomes of nurse-sensitive indicators such as skin breakdown and falls with injury. For providers, hospital-acquired skin breakdown and falls with serious injury can result in nonpayment for services rendered for either of those conditions. Care must still be rendered, but there is no offset for the cost of care in terms of additional reimbursement to treat the undesirable outcome. For payors, these outcomes may signal issues with quality of care, which can drive the level of reimbursement that they will pay for certain services.

Understanding that improvement versus measurement is the goal, selecting indicators for measurement is dependent on knowing the goal of the improvement process. Given that outcomes of interest are different to different stakeholders, consideration must be given to who the stakeholder is in order to measure what matters to each stakeholder.

## ■ SELECTION OF INDICATORS

If the goal of measuring outcomes is to manage practice that achieves desired results, then outcomes management is accomplished through quality improvement efforts. Central to any

**TABLE 14.1   Progression of Perspectives of Interest by Stakeholder**

|  | CHF | DM | Nurse Staffing |
|---|---|---|---|
| Individuals | Quality of life related to activities of daily living | Perceived disease burden in patients with Type 2 diabetes | Nurse burnout |
| Providers | Treatment adherence related to medications, diet, and daily weight | Perceptions of treatment compliance in patients with Type 2 diabetes | Quality of care and nurse sensitive indicator performance (i.e., falls with injury and health care–acquired skin breakdown) |
| Payors | Cost of care, morbidity and mortality and hospital readmission rate in the congestive heart failure patient population | Preventive care in diabetics: avoidance of hospital admissions | Nurse sensitive indicators, nurse driven serious reportable events (i.e., falls with injury, health care–acquired skin breakdown) |
| Regulators/ accreditors | Core measure performance | Change in oral agent compliance related to Medicare prescription drug coverage | The Joint Commission staffing effectiveness and standards compliance |

quality improvement process is the selection of the correct or appropriate indicators that inform the process under study.

There are many different types of indicators. There are financial indicators, quality indicators, safety indicators, and patient experience indicators, to name a few. Focusing on only one or two types of indicators may give an incomplete picture of the overall success of a given process (Lloyd, 2004). A balanced approach to indicator selection and measurement is required to truly reflect the success of care processes. Donabedian first proposed that indicator selection should be balanced and indicators of structures, processes, and outcomes should be selected and monitored together in order to give a complete picture of the health of a process (Lloyd, 2004). Since then, other organizations have suggested multiple dimensions from which to select indicators for measurement.

In 2001, the Institute of Medicine's report, *Crossing the Quality Chasm*, identified six aims for improvement, which could be used to categorize indicators. The six aims are safety, effectiveness, patient-centeredness, time lines, efficiency, and equity (Institute Of Medicine, 2001; Lloyd, 2004).

In November of 2010, TJC proposed an approach to indicator measurement that focuses clearly on maximizing health benefits to patients (Chassin et al., 2010). This initiative refines the approach initially used in the ORYX initiative by identifying four criteria that each measure must meet, the purpose of which is to separate the measures that advance the goal of maximizing health from those that do not. The four criteria are

*(1) Research:* Strong scientific evidence base showing that the care process leads to improved outcomes.

*(2) Proximity:* The measure accurately captures whether the evidence-based care process, has, in fact been provided.

(3) *Accuracy:* The measure addresses a process that has few intervening care processes that must occur before the improved outcome is realized.

(4) *Adverse Effects:* Implementing the measure has little or no chance of inducing unintended adverse consequences. (TJC, 2011)

Core measures meeting these criteria are now considered accountability measures, and those not meeting these criteria are considered nonaccountability measures. Nonaccountability measures are care processes that are considered "good advice" for patient care but not necessarily contributing directly to the outcome of interest (TJC, 2011). All but six of TJC's core measures are accountability measures. This move by TJC to separate core measures according to these criteria supports the notion that process indicators should be measured in conjunction with outcomes indicators.

Regardless of the types of indicators that are identified to measure, the important idea is to use a balanced approach to indicator selection. Once you have identified the types of indicators appropriate to measure for a given process or outcome, it is then necessary to select specific indicators that reflect the specific aspect of the process. For example, if you are working on fall prevention, specific indicators for the processes of care associated with falls will include number of patient falls, fall rate (in falls per 1000 patient days), or percent of patients that fall. These are outcome measures; a balanced approach would also include process indicators such as nursing interventions intended to prevent falls (e.g., frequent toileting, call bell within reach, communication to care team members about fall risk). Using Donabedian's model, you could also collect indicators of structure, such as number of nursing and ancillary staff on at the time of the fall. Collecting measures that reflect structure, process, and outcomes simultaneously provides the balanced approach that is necessary to truly inform improvement processes in health care.

## ■ DATA USE

Once you have determined the appropriate indicators to collect to inform care processes, the data needs to be available and understandable to health care professionals working to improve the delivery of care. Central to this concept is understanding variation in data.

In order to understand variation, one must first understand the concept of variation and also understand how some simple statistical methods and tools can assist in the understanding of variation (Lloyd, 2004). Webster's New Collegiate Dictionary (2010) defines variation as "(a) the act, fact, or process of varying; change or deviation in form, condition, appearance, extent, etc. from a former or usual state, or from an assumed standard; (b) the degree or extent of such change." While the definition or variation seems clear, the interpretation of it may not. A major factor in the accurate interpretation of variation is the manner in which data is displayed.

In health care, data is often displayed in aggregate form. Examples of aggregated data include tools like pie charts, bar charts, and tables with summary statistics, to name a few. Clinical dashboards often contain monthly average scores for selected quality indicators. Data displayed in aggregated form can lead only to judgment, and sometimes to inaccurate judgment. It is not useful in determining if improvement processes are achieving goals. Aggregated data doesn't display variation in data and will not help in determining if variation is due to random or natural faults in a system (common cause variation) or due to special circumstances that enter a system for a short period of time and have an effect that cannot be explained by random variation (Lloyd, 2004; Nelson et al., 2007).

Figure 14.1 is a bar graph of average length of stay in an emergency department for FY11 Quarter 2. This figure illustrates summary data that is displayed in a bar graph. One possible judgment from this graph is that the length of stay in April was better than that in either May or June. This approach does not provide information about the processes related to length of stay in the ED over time. Table 14.2 provides the raw data that was aggregated to produce the bar graph in Figure 14.1.

If we change the way that the data is displayed, we can see something very differently (see Figures 14.2–14.4).

When you plot the data over time and by month, what conclusions do you now make? If you were using the summary data in Figure 14.1, you may be led to believe that in April, emergency department length of stay (ED LOS) was better than in either May or June. When you look at the line charts by month, you can see a very different story. In fact, the median ED LOS was lowest for the month of June. You cannot tell that from the summary data presented in Figure 14.1. For the three graphs that show data in a time series, you can see that there are days when the LOS is very high and those where it is either at or below the goal of 180 minutes. Further analysis would reveal that the days when the LOS is high are weekend days. This data is now useful for performance improvement. It provides clues as to where there are opportunities for improvement in existing processes. When you overlay the results for all 3 months in the quarter, you can see how each month's performance compares to the goal of 180 minutes.

In Figure 14.5, you can easily see that the months of May and June had most of its data points below the goal line. The month of April had none of its data points below the goal line. This information tells you that for most of the days in May and June, the LOS was at or below the goal of 180 minutes. When looking at the days when LOS was higher than desired, you can drill down to the potential causes in the process. It will allow an improvement team to look at all the variables in the process and to implement countermeasures to improve the performance on the days that are not meeting the goal.

Figures 14.2–14.4 are examples of a simple statistical tool that is important to use in understanding if the changes we make to processes or systems over time lead to improvement: a run chart. A run chart is a plot of data over time with the unit of time plotted on the horizontal x-axis. The data is arranged in chronological order, and the centerline of the chart is the median. Objective analysis of run charts is important to avoid overreacting to single data points. There are three basic rules to use in interpreting run charts: shifts, trends, and runs. A shift is six or more consecutive points either above or below the median (Perla, Provost, & Murray, 2011). Points that fall on the median do not count in the shift. A trend is five or

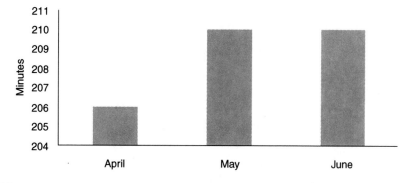

**FIGURE 14.1** Bar graph of ED LOS for 3 months.

**TABLE 14.2 Example of Raw Data for ED LOS by Days for 3 Months**

| Day | ED LOS (Goal: 180) | | |
| --- | --- | --- | --- |
| | Apr-11 | May-11 | Jun-11 |
| 1 | 206 | 300 | 150 |
| 2 | 206 | 160 | 160 |
| 3 | 206 | 235 | 340 |
| 4 | 206 | 165 | 340 |
| 5 | 206 | 160 | 160 |
| 6 | 206 | 165 | 165 |
| 7 | 206 | 308 | 150 |
| 8 | 206 | 300 | 150 |
| 9 | 206 | 180 | 160 |
| 10 | 206 | 180 | 340 |
| 11 | 206 | 180 | 340 |
| 12 | 206 | 160 | 165 |
| 13 | 206 | 160 | 160 |
| 14 | 206 | 310 | 165 |
| 15 | 206 | 340 | 160 |
| 16 | 206 | 160 | 170 |
| 17 | 206 | 165 | 340 |
| 18 | 206 | 165 | 340 |
| 19 | 206 | 160 | 160 |
| 20 | 206 | 160 | 165 |
| 21 | 206 | 308 | 180 |
| 22 | 206 | 300 | 180 |
| 23 | 206 | 170 | 160 |
| 24 | 206 | 189 | 340 |
| 25 | 206 | 180 | 340 |
| 26 | 206 | 165 | 165 |
| 27 | 206 | 170 | 150 |
| 28 | 206 | 300 | 165 |
| 29 | 206 | 310 | 160 |
| 30 | 206 | 160 | 180 |
| 31 | – | 160 | – |
| AVG | 206 | 210.48 | 210.00 |

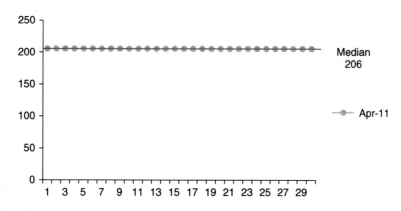

**FIGURE 14.2** Run chart of ED LOS, April 2011.

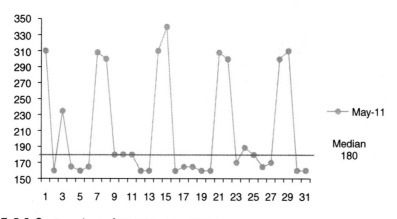

**FIGURE 14.3** Run chart of ED LOS, May 2011.

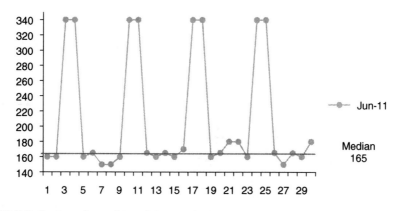

**FIGURE 14.4** Run chart of ED LOS, June 2011.

more consecutive points all going up or down (Perla et al., 2011). If two or more consecutive values are the same, count only one and ignore the repeating values when determining a shift. Like values do not make or break a trend. A run is a series of points in a row on one side of the median. Too many or too few runs signals special cause variation (Lloyd, 2004). In order to determine if the number of runs is appropriate, count the number of times that the line connecting the data points crosses the median and add one. You must also determine the number of useful observations. Useful observations are data points that do not fall exactly on the median. Data points on the median line are subtracted from the total number of observations to determine the useful observations. Tabled critical values can then be used to determine if the number of runs is appropriate. If the number of runs falls between the minimum and maximum, you do not have special cause variation. Table 14.3 provides upper and lower limits for number of runs based on useful observations. If there are too few or too many runs, variation in the data is due to a special cause. When the number of runs falls below the upper and lower limits, variation is from common cause or random variation in processes (Lloyd, 2004).

There are other useful tools and techniques to guide the use of data. The control chart offers another method to display data over time. The major difference between a run chart and a control chart is that the centerline is the mean (vs. median) and there are both upper and lower control limits in the control chart. The control limits define the boundaries of variation around the mean (Lloyd, 2004). Points between the boundaries represent normal variation around a mean and points outside the limits signals a special cause (Lloyd, 2004). The method to construct a control chart is beyond the scope of this chapter. Further information can be obtained in classical statistics textbooks.

## ■ MEASUREMENT FOR IMPROVEMENT: WHERE THE RUBBER MEETS THE ROAD

We learned earlier in this chapter that the driving force for measurement in practice is to inform improvement processes. It is important to understand if changes we make to processes result in actual improvements. The Institute for Healthcare Improvement (IHI) provides a framework for this.

The IHI's Model for Improvement (See www.ihi.org/knowledge/Pages/HowtoImprove/default.aspx) outlines a structure for testing change ideas that are expected to result in improvements. The model starts with three questions that help to focus the improvement project: "What are we trying to accomplish?" or "What is the aim of the work?"; "How will we know that a change is an improvement?" or "What are the Measures for the project"; and

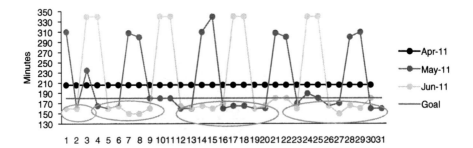

**FIGURE 14.5** Line graph of ED LOS for FY11 Quarter 2.

**TABLE 14.3  Test for Too Many or Too Few Runs on a Run Chart**

| Total Number of Data Points That Do Not Fall on the Median | Lower Limit for the Number of Runs | Upper Limit for the Number of Runs |
|:---:|:---:|:---:|
| 10 | 3 | 9 |
| 11 | 3 | 10 |
| 12 | 3 | 11 |
| 13 | 4 | 11 |
| 14 | 4 | 12 |
| 15 | 5 | 12 |
| 16 | 5 | 13 |
| 17 | 5 | 13 |
| 18 | 6 | 14 |
| 19 | 6 | 15 |
| 20 | 6 | 16 |
| 21 | 7 | 16 |
| 22 | 7 | 17 |
| 23 | 7 | 17 |
| 24 | 8 | 18 |
| 25 | 8 | 18 |
| 26 | 9 | 19 |
| 27 | 10 | 19 |
| 28 | 10 | 20 |
| 29 | 10 | 20 |
| 30 | 11 | 21 |
| 31 | 11 | 22 |
| 32 | 11 | 23 |
| 33 | 12 | 23 |
| 34 | 12 | 24 |
| 35 | 12 | 24 |
| 36 | 13 | 25 |
| 37 | 13 | 25 |
| 38 | 14 | 26 |
| 39 | 14 | 26 |
| 40 | 15 | 27 |

*Source:* Adapted from Perla et al. (2011).

"What changes can we make that will result in an improvement?" or "What are the changes that will be implemented and tested?" The second part of the model provides the structure for executing small tests of change using the plan–do–study–act or PDSA method, pioneered by Walter Shewhart and promoted by W. E. Deming (Nelson et al., 2011). The planning phase is where the objective and specific changes to be tested are outlined. It details all of the steps necessary to carry out the test, including roles, functions, education needed, how data will be collected, and how long the test will last. In the "do" phase, execution of the test is carried out, and the "study" phase is used to analyze the data collected during the "do" phase. When conclusions from the data are drawn, the act phase occurs and modifications to the plan are made if expected results are not achieved. If desired results were achieved, plan for dissemination can then be made.

It is extremely important to select a balanced set of measures to inform improvement processes. A scorecard that incorporates process, outcome, and balancing measures will provide a comprehensive set of data to inform the effectiveness of the improvement effort (IHI, 2011).

Regardless of the framework used for improvement, measurement and analysis of data in a systematic way should be what drives improvement. It is important for DNP-prepared nurses to be competent in the techniques and tools used to evaluate the performance of processes and to then translate that knowledge to inform improvements in care.

■ SUMMARY

This chapter discusses various concepts in outcomes measurement. It is important to understand the purpose of measurement in order to select appropriate measures. Measurement for research differs from measurement for judgment or improvement. We use measurement in research as the platform for evidence-based practice. In practice, measurement is used primarily to drive improvement. Translating research into practice requires the use of basic performance improvement frameworks and concepts. Identifying best practices through research and comparing the outcomes of research to those in practice will help to identify areas in need of improvement. Use of an improvement framework, such as the IHI's Model for Improvement, provides structure for improvement work. Selecting balanced metrics to reflect the effectiveness of the improvement effort raises the probability of success. Knowledge of some basic statistical tools and analysis are important competencies for the DNP-prepared nurse to have in order to lead improvement efforts in practice.

It is important to remember that the goal is not measurement; rather, the goal is improvement. Measurement provides information to inform processes of care that will result in better outcomes for patients in both quality and safety arenas.

■ REFERENCES

American Association of Colleges of Nursing. (2006). *The essentials of doctoral education for advanced practice nursing*. Retrieved from http://www.aacn.nche.edu/publications/position/dnpessentials.pdf

Centers For Medicare & Medicaid Services. (2011, June 27). *Hospital value-based purchasing*. Retrieved June 27, 2011, from http://www.cms.gov/Hospital-Value-Based-Purchasing

Chassin, M. R., Loeb, J. M., Schmaltz, S. P., & Wachter, R. M. (2010). Accountability measures: Using measurement to promote quality improvement. *The New England Journal of Medicine, 363*(7), 683–688.

Donabedian, A. (1988). The quality of care: How can it be assessed? *The Journal of the American Medical Association, 260*(12), 1743–1748.

Donabedian, A. (2005). Evaluating the quality of medical care. *The Milbank Quarterly, 83*(4), 691–729.

Hamric, A. B., Spross, J. A., & Hanson, C. M. (Eds.). (2009). *Advanced practice nursing: An integrative approach* (4th ed.). St. Louis, MO: Saunders Elsevier.

Institute of Healthcare Improvement (2011). *Science of improvement: Establishing measures.* Retrieved May 27, 2011, from http://www.ihi.org/knowledge/Pages/HowtoImprove/ScienceofImprovementEstablishingMeasures.aspx

Institute Of Medicine (2001). *Crossing the quality chasm: A new health system for the 21st century.* Washington, DC: The National Academies Press.

John Wiley & Sons (Eds.). (2010). *Webster's new collegiate dictionary.* Cleveland, OH: Wiley Publishing.

Kleinpell, R., & Gawlinski, A. (2005). Assessing outcomes in advanced practice nursing practice: The use of quality indicators and evidence-based practice. *AACN Clinical Issues, 16*(1), 43–57.

Lloyd, R. (2004). *Quality health care: A guide to developing and using indicators.* Sudbury, MA: Jones & Bartlett Learning.

Longwoods Publishing Corporation (n.d.). *Donabedian's framework of structures and outcomes.* Retrieved July 1, 2011, from http://www.longwoods.com/articles/images/HQ82FEl-JardaliMLagaceF1.jpg

Nelson, E. C., Batalden, P. B., Godfrey, M. M., & Lazar, J. S. (Eds.). (2011). *Value by design: Developing clinical microsystems to achieve organizational excellence* (1st ed.). San Francisco: Jossey-Bass.

Oermann, M. H., & Floyd, J. A. (2002). Outcomes research: An essential component of the advanced practice nurse role. *Clinical Nurse Specialist, 16*(3), 140–144.

Perla, R. J., Provost, L. P., & Murray, S. K. (2011). The run chart: A simple analytical tool for learning from variation in healthcare processes. *BMJ Quality & Safety, 20*, 46–51.

Solberg, L. I., Mosser, G., & McDonald, S. (1997). The three faces of performance measurement: Improvement, accountability, and research. *Joint Commission Journal on Quality Improvement, 23*(3), 135–147.

The Joint Commission (2011, January 27). *Facts about ORYX for hospitals (National hospital quality measures).* Retrieved January 25, 2011, from http://www.jointcommission.org/facts_about_oryx_for_hospitals

# PART V

## Policy, Politics, and the DNP

*America's present need is not heroics but healing; not nostrums but normalcy;*
*not revolution but restoration.*

—Warren G. Harding

Given the newness of the doctor of nursing practice (DNP) degree, questions abound relative to the need to transform specialty education to the doctoral level, the rigor of DNP programs, and the value of practice scholarship. As new DNP graduates migrate into the work setting, employers, both clinical and academe, are seeking to understand how the degree will impact existing roles for nurses engaged in advanced practice within their organizations. DNPs have similar questions—are DNP faculty provided tenure, what is the role of the DNP in research, or perhaps what is the impact of doctoral education upon licensure, certification, and titling? In this context, the establishment of a community for DNPs becomes a critical tool for the development and advancement of DNP education, practice, and policy.

In September, 2009, in Miami, Florida, a group of new DNPs and interested parties gathered for the second national DNP conference and engaged in a discussion around such issues. This process allowed the DNP-prepared nurse to be engaged meaningfully in the dialogue, rather than deferring to the discipline to decide the answers. Further, the group engaged national nursing leaders around topics of interest as we sought to define ourselves, our practice, and our place within the larger nursing agenda. This exercise was repeated in 2010 and again in 2011 at the national DNP conferences. Themes have been recorded and are presented in this part as a national DNP agenda.

In addition to being conversant in policy issues related to practice, the DNP-prepared leader must think beyond the bedside and the boardroom to larger health care issues. In the current context of an economic recession, the number of Americans without access to employer-based health insurance has risen dramatically. Washington engages the nation in debate around payment reform and the movement to integrate quality measures into care delivery with the development of accountable care organizations (ACOs). It is clear that the American health care landscape is undergoing rapid change. DNPs, through their diverse roles, must be not only able to speak to such issues, but they must also be positioned to make an impact through participation in policy development and the larger legislative process. Further, given nursing's social contract with society, such efforts should not be limited to home. Effective DNPs must be able to translate this skill set to the global arena, seeking to impact larger public health agendas.

# CHAPTER 15

# Building the DNP Professional Nursing Community: Reflections and Expectations

David G. O'Dell

The rate of growth of the Doctor of Nursing Practice (DNP) degree is unparalleled with any other degree seen within the discipline of nursing (American Association of Colleges of Nursing [AACN], 2010). As a result of this growth, many challenges surface, including the ability to communicate issues and trends in rapidly changing education and practice environments. How will a nursing professional in a relatively new role learn the latest in practice? What opportunities are available for professional growth? How are colleagues networking in order to develop optimum outcomes for their respective patient populations? The ability to communicate, share, and build a community of providers is one method of growing professionally. This chapter explores the importance of building community for the professional development of nurses who have earned the DNP degree. The chapter also describes one organization's efforts to build community for the DNP-prepared nurse to enhance the nursing profession and promote the growth and development of the nursing profession in the United States and internationally.

## ■ DEFINITIONS OF COMMUNITY

Though the common definition of community implies a group of people living in the same locality under the same government, or a district or locality in which such a group lives, the functional definition is much broader. A group of professionals with common interests reflects the definition of the growing DNP community. We may all belong to a number of different communities simultaneously. The concept of community has grown and evolved as a result of changes in the Internet. Technology provides access to networks and cyber communities that link individuals and organizations around the globe without regard to national boundaries (Boyles, 1997).

Evaluating the concept of community from a sociologist's perspective illustrates the facets and dimensions of community growth and development in the world of the DNP. Community is a sociological construct. It is a set of interactions and human behaviors that have meaning and expectations between its members. These interactions and actions are based on the shared expectations, values, beliefs, and meanings between individuals (Bartle, 2010).

The act of building community is reflective of the perceived need and urgency by members of the community. Recognizing the nebulous end result of community as social capital places the concept in perspective specific to DNP community growth. Whereas physical capital refers to physical objects and human capital refers to the properties of individuals, social capital refers to connections among individuals—social networks and the norms of reciprocity and trustworthiness that arise from them. In that sense, social capital is closely related to what some have called civic virtue. The difference is that social capital calls attention to the fact that civic virtue is most powerful when embedded in a network of reciprocal social relations. A society of many virtuous but isolated individuals is not necessarily rich in social capital (Smith, 2002). These concepts of community building reflect the value, need, and urgency for a perception of social capital as a result of a coordinated effort. This is one of the driving forces behind the development of community within and among the DNP-prepared professional nurse and the nursing community as a whole.

Social capital can be seen as an end product, or as a means to an end. The DNP community's growth and development goal is the evolution of skills and talents to a desired end product of improving practice and health care outcomes, and further, meaningful recognition of such contributions by the discipline. Exploring and appreciating the dimensions of community, and reflecting on the history of past community growth within the nursing discipline will shed light on the future of the DNP community.

As nursing continues to grow in numbers and scope of services, the complexity of nursing practice continues to expand. In this context, a practice doctorate seems like a logical evolution for the discipline. However, there have been some who question what the degree can offer (Edwardson, 2010; Hawkins & Nezat, 2009), while others question the rigor required to obtain the degree (Catalona, 2008; Florczak, 2010; Webber, 2008). Is the growth and development of the DNP degree reflective of the growth and development of the discipline in response to the needs of society? Do DNP students, faculty, and graduates realize their potential in terms of outcomes? Does the DNP-degreed nursing professional recognize the opportunities for impacting the delivery of health care and the growth of the nursing discipline? These questions are best answered by the collective voice of those involved in DNP education and practice. In order for such questions to be adequately addressed, a community of DNP-interested professionals must share and mature together through ongoing communication.

## ■ DEVELOPMENTAL STAGES OF CREATING COMMUNITY FOR THE DNP

### Nursing Research Evolution

One example of how community was built and evolved within the profession of nursing is the evolution of research in nursing academia. In January 2010, Dr. Pamela H. Mitchell, the Associate Dean for Research at the University of Washington School of Nursing (UWSON) outlined the steps of community building as it relates to nursing research including: (1) commitment of administrative leadership, (2) awakening, (3) tender phase, (4) coming of age, (5) maturity, and (6) generativity. These stages of development spanned over 50 years of effort and provide a good backdrop and foundation to discuss the evolution of the DNP degree (P. Mitchell, personal communication, January 30, 2010).

Mitchell recalled that in the 1950s the administration of UWSON recognized the significance of research to the development of knowledge essential to nursing science and practice. At this stage, university administration was beginning to make a commitment to foster the incorporation of research into the faculty role. Ten to twenty years later, she described an awakening or recognition of the potential of their efforts. This resulted in improved individual faculty development, faculty research development grants, and nurse scientist training grants. Within another 10 to 20 years, she described a tender phase when ideas began to coalesce and the efforts of nurse researchers began to be realized. There was an emphasis on the entrepreneurial spirit. Departments of research facilitation were developed; research was successfully attributed to the faculty's role. Still, 10 years following the tender phase, researchers began to experience a coming of age stage. During this phase of evolution, the participants perceived a greater sense of team building and integration with other resources and improved collegiality began to take place. There was a greater sense of integration and collaboration in the context of increased technology and computerization. Finally, the stages of research development evolved into a maturity phase. Recognition for these efforts was appreciated along with the maturity of the researchers. There was an alignment of rewards, and also a consolidation of programs. Interdisciplinary research was also seen along with increased productivity. Finally, generativity and sustainability evolved again through interdisciplinary efforts, the development of new faculty, and the beginnings of translation of research into practice (P. Mitchell, personal communication, January 30, 2010).

There are uncanny parallels between the evolution of a sustainable research program by PhD-prepared nurses and the inception and development of the DNP degree. The DNP-prepared professional nurse strives for improved outcomes through similar stages of growth and development as outlined by the evolutionary processes accomplished by PhD colleagues with their emphasis on research.

## Stages of DNP Community Development: Parallels

Although the stages of nursing research as outlined by Mitchell parallel the development of the growth of the DNP in practice and education, the stages of community development are not concise and easy to identify. For example, the first stage of commitment of administrative leadership may be realized in many universities, yet according to discussions in an on-line community for DNPs and interested parties, not all health care organizations or legal entities acknowledge the DNP degree and the use of the title of doctor in nursing practice (http://www.doctorsof nursingpractice.org/DNP_NON-Supporters.htm). Still, progress is being made and the community of DNPs and those committed to witness the continued evolution of nursing roles impacted by the DNP degree continue to communicate and share information. Academic institutions and health care organizations are still adjusting to the concept of the DNP-degreed professional. Some have embraced the concept, integrating The Essentials of Doctoral Education for Advanced Nursing Practice (2006) into the curriculum as outlined by the AACN. Jointly, the dialogue continues through peer-reviewed journals and online as the community continues to expand.

Has the DNP degree evolved into the stage of awakening? The history and stages of nursing research and the integration into academia evolved over 10 to 20 years before an awakening took place. The DNP evolution is still at a young phase of development. Though the circumstances and evolution of nursing research at UWSON cannot be compared with the evolution of a degree on a macrolevel, the phase of awakening as anticipated for the DNP degree has still not occurred. We can anticipate that after the transition from MSN to DNP for all NP graduates occurs, there will be greater commitment and awakening. Nevertheless, the stage of coming of age, as of this writing, has not yet been actualized.

Regardless, there is "administrative commitment" appreciated by many entities, including new grassroots organizations dedicated solely to growth and development of this degree. The fruits of its collective efforts will no doubt evolve into an awakening. A tender phase is soon to follow. From a community-building perspective, this tender phase is reflected in the struggle to self-identify. Similarly, along with self-identification is differentiation of contributions and outcomes. As the DNP community evolves, these issues will be addressed, leading to a stage of maturity. It is beyond the scope of this author to predict the possibilities of what can occur as a result of these stages of development. However, having been a part of the process for close to a decade, there is recognition that the rate of change and confluence of social and financial factors are moving fast. Multiple elements are now in play to help the evolution of the DNP-degreed nursing professional to make a collective impact on the health care system, including the acceptance and integration of the DNP-prepared nursing professional into systems of care, the continued growth of DNP university and college programs, and the growing numbers of DNP-prepared nurses graduating every year. These influences will lead us to stages of maturity and ultimately generativity.

## Application and Evolution of Technology to Community Evolution

The building of the DNP community from the inception of the degree has been influenced by many factors, including the Internet and technology in general. These tools of communication that have become ubiquitous have had, and will continue to impart, an influence on the development of communities. Concepts of communication that are standard vernacular today began with concepts that allowed the growth and dissemination of information. For example, the concepts of Web 2.0 have influenced the way we communicate today. The term Web 2.0 can be attributed to O'Reilly Media during a conference in 2004 (O'Reilly, 2005). The concepts originally related to a new web-based application platform designed to share and collect data. Thus began an evolution of new and rapidly growing concepts that allowed for information sharing by all. Examples include Wikipedia and democratic sharing of information that have evolved into large social media applications like Facebook, YouTube, and Twitter. Google, the powerful search engine, may be considered the consummate Web 2.0 company. Yet, the foundational power of the Internet as a result of the Web 2.0 concept is manifested in the ability for all to communicate equally. Top links for news may direct the user to an individual's site rather than a media company. All who participate can share information, and it is essentially free (Graham, 2005).

The core characteristics of Web 2.0 services that have applicability to the building of community include a user-centered design, crowd-sourcing, web as platform, collaboration, power decentralization, dynamic content, cloud computing, and a rich user experience (Sharma, 2009). These constructs of decentralized power and democracy of communication circle around an experience by the user to have easy access to information and the ability to contribute to the conversation as well. The Internet and technology development contribute to the development of a community and may potentiate beneficial growth, while simultaneously creating forces that no individual could predict. Individual voices can be heard when joining with others who have similar interests. The power of aggregation of interests and collection of voices cannot be minimized.

For example, the aggregation of conversations has the potential of illustrating common beliefs and perceptions. A popular book was written almost entirely by an aggregation of comments collected from one web log (blog). Anderson (2006) demonstrated a phenomenon of culture and commerce through such a technique. His book is a compilation of discussions over a number of years addressing issues of the Internet market. The collective wisdom gleaned from these conversations produced themes and insights that could not have been appreciated from isolated and fragmented discussion. If his aggregation of blog entries could evolve into a book reflecting a timely phenomenon, then there is no reason to doubt that a collection of thoughts and dialogues by DNPs or those interested in doctorally prepared practice would provide similar substance. The collection of shared thoughts could enhance DNP practice and ultimately outcomes.

## Dimensions of Communities: A Conceptual Framework

Is there a theoretical foundation for the creation and evolution of the concept of community? One such framework is offered through a sociological perspective of community. This structure and identification of dimensions sheds light on the parameters and expectations of forming and growing a community of DNPs. According to Bartle (2010), there are six dimensions to every community, no matter how small, large, simple, or complex. These dimensions consist of technology, economic, political, institutional, esthetic value, and belief.

### Technology
The technology dimension of community refers to the facilities, infrastructure, and tools used by the community. It suggests the complexity of the environment in which the community exists. In any community, elements can be introduced to augment the technology, such as a new system of communication or the addition of an organization or entity that will ultimately expand the community. In essence, technology addresses the nuts and bolts of the community (Bartle, 2010).

### Economic
The economic dimension is the capital of the community. It describes what the community has to offer and includes what services or goods are made available as a result of the community. This dimension does not refer to cash—rather, the value is what the community ascribes as valuable for itself.

### Political
The political dimension of community describes how the community identifies and values power and influence. It is about the management of the communication system of the community. It also describes how people make decisions. For example, a change agent must be able to develop the existing power and decision-making system to promote community unity and group decision making that benefits the whole community—not just the vested interests. The political dimension of community addresses power and influence.

### Institutional
The institutional or social dimension of community described how members of the community act in relation to each other. This includes their expectations, assumptions, judgments, predictions, responses, and reactions. Institutional dimension refers to patterns of relationships, which could be considered roles and status. This social dimension is not about power and influence. Rather, it is about the depth and breadth of the community. The more organized the institutional dimension of a community, the more capacity it has to achieve its communal or organizational objectives.

### Esthetic Value

The esthetic-value dimension of community addresses judgments between right and wrong, good and bad, and beauty and ugliness. These are based on community values that can change according to the community. The degree to which community or organizational members share values and/or respect for values is an element of strength and capacity. Values result from changes in technology and social organization—not by lecturing or trying to promote change. Therefore, building capacity in terms of infrastructure and how people communicate will promote change rather than imposing or trying to persuade a group to accept a value. The group generates its own values and esthetics as it forms and matures.

### Belief

The belief dimension of community addresses the conceptual dimension of community. It refers to a shared belief in how the world should operate—the nature of the universe. This is different from the esthetic-value dimension in that beliefs are guiding principles of the community, not the product of the group. Guiding principles are not typically changed internally. Instead, these belief systems are the overarching philosophies of the larger community/society.

These dimensions can be identified in the existing and evolving community of the DNP-degreed professional. The technology of the group includes mechanisms of communication with colleagues, either classmates or business colleagues in any process, including email, phone calls, and publications. The economy of the DNP community is in process as the collective efforts of universities, students, graduates, and organizations realize the impact and potential outcomes of efforts initiated or supported by the DNP. The politics of DNP community is also evolving, as there are many leaders, supporters, sponsors, and change agents within the health care community at large and the nursing community in general, and the DNP community more specifically. These leaders and processes of power and influence are being created by the DNP community, for the DNP community with influence from outside the group.

The institutional/social dimension of the DNP community is also in process as graduates begin to interact, communicate through multiple venues, publish, and establish roles within organizations and systems in order to demonstrate the skills learned at universities and other institutions of higher learning, as the DNP numbers grow and influence the trends of nursing education. As a result of this particular social dimension, the esthetic-value system of the community will surface and make itself known. The value system and structure will reflect the talents and collective directives of the DNPs that participate in the community. These values can be appreciated in the context of the belief system of the DNP community, which consists of members of the greater nursing organization, general health care community, and society. The dynamics of the DNP community's inception, growth, and maturation are tremendous as it forms and begins to generate its own lexicon of information and product. The expected outcomes of improved patient care will be the result of a DNP community that is aware of the interactions and descriptions of these dimensions of community.

### ■ APPLICATION: EXAMPLE OF ONE DNP COMMUNITY BUILDING EFFORT

One organization that saw the value of community development while the DNP degree was still in a nascent phase is Doctors of Nursing Practice, LLC (DNP, LLC). This organization was formed by a group of DNP students at the University of Tennessee Health Science

Center College of Nursing in Memphis. In 2005, during one of the first courses in the program, a discussion began relative to the growth of the DNP degree among nurses and the ability to share information specific to the DNP's activities. There were less than 10 universities offering the DNP degree at that time, and the classmates recognized that, as a cohort, there were few colleagues nationally to connect and grow with professionally. In the fall of 2006, during an advanced leadership class, classmates agreed to develop a business plan with the mission of promoting the DNP degree. By the end of November 2006, the corporation was formed. By February 2007, the DNP web site was launched. The founding board members are Nancy Cabelus, DNP, MSN, RN; Amelie Hollier, DNP, APRN, BC, FAANP; LaRae Huycke, DNP, MS, APRN, BC; David G. O'Dell, DNP, FNP-BC; Sally R. Schafer-Beltz, DNP, APRN, BC; and Joyce Williams, DNP, MFSA, RN. Later, another classmate, Margaret "Peggy" Pierce, DNP, APN, BC, joined the board.

The original goals were to create a venue to demonstrate the contributions of nurses with the DNP practice degree. A scholarly, peer-reviewed journal was the intent, yet the preliminary steps required the development of an online presence to determine the market and interest in the nursing community for such a venture. The mission of the organization was and remains the development of a forum that permits the communication of information, ideas, and innovations to promote the growth and development of the practice doctorate degree in nursing. The vision of DNP, LLC is grounded in the following principles: The organization is dedicated to (1) providing accurate and timely information; (2) supporting, developing, and disseminating professional practice innovations; (3) collaborating in a professional manner that demonstrates universal respect for others, and honesty and integrity in communications; and (4) responding with open discussions and dialogues that promote the evolution of advanced nursing practice and the growth of the DNP degree.

These plans materialized while the founders were students and evolved over a year before there was a realization of the beginnings of a community. The expectations for growth were tremendous, while the reality of community growth included the knowledge that that information is shared slowly. The board members soon realized that just because a web site was built, there was no guarantee that visitors would come. The naïveté of the board was soon realized and consultants were sought to address the best way to utilize the technology to garnish input and ultimately to build community. A measure of success was realized within the first 10 months of the company's existence as the second generation of the web site evolved. The site was modular in structure with multiple pieces in place from open source code features. For example, a programmer who provided HTML code for free designed a bibliography feature. All modules required extensive work to address our growing needs. After about 12 months, it was obvious that the system would not work. Through the personal investment of board members, the web site was modified to address growing needs and to assist in gathering and disseminating information about an annual conference. One of the goals of DNP, LLC is to build community through a natural progression of conversation, then a collection and aggregation of data web site participants. This conceptual foundation for choosing this tact is reflected by Kaminski (2003):

> Self-organized communities potentiate the development of a group identity and even, a group consciousness. A community memory and awareness can be created which facilitates decision-making, brainstorming, sharing and dialogue. These communities potentially elicit a number of empowering benefits including: community consciousness, innovation amplification, social capital, access, collective knowing and a context for exchange. (Self Organizing Cyber Communities, para. 1)

As the organization and the web site grew, new areas of services were added on to meet the growing needs and desires of the DNP community, including students, graduates, faculty, and others interested in the development of this degree. The first National DNP Conference took place October 9–11, 2008, in Memphis, TN. This site was selected as a tribute to the University of Tennessee Health Science Center College of Nursing and the city of Memphis, as this is where the organization began. A surprising number of attendees participated in this inaugural conference. About 100 registrants were expected, and over 140 attended. This conference marked the beginning of a unified, national voice for DNPs to share, contrast, and evolve professionally. The second conference took place September 29–October 2, 2009, in Miami. It too was a great success, with over 185 in attendance. The number of DNP students in attendance increased, along with an increase in the number and caliber of presentations, both podium and poster. During that conference, attendees identified the key aspects of DNP practice and began to form a national agenda for growth. The DNP community began to gain its footing and the foundation for the community to mature had been laid.

The third National DNP Conference took place between September 29 and October 1, 2010, in San Diego. The registrants exceeded 240 and the caliber of presentations and discussions again revealed the need to continue a communication effort by and for DNP graduates, students, and faculty. The fourth National DNP Conference took place September 28–30, 2011, in New Orleans. Over 350 were in attendance. The content reflected an understanding of the need for collective growth in the discipline and by those with the DNP degree, as policy is the central theme. All conference archives including a description of presenters can be found at www.DoctorsofNursingPractice.org.

The efforts of DNP, LLC included the creation of an infrastructure that could accommodate the growth and development of the DNP community. After exploring options of applications and types of sites that could address our anticipated needs, a social networking site that had a similar look and feel to Facebook was selected. The online community site moved quickly from 400 members to over 1,500 in the first few months of existence. It continues to grow as more and more people involved in DNP practice, education, or policies join the site for discussions and sharing. During its inception, discussions reflected an acknowledgement that others existed, as there were a lot of comparisons of practice and education between members around the country. Later, issues such as titling, independent practice, educational expectations, and disparities evolved. As of this writing, there are over 2,800 members on the online community, with 8 forums and over 225 discussion threads. There are also an additional 64 blog posts, and groups have formed on the community web site. This may seem small compared with other social networks, blogs, and forums; however, this has been considered active and robust considering the size of the DNP community overall. A page dedicated to educational events that may interest the DNP-prepared nursing professional is also available for all to view and contribute to. Regional, national, and international seminars are posted by members reflecting numerous specialties and types of practice.

Another aspect of the community that has grown without encouragement is the Groups page. Over 65 groups have formed spontaneously reflecting university affiliation, type of practice, and geographic proximity. Members within these groups can communicate quickly and can also easily communicate with other groups. These groups are able to compare observations, best practices, policy obstacles, successes, and recommendations for professional growth at a speed and accuracy that was not available 10 years ago. The potential for an individual to communicate with colleagues and peers across the country and next door is now available with the infrastructure of communication that is available through the DNP web site. Groups can coalesce and develop and communicate with members of that particular group through the larger web site, while at the same time sharing their activities, challenges, obstacles, and triumphs more-or-less "real time" with others on the site around the world.

Most members are from the United States, yet there are some from Canada, the United Kingdom, Australia, New Zealand, Thailand, Vietnam, Japan, and Hong Kong. The community is growing in geographical diversity as it stretches to meet members' needs. A weekly broadcast email describing issues that may impact the DNP along with conference updates keep the community informed of issues, trends, activities, and opportunities. In essence, the DNP web site and organization has become a communication tool as it helps to promote the DNP degree, so that it can coalesce and improve patient outcomes.

Future expectations for the DNP, LLC organization reflect the evolution and augmentation of those with the DNP degree as we individually and collectively strive to enhance health care outcomes. The efforts of the organization are shifting to work with other organizations in creative and constructive ways to meet similar goals and missions. To this end, the organization is developing its nonprofit company, anticipating a name change, and applying for 501(c)(3) nonprofit status. Several members and supporters are working to explore the opportunities for grants to enhance the services of the organization, as the structure of the organization becomes more refined and able to meet the shifting needs and growing demands of promoting professional development, communicating DNP skills and talents, providing modalities of DNP education, and demonstrating the best practice techniques to improve patient outcomes individually, in the aggregate, systematically, and internationally.

A developmental and educational step that the DNP, LLC organization took in 2010 was the generation of a National DNP Outcomes survey. This survey was planned and developed by volunteers and colleagues of DNP, LLC/Doctors of Nursing Practice Professional Development, Inc. The goal was to determine the "state of the practice" of DNP graduates on an annual basis. The initial plan was to collect and analyze data on an annual basis and then disseminate these findings first at the 2010 DNP Conference and then annually thereafter. The survey has two arms: (1) DNP Graduate outcomes data and (2) DNP University Program data. The development team members were: Stephanie Ahmed, DNP, FNP-BC; Catherine S. Bishop, DNP, NP, AOCNP; Karen Crowley, DNP, APRN-BC, WHNP, ANP; Donald Grimes, DNP, RN; Star Evangelista Hoffman, DNP, MEd, CNL; David G. O'Dell, DNP, FNP-BC; and Marie G. Young, DNP, MSN, MPH, FNP, PMHNP. Selected findings from the 2010 survey are in Exhibit 15.1.

The future is bright for the DNP regardless of perceived or real obstacles and barriers to growth. As a community, the numbers of DNP graduates will soon create a critical mass of doctorally prepared nurses engaged in advanced practice. The rate of DNP graduations has exceeded the rate of PhD nursing graduates (AACN, 2010). These numbers do not have meaning unless there is a coordinated effort to demonstrate value in the degree. The formation and growth of the DNP community through such organization as DNP, LLC will assist in this development.

DNP, LLC has developed a place and infrastructure to support, endorse, and promote all efforts from all groups that aim to grow the DNP-prepared professional and it is important to note that this organization is not the only DNP-supportive entity. At present, in various geographies throughout the United States, there are similar organizations in development that share DNP, LLC goals and missions.

---

## EXHIBIT 15.1

### Selected Results from the 2010 Survey

---

DNP university/college program comparison: 131 programs
  44% have BSN–DNP entry
  66% MSN–DNP entry

APRN requirements
  73.3% NP entry
  51.0% CNS entry
  40.5% CNM entry
  36.6% CRNA entry

Role concentration
  29.5% no specific role concentration
  29.7% nurse executive
  14.5% educator
  0.05% health policy
  0.05% informatics
  Others: Scientist, CNL, public health, clinical research management

Credit hours
  BSN–DNP average: 97
  MSN–DNP average: 41

Clinical hours
  BSN–DNP: up to 1,260
  MSN–DNP: up to 1,125

A survey of DNP graduates revealed the following:
Total number of DNP graduate respondents to the survey: 292 (n = 292)
Demographics
Age
  25–30: 1%
  31–35: 7%
  36–40: 8%
  41–45: 14%
  46–50: 22%
  51–55: 31%
  56–60: 12%
  61–65: 4%

Gender
  Female: 88%
  Male: 12%

Practice area
  APN: 78%
  Nurse executive: 9%
  Nurse educator in an academic setting: 31%
  Policy/legislation: 3%
  Researcher: 3%
  Other: 7%

Work environment
  Primary care: 39%
  Acute care: 30%
  Long-term care: 3%

*(Continued)*

## EXHIBIT 15.1

### Selected Results from the 2010 Survey (*Continued*)

Rehabilitation: 2%
Community-based care: 11%
Public health: 5%
Academia: 38%
Other: 18%

Percentage of DNP-prepared nurse educators in an academic setting:
47% are NPs (FNP, ANP, CNM, CRNA, CNS)

Universities that have a tenure track (reported by DNP-prepared academics): 22%

Since earning the DNP degree, has your practice area changed?
Yes: 34%
No: 66%

Since earning the DNP degree, has your practice setting changed?
Yes: 26%
No: 74%

The reason why I pursued a DNP degree
Job requirement: 9%
Personal goal: 88%
Peer pressure: <1%
Professional advancement: 76%
Other: 5%

Income/salary
Since earning the DNP degree, salary has:
Increased: 30%
Remained the same: 66%
Decreased: 3%

Survey responses that correlate with the eight essentials:
AACN Essential II: Organizational and system leadership
30% function as an administrator
29% develop, implement, and evaluate business plans
23% have initiated a program to address disparities
20% have a leadership role in a specialty nursing organization
16% have a leadership role in a national nursing organization
20% have a leadership role in a state nursing organization
10% are currently involved in a nation-wide policy
29% are currently involved in a statewide policy

AACN Essential III: Clinical scholarship and analytical methods of evidence-based practice (EBP)
86% utilize EBP skills more
75% translate and disseminate relevant research into practice
70% utilize EBP skills to develop/translate practice guidelines
67% are able to translate research to identify gaps
45% actively translate EBP skills outside of their practice

AACN Essential IV: Information systems/technology
24% develop, implement, and evaluate information systems
52% utilized available technology to promote a change in practice

AACN Essential V: Heath care policy

*(Continued)*

---

***EXHIBIT 15.1***

**Selected Results from the 2010 Survey (*Continued*)**

---

42% are actively involved in health policy issues
23% initiated a program addressing health disparities
53% are active members in a specialty nursing organization
75% are active members in a national nursing organization

AACN Essential VI: Interprofessional collaboration
60% lead and participate in an interdisciplinary team
66% are able to implement practice changes
61% actively participate in interprofessional activities
55% purse practice change initiatives

AACN Essential VII: Clinical prevention and health promotion
74% incorporate health promotion and disease prevention
23% initiated a program addressing health disparities
58% are more aware of the impact of culture in their practice
55% utilize their understanding of cultural differences

AACN Essential VIII: Advanced nursing practice
62% develop, implement, and evaluate practice initiative
51% have increased the scope of their practice
61% function to the fullest capacity for their role

*Source:* Study summary reprinted with permission from DNP, LLC/DNPPD, Inc.
(www.DoctorsofNursingPractice.org).

## Future Efforts and Expectations for DNP Community Evolution

The roles of DNPs are diverse, and in this context some have begun to consider the need for organizational representation for the DNP, as opposed to specialty representation. At present, other than DNP, LLC, there is no single organization representing all doctorally prepared nurses in advanced practice. APRNs generally belong to a specialty organization and the national organizations such as the American Academy of Nurse Practitioners. Executives belong to the American Organization of Nurse Executives, Nurse Midwives to the American College of Nurse Midwives, and the like. However, until the time when nurses engaged in advanced practice are uniformly required to have a doctoral degree, we will continue to have fragmented membership. Community building and networking through DNP organizations will remain critical for DNPs to continue to mature and grow as a distinct discipline within nursing—in order to reach the mature and generative stages of development. We are confident that the DNP movement is on its way. There are parallels with the elements of community from a sociological perspective, and also parallels to how other communities have developed both within and outside of the discipline of nursing. The growth of community is propelling the DNP into a position of required contribution to impact the health care delivery system.

The DNP degree is young, yet growing quickly. Measured understanding of educational process, practice expectations, standards of care in doctoral practice, and demonstrated outcomes may be the result regardless of obstacles. The building of community is one step in the process that should not be overlooked or minimized. Collectively, and with a clear approach, the potential for the DNP community will exceed the expectations of the original stakeholders.

## ■ REFERENCES

AACN. (2010). *Amid calls for more highly educated nurses, new AACN data show impressive growth in doctoral nursing programs.* Retrieved from http://www.aacn.nche.edu/media/newsreleases/2010/enrollchanges.html

Anderson, C. (2006). *The long tail: Why the future of business is selling less of more.* New York: Hyperion.

Bartle, P. (2010). *What is community? A sociological perspective.* Retrieved from http://www.scn.org/cmp/whatcom.htm

Boyles, A. (1997). *The meaning of community. Bahai topics.* Retrieved from http://info.bahai.org/article-1-9-1-1.html

Catalona, J. T. (2008). DNP degree: Do we really need it? (Editorial). *American Nurse Today, 3,* 5.

Edwardson, S. R. (2010). Doctor of philosophy and doctor of nursing practice as complementary degrees. *Journal of Professional Nursing, 26,* 137–140.

Florczak, K. L. (2010). Research and the doctor of nursing practice: A cause for consternation. *Nursing Science Quarterly, 23,* 13–17.

Graham, J. (2005). *Web 2.0.* Retrieved from http://www.paulgraham.com/web20.html

Hawkins, R., & Nezat, G. (2009). Doctoral education: Which degree to pursue? *AANA Journal, 77,* 92–96.

Kaminski, J. (2003). *Self organizing communities as educational structures.* Retrieved from http://www.nursing-informatics.com/educcommunities.html

O'Reilly, T. (2005). *Design patterns and business models for the next generation of software.* Retrieved from http://oreilly.com/web2/archive/what-is-web-20.html

Sharma, P. (2009). *Core characteristics of Web 2.0 services.* Retrieved from http://www.techpluto.com/web-20-services/

Smith, M. K. (2002). *Community.* Retrieved from http://www.infed.org/community/community.htm

Webber, P. B. (2008). The doctor of nursing practice degree and research: Are we making an epistemological mistake? *Journal of Nursing Education, 47,* 466–472.

CHAPTER 16

# DNPs: Finding Our Voices and Defining Ourselves

Stephanie W. Ahmed and David G. O'Dell

In September of 2009, as aggressive discussions around a national health reform agenda were taking place in Washington, DC, an audience of 185 participants largely comprising new Doctors of Nursing Practice (DNPs) and nursing faculty gathered in Miami, FL, for the second annual DNP conference entitled, Exemplars of DNPs in Practice and Nursing Education: Defining Ourselves. Content for the 3-day conference addressed topics on advanced practice, quality and safety, evidence-based practice (EBP) initiatives, technology, education, and nursing education. The session culminated in a session moderated by Stephanie Ahmed, DNP, FNP-BC, entitled National Organizations: Exploring Roles for DNPs. Given the newness of the degree and the relatively small numbers of DNPs across the country, the spectrum of specialty practice nursing roles was not fully accounted for but participants represented the following specialties: Certified Registered Nurse Anesthetists, Certified Nurse Midwifes, Nurse Practitioners (NP), Clinical Nurse Specialists, and Nurse Executives.

National organization participation included:

- The American Association of Colleges of Nursing (AACN), represented by Poly Bednash, PhD, RN, FAAN;
- The American Academy of Nurse Practitioners (AANP), represented by Jan Towers, PhD, NP-C, CRNP, FAANP, FAAN, and Tim "TK" Knettler, MBA;
- The American College of Nurse Practitioners (ACNP), represented by Susan Apold, PhD, ANP;
- The American Organization of Nurse Executives (AONE), represented by Carol Watson, PhD, RN;
- National Organization of Nurse Practitioner Faculty (NONPF), represented by Mary Anne Dumas, RN, PhD, CFNP, FAANP; and finally
- The Honor Society of Sigma Theta Tau International (STTI), represented by Gwen Sherwood, PhD, RN, FAAN. (DNP LLC, 2009)

The aforementioned organizations are reflective of, but a sampling of, those serving nurses in the United States; however, despite limitation, the exchange was both interactive and significant. Conference attendees demonstrated an eagerness to engage national nursing leaders around topics of interest including certification, licensure, titling, practice models, scholarship, leadership, and the role of the DNP in academe. Building upon the previous outcomes of a small DNP-led focus group conducted in New England, Ahmed engaged the Miami conference attendees in an exercise that strategized to identify core elements and ideas from the morning session that would serve as the foundation for a national agenda for DNPs around education, practice, and policy (Tables 16.1–16.3). While national discussions about a practice doctorate for nursing had been robust both internal and external to the discipline, conference attendees recognized that the voice of the DNP was missing from the discussion and conference attendees sought to be heard. Deferring to be defined externally, DNPs from various regions across the United States were engaged in a discussion that has been repeated in similar fashion at both the third national DNP conference entitled Leadership and Innovation in San Diego, CA, during September of 2010 (DNP LLC, 2010), and the fourth national DNP conference held in New Orleans, LA, entitled Impacting Healthcare

### TABLE 16.1  DNP Agenda for Education

| Curriculum | Create consistency with admission standards and credit hours across DNP programs |
| | Partner with specialty organizations to develop competencies for clinical and non-clinical roles.  Integrate content into curriculum. |
| | Develop guidelines for "practice hours" and final projects across all DNP roles |
| | Integrate pedagogy into DNP curriculum and prepare DNPs for faculty roles |
| Faculty | Augment the presence of DNP-prepared faculty teaching in DNP programs |
| Scholarship | Recognition from the discipline of nursing relative to the value of the scholarship of practice |

*Source:* DNP, LLC (2009, 2010), reprinted with permission.

### TABLE 16.2  DNP Agenda for Practice

| Clinical roles | Expand clinical opportunities for DNP-prepared clinicians |
| | Provide DNP-prepared APRNs who practice in academic medical centers with faculty appointments |
| | Develop meaningful academic practice partnership opportunities and develop career trajectories for DNP-prepared APRNs that support both a clinical and faculty appointment |
| Academia | Develop academic/practice partnerships that encourage DNP-prepared faculty to remain active in practice |
| | Realign outdated tenure criteria and methods of faculty promotion with those consistent with the current culture of interdisciplinary work and practice-based scholarship |
| Leadership | Enhance opportunities for nursing representation on boards and other key positions in health care organizations |

*Source:* DNP, LLC (2009, 2010), reprinted with permission.

**TABLE 16.3   DNP Policy Agenda**

| | |
|---|---|
| Credentialing and licensure | Universal participation in the APRN Consensus Model—creating a uniformity for nursing education, credentialing, licensure, and practice |
| Remove barriers to APRN autonomy | Create uniformity around APRN prescriptive practice and autonomy Remove barriers that limit the ability of APRNs to generate revenue and be reimbursed for care |
| Titling | Clarify use of academic title "doctor" in clinical settings |

*Source:* DNP, LLC (2009, 2010), reprinted with permission.

Policy during September of 2011 (DNP LLC, 2011). Themes from the "DNP National Agenda" sessions from the 2009 and 2010 conferences have been identified and are discussed in the following chapter. Content is occasionally supported by a selection of conference transcript excerpts that offer relevance and are provided to document the history and the rich dialogue that occurred between participants and national nursing leaders as new DNPs were seeking to establish their place within the national nursing agenda.

### ■ TRANSFORMING SPECIALTY EDUCATION IN NURSING

With a statement that counters the debate raised by national nursing leaders who have challenged the movement of specialty education in nursing to the DNP (Cronenwett et al., 2011; Dracup, Cronenwett, Meleis, & Benner, 2005; Meleis & Dracup, 2005), Towers' (2009) words were powerful when she stated "this is an idea whose time has come." Indeed, the current US health care crisis supports her thoughts, creating a strong case for greater leadership and an expanded tool box for those nurses engaged in advanced practice and who are most likely to play a larger role in care delivery models of the future.

While the degree is not yet uniformly offered across all US states, Bednash (2009) reports that there has been significant interest in DNP programs from both students and academic institutions alike. In 2009, there were 102 programs conferring the degree (Bednash, 2009), a number that has grown to 153 programs at the time of the 2011 DNP conference (AACN, 2011a, 2011b) and supports a growing interest in a practice doctorate for nursing nationally.

Addressing the DNP degree, Bednash (2009) referenced the landmark Flexner Report which called for the restructuring of US medical education and stated that the movement of specialty education in nursing to the doctoral level offers nursing a reconstruction of the highest level of education for practice. Physical therapy, optometry, osteopathy, public health, and pharmacy have arrived at this same juncture and successfully paved the way (Brown-Benedict, 2008). Such movement toward a terminal degree for practice would not only provide nurses with competencies in topics such as leadership, technology, and aggregate care but also further serve to establish parity among health care peers whose disciplines have likewise made the transition to prepare graduates at the doctoral level (AACN, 2009).

### ■ A DEGREE, NOT A ROLE!

The DNP is the newest nursing degree—not a role (Dumas, 2009). While there is no question that education has a strong impact upon practice and roles, and further that some DNPs may experience a role change as a result of obtaining the DNP degree, it is important to note that it is not the intention for the degree to prepare nurses for new roles or to expand the scope of advanced practice (AACN, 2011a, 2011b). History bears witness that such changes in nursing education and practice have long been shaped by societal demands and, with this in mind, there is no question that the current U.S. health care challenges coupled with the complexities of a modern health care system would again demand a response from the discipline of nursing. With a documented need to augment the number of doctorally prepared nurses (Institute of Medicine [IOM], 2011) and to further ensure that nurses engaged in advanced practice are better prepared for the future (AACN, 2011a, 2011b), this educational shift toward doctoral preparedness represents a logical response to a national call to action around contemporary health care agendas. However, despite the aforementioned, some have voiced concern that the development of DNP programs would result in a decrease in the number of nurses seeking to enroll in PhD programs, thereby reducing the number of nurse scientists engaged in advanced practice (Dracup et al. 2005). Bednash (2009) however dispelled such a myth by reporting to conference attendees that the enrollment in PhD programs has in fact increased. Further, with the addition of a practice doctorate, nursing is being framed as a discipline with an intellectual base and demonstrates acknowledgment of a need for a terminal degree (Bednash, 2009). With the integration of what are projected to be foundational competencies for all health care providers, including topics such as interdisciplinary practice, information systems, quality improvement, and patient safety into "The Essentials of Doctoral Education for Advanced Nursing Practice" (AACN, 2006), nursing is not expanding the scope of practice but rather seizing an opportunity to contemporize competencies. With such a strategy, doctorally prepared nurses engaged in advanced practice will be academically prepared to be leaders in the delivery of patient care and, further, to assume responsibility for both patient and organizational outcomes in complex and evolving health care arenas. DNP National Conference participants have consistently recognized this responsibility, and their comments and recommendations have evolved into the following themes for professional growth in the discipline of nursing specific to the roles and contributions of the doctor of nursing practice professional.

## ■ DNP EDUCATION

### DNP Curriculum

#### DNP-Recommended Agenda: Create Consistency with Admission Standards and Credit Hours Across DNP Programs

Conference attendees expressed concern that variation may exist in the admission requirements of DNP programs across the country (DNP, LLC, 2009). Citing specific concerns about the impact that variability in admission standards and credit hours might have upon the value of the DNP degree, attendees identified a desire to see greater standardization and a focus upon scholarliness (DNP, LLC, 2009). AACN (2009) has outlined the key DNP curricular elements and structure, which theoretically should standardize academic objectives and eliminate wide variability. The degree is evolving, and early programs have recruited master's-prepared nurses engaged in advanced practice; however, over time it is anticipated that these same programs will accept the post-baccalaureate DNP candidate. With this in mind, the AACN allows for some interpretation, stating logically that the post-master's DNP program design should account for the candidate's education, experiences, and area of specialty while ensuring that both the post-master's and post-baccalaureate candidates achieve the same end-of-program competencies. In this context, some variability is inevitable and, further, there are a multiple other variables that have the potential to impact a student's educational experience including institutional, state, and accrediting agency policies (AACN, 2009). While acknowledging the aforementioned, conference participants strongly voiced that implementing academic rigor, which includes structure for admission standards, scholarliness, and defined professional outcomes, is essential to the successful integration and, ultimately, the acceptance of the practice of the DNP-prepared nurse (DNP, LLC, 2009).

## Practice Experiences and Final Projects

### DNP-Recommended Agenda: Develop Guidelines for "Practice Hours" and Final Projects Across All DNP Specialties

Conference attendees report experiencing variability across DNP programs around how practice hours and final projects, often referred to as "capstone projects," are both defined and operationalized academically (DNP, LLC, 2009). The capstone project provides an opportunity for the student to demonstrate synthesis and mastery of content, and differs from a research thesis in that it is not aimed at generating new knowledge. Like the DNP, such projects should be a practice-focused experience (AACN, 2006).

Practice hours are incorporated into the curriculum to assist the student to achieve competency with respect to the "Essentials" and, more specifically, the role-specific content. At the post-baccalaureate level, students are required to complete a minimum of 1000 "practice hours" through a mentored experience (AACN, 2006). A review of DNP programs demonstrates that a variety of terms are used to describe the practice experience including; residency, mentorship with faculty, clinical practicum, and clinical experiences (Neilheisel & Kaplan, 2011). Describing a post-graduate clinical experience that is often used by other disciplines and may even imply a salaried experience could contribute to confusion, particularly when considering that many DNPs are anticipated to be engaged in non-direct care roles. Based on this, a call has been issued for consistency to suggest the term "practicum" to best describe DNP practice hours (Neilheisel & Kaplan). Dumas (2009) appropriately advises conference attendees that when considering knowledge and skill acquisition, there is variation in how students learn and therefore it is essential that learning be competency-based rather than hours driven. Education that is hours driven does not provide assurance that the student would achieve the expected competencies in the prescribed number of hours (Dumas, 2009). Conference participants recognized the value of competency-based learning experiences as a mechanism for measuring student achievement of competencies (DNP LLC, 2009). Further, they expressed concern that some DNP programs may lack structure and academic rigor (DNP LLC, 2009). National nursing organizations engaged in setting education and practice standards for CNMs, CRNAs, and CNSs must develop guidelines for practice hours and final projects for their respective advanced practice roles as NONPF has done for the NP. Additionally, if DNPs are to be prepared for non-direct care roles, such as executive nurse leadership roles, similar guidelines must be developed. The aforementioned provides an opportunity for the American Organization of Nurse Executives and others to set such standards.

## Meeting Essential Eight

### DNP-Recommended Agenda: National Specialty Organizations Must Define Doctoral-Level Content, Competencies, and Practica

With respect to programs engaging in the development of the advanced practice registered nurse (APRN), it has been suggested that "The Essentials" document may have some inherent limitations (NONPF, 2006). Successful attainment of "Essential Eight" requires the incorporation of specialty-focused competencies into DNP curricula (AACN, 2006). Such integration and defining of the advanced practice role necessitates national specialty organizations develop content, competencies, and practica, which a DNP-prepared nurse is then required to meet (http://www.aacn.nche.edu/dnp/dnpfaq.pdf). NONPF has taken the lead in the development of DNP competencies for NPs, including criteria and exemplars for DNP scholarly projects for the nurse practitioner DNP degree (Dumas, 2009; NONPF, 2007). Other advanced practice role standards setting bodies have yet to develop competencies or guidelines for the respective roles. Until there is a uniform acceptance of the DNP as the education standard for entry into advanced practice, and further, the subsequent development of role-specific doctoral competencies, variation in how such content will be integrated into DNP curricula is likely to continue. This has the potential to create a significant gap in the educational experience of DNP students and could potentially devalue the degree. Under such circumstances, there is an obvious benefit to distinguishing doctoral-level competencies across all DNP-advanced practice roles.

## Role Acquisition

### DNP-Recommended Agenda: Augment the Presence of DNP-Prepared Faculty Teaching in DNP Programs

DNP conference participants voiced a desire to have more DNP-prepared faculty teaching in DNP programs (DNP LLC, 2009). With the relative newness of the DNP degree, faculty teaching in DNP programs are likely to be PhD, EdD, or DNSc-prepared and thus likely to be geared more toward research than to practice. The generation of new knowledge significantly diverges from the intended objectives of the practice-focused DNP to whom EBP and translational research are foundational. Without question, the DNP student benefits from a broad exposure to faculty with educationally diverse backgrounds and roles, however successful role attainment further requires exposure to practicing DNPs, particularly in the specialty areas. Integration of DNP-prepared faculty into the academic experience of DNP students should not be restricted to mentoring for practice hours, but also should be integrated into both the classroom and project committees, thus enhancing the likelihood that students will be socialized appropriately to the practice objectives of the degree and further ensuring that capstone projects remain practice oriented.

With acknowledgment that neither the PhD nor the DNP is specifically prepared toward assuming the role of an educator (AACN, 2006), conference participants desire that opportunities to develop the necessary skill set for pedagogy must be meaningfully integrated into the DNP curricula. The IOM has issued a call to double the number of doctorally prepared nurses by 2020 (ANA, 2011). Without the DNP, attainment of such a goal seems unlikely. Further, in the setting of a documented nursing faculty shortage (AACN, 2011a, 2011b), failure to integrate meaningful pathways that prepare doctoral candidates for pedagogy seems illogical.

## ■ DNP PRACTICE

### Tenure

### DNP-Recommended Agenda: Revise Tenure Criteria and Methods of Faculty Promotion to Be Consistent With the Current Culture of Interdisciplinary Work

Dumas (2009) reports a significant faculty shortage across all levels of nursing education. Comparing clinical practice and academe, wide salary discrepancies are thought to contribute to the difficulty in recruiting nursing faculty (Dumas, 2009). In the setting of such a shortage, it has been suggested that the new DNP may offer a solution to filling vacant faculty roles (AACN, 2006). However, questions have arisen nationally around the parity of DNP-prepared faculty in academic settings where the tenure-eligible has historically been prepared at the PhD or EdD level (AACN, 2006). Some state that schools with both practice doctorate and research-focused doctorate prepared faculty may exclude the practice-oriented DNP from the university "Senate," thereby restricting the DNP's ability to participate in the decision-making processes of the university or to achieve tenure (Meleis & Dracup, 2005). Central to any discussion of tenure is the threefold academic mission of research, teaching, and service, in which greater value may be placed upon research secondary to its potential to generate revenue for the university. In such a context, the practice-focused DNP is at risk to be devalued in academia. However, the significant gap from the bench to the bedside supports that as a discipline nursing must broaden its thinking beyond the generation of new knowledge.

Boyer (1990) articulated a paradigm for faculty scholarly activity that expanded the concept of scholarship, traditionally viewed as the scientific discovery of new knowledge, to include three other equally important areas: the scholarship of integration, the scholarship of application, and the scholarship of teaching. The scholarship of integration involves making connections across the disciplines, placing the specialties in larger context, and illumination of data in a revealing way (Boyer, 1990, p. 17). The scholarship of integration is the synthesis of knowledge from isolated facts or other disciplines into a new meaning. The scholarship of application includes professional practice and involves the use of knowledge or creative activities for development and change. Clearly, the essentials of DNP education and practice capture these elements of scholarly expectations, reflecting the critical need for DNPs to be involved in both practice and nursing education.

Sneed et al. (1995) state that the "scholarship of application" provides a broadened view on what it means to be a scholar, and encourages innovative approaches to the evaluation and remediation of problems in the health care system. Faculty who engage in the scholarship of application further demonstrate the potential to minimize the boundaries between education and practice (Sneed et al., 1995), which is not insignificant when considering the chasm that currently exists with respect to transporting new knowledge from the bench to the bedside. With an academic grounding in EBP and translational research, the practice-oriented DNP is uniquely prepared to engage in such scholarship of integration and application. The DNP-prepared nurse is positioned to compliment the PhD, creating a research–practice continuum that ensures that the divide between the bench and the bedside is reduced.

With respect to the scholarship of teaching, while some DNPs may be inclined to teach, there will be little incentive if academic institutions do not revisit current models of faculty promotion and tenure criteria. In this setting, there would be no meaningful alleviation of the existing faculty shortage. Nursing is a practice-focused discipline, and the DNP provides an opportunity to reframe the academic mission of scholarship, teaching, and service into a contemporary context, reflective of the current culture in which health care professionals are engaging in interdisciplinary work. Achieved successfully by physician colleagues, creative academic promotional pathways can be developed for DNPs who seek to straddle both clinical practice and academia. Faculty appointments for DNPs practicing in academic medical centers and academic/practice partnerships which encourage the DNP to remain clinically engaged as well as teach are some of the solutions that have been identified by conference participants. Ultimately, DNP conference attendees expressed a clear expectation for parity among their peers—both internal and external to the discipline (DNP, LLC, 2009). Such parity will demand the restructuring of outdated tenure criteria and methods of faculty promotion while creating a new culture that is supportive of practice.

## ■ DNP POLICY

### Certification

Conference attendees have voiced concern about suggestions that they may be required to re-take certification exams (DNP, LLC, 2009). With health reform positioning the NP toward independent practice, particularly in the area of primary care, NONPF (2006) reports that the DNP represents an important evolutionary step for the preparation of the NP. Banding together with the other NP organizations, a joint statement was issued entitled Nurse Practitioner DNP Education, Certification and Titling: A Unified Statement (AANP et al., 2008). Bednash (2009) acknowledged that such a movement of specialty education toward the DNP degree has strong policy implications. Questions relative to the regulation and licensure of the DNP-prepared nurse are being debated (Guadagnino & Mundinger, 2008). National nursing leaders and physician organizations are engaging in discussions relative to the titling and credentialing of DNP-prepared APRNs, at one point even suggesting the United States Medical Licensure Exam as an effective measure of competence for advanced clinical practice (ACNP, 2008). At present, the DNP-prepared nurse engaged in clinical practice is board certified through a nationally recognized certifying entity and therefore should not be subjected to further exam requirements. Further, nursing is responsible for establishing the standards around nursing practice and should not look externally to the discipline to measure nursing competency. To this extent, there is an opportunity to remove the joint oversight for advanced nursing practice from Boards of Medicine and Boards of Pharmacy, which still exists in some states throughout the country (NCSBN, 2011). And further, as the number of DNPs in practice increases, an evaluation of practice and subsequent task analysis will serve as a foundation to drive future changes to the national certification processes (Towers, 2009).

### The Impact of State Policy on the DNP

As nurse practice acts are known to vary widely, similar variances have been identified at the state level with respect to nursing education, which are likely to impact the DNP (Bednash, 2009; Towers, 2009). In time, nursing students will move directly from the baccalaureate through to the doctoral level. However, such a transition will not be without complication (Bednash, 2009). Citing California state law as an example of state-based restriction, Bednash (2009) discussed a mandate that allows only University of California institutions to confer a doctoral degree. While many academic institutions throughout the state are actually engaged in educating nurses for advanced practice, the aforementioned will likely limit the development of DNP programs within that state. Similar circumstances have been witnessed in other states, including Minnesota, where the AACN successfully partnered with colleagues to change similar legislation that restricted the awarding of doctoral degrees (Bednash, 2009). Attention must be given to reduce any state-based restrictions that would limit the development of DNP programs across the country.

### The DNP and APRN Billing

Similarly, national restrictions exist that may contribute to the inability of DNP-prepared APRNs to be appropriately reimbursed for care they provide to patients. AACN has actively been engaging the Center for Medicare and Medicaid Services (CMS) around reimbursement issues for advanced practice (Bednash, 2009). CMS regulation defined reimbursement-eligible APRNs as those with a master's degree in nursing, thus excluding from reimbursement those who possess only doctoral-level preparedness. While Bednash (2009) attempted to convey to CMS that a doctoral degree exceeded their requirements and therefore the provided services should be reimbursed, ultimately, the involvement of AACN legal counsel was required to successfully change the regulation.

In anticipation of independent practice and the larger role that DNP-prepared APRNs will likely assume in the future, policy language must move away from restrictive language that cites the master's degree as a requirement for practice and billing, moving toward a more universal language that cites a requirement of graduate education (Bednash, 2009; Towers, 2009).

## The DNP and the Title Doctor

As the number of doctorally prepared nurses continues to increase in the clinical setting, questions around title will likely arise for DNPs, their patients, and for the organizations in which they are employed. Towers (2009) addressed inquiries around DNP utilization of the credential "doctor" by stating the title represents an academic credential and therefore its use is not protected. While the aforementioned may be true, with respect to how DNPs will communicate title, educational preparation, and role competency to patients and colleagues, it is also essential to note that academic titles indicate successful completion of a requisite course of study, but do not validate role competencies (AANP et al., 2008). Further, the state in which the DNP-prepared nurse is licensed may also impose restrictions on the use of the title "doctor" by non-physicians (Harris, 2011). Institutional restrictions may also apply as hospitals have the right to restrict the professional use of the title "doctor" by individuals with an academic title, as there is no case or statute that currently prevents them from doing so (Buppert, 2011). The DNP is licensed for practice as a registered nurse, or an APRN, and must be aware of any legislative or policy restrictions.

## ■ CONCLUSIONS

The 2009, 2010, and 2011 national DNP conference dialogues demonstrate that DNP-prepared nurses are seeking to understand the impact of this new degree upon existing nursing roles and, further, to understand themselves in the context of the larger health care community. The transformation of specialty education from the master's to the doctoral level provides an opportunity to integrate into advanced practice education what will be considered foundational competencies for members of contemporary health care teams. National specialty organizations across all advanced practice roles must evolve with the change in education, developing doctoral-level competencies and outcomes. Further, such organizations should play a role in advocating for the limitation of state-based variations in both education and legislation that will have an impact on the DNP-prepared nurse. If APRNs are to have significant and independent roles in the provision of health care in the future, a foundation that supports education, practice, and reimbursement must be established. Clearly, the DNP professional has the opportunity to impact health care outcomes and to self-direct the development of their professional practice. The intended integration of the DNP-prepared nurse from the bedside to the boardroom will be successfully realized when DNPs have secured their rightful positions within national health care organizations, policy boards, academia, and clinical practice settings.

■ REFERENCES

American Academy of Nurse Practitioners (AANP), American College of Nurse Practitioners (ACNP), Association of Faculties of Pediatric Nurse Practitioners, National Association of Nurse Practitioners in Women's Health, National Association of Pediatric Nurse Practitioners, National Conference of Gerontological Nurse Practitioners, & National Organization of Nurse Practitioner Faculties. (2008, June). *Nurse practitioner DNP education, certification, and titling: A unified statement.* Retrieved October 29, 2011, from http://www.acnpweb.org/files/public/DNP_GROUP_LETTER_6-08_w_copyright.pdf

American Association of Colleges of Nursing (AACN). (2006, October). *The essentials of doctoral education for advanced nursing practice.* Retrieved July 10, 2011, from http://www.aacn.nche.edu/dnp/pdf/essentials.pdf

American Association of Colleges of Nursing (AACN). (2009, October). *Doctor of nursing practice (DNP) programs frequently asked questions.* Retrieved October 29, 2011, from http://www.aacn.nche.edu/dnp/DNPfaq.pdf

American Association of Colleges of Nursing (AACN). (2011a, April). *DNP fact sheet.* Retrieved October 29, 2011, from http://www.aacn.nche.edu/media/FactSheets/dnp.htm

American Association of Colleges of Nursing (AACN). (2011b, April). *Faculty shortage.* Retrieved October 29, 2011, from http://www.aacn.nche.edu/media-relations/fact-sheets/nursing-faculty-shortage

American Association of Colleges of Nursing (AACN), The American Academy of Nurse Practitioners (AANP), The American College of Nurse Practitioners, The American Organization of Nurse Executives (AONE), National Organization of Nurse Practitioner Faculty (NONPF), & The Honor Society of Sigma Theta Tau International (SSTI). (2009, September–October). *National organizations: Exploring roles for DNPs* [Audio podcast]. Paper presented at the Fourth National Doctors of Nursing Practice Conference on Exemplars of DNPs in Practice and Education: Defining Ourselves, Miami, FL.

American College of Nurse Practitioners (ACNP). (2008, March). *NBME development of a certifying examination for doctors of nursing practice.* Retrieved October 29, 2011, from http://www.acnpweb.org/files/public/DNP_GROUP_LETTER_6-08_w_copyright.pdf

American Nurses Association (ANA). (2011, March). *ANA, CMA and OA activities reflected in the IOM recommendations.* Retrieved October 29, 2011, from http://www.nursingworld.org/ANA-Activities-IOM-Report

Bednash, P. (2009, September–October). *National organizations: Exploring roles for DNPs.* Paper presented at the Fourth National Doctors of Nursing Practice Conference on Exemplars of DNPs in Practice and Education: Defining Ourselves, Miami, FL.

Boyer, E. L. (1990). *Scholarship reconsidered: Priorities of the professoriate.* Princeton, NJ: Carnegie Foundation for the Advancement of Teaching.

Brown-Benedict, D. J. (2008). The doctor of nursing practice degree: Lessons from the history of the professional doctorate in other health disciplines. *Journal of Nursing Education, 47,* 448–457.

Buppert, C. (2011, February). *What legal issues lead a hospital to deny DNPs "Dr." title?* Retrieved October 29, 2011, from http://www.medscape.com/viewarticle/737862

Cronenwett, L., Dracup, K., Gray, M., McCauley, L., Meleis, A., & Salmon, M. (2011). The doctor of nursing practice: A national workforce perspective. *Nursing Outlook, 59,* 9–17.

Doctors of Nursing Practice, LLC (DNP, LLC). (2009, September–October). *Paper presented at the Second National Doctors of Nursing Practice Conference on Exemplars of DNPs in Practice and Education: Defining Ourselves, Miami, FL.* Retrieved from http://www.doctorsofnursingpractice.org/2009ConfPresentations.htm

Doctors of Nursing Practice, LLC (DNP, LLC). (2010, September–October). Paper presented at the Third National Doctors of Nursing Practice Conference on Leadership and Innovation, San Diego, CA. Retrieved from http://www.doctorsofnursingpractice.org/schedule.html

Doctors of Nursing Practice, LLC (DNP, LLC). (2011, September). Paper presented at the Fourth National Doctors of Nursing Practice Conference on Impacting Health Policy, New Orleans, LA. Retrieved from http://www.doctorsofnursingpractice.org/2011Conference.htm

Dracup, K., Cronenwett, L., Meleis, A. I., & Benner, P. (2005). Reflections on the doctorate of nursing practice. *Nursing Outlook, 53,* 177–182.

Dumas, M. A. (2009, September–October). *National organizations: Exploring roles for DNPs.* Paper presented at the Fourth National Doctors of Nursing Practice Conference on Exemplars of DNPs in Practice and Education: Defining Ourselves, Miami, FL.

Guadagnino, C., & Mundinger, M. O. (2008, May). *Growing role of nurse practitioners.* Retrieved from http://www.lifeupenn.org/Growing%20role%20of%20nurse%20practitioners.pdf

Harris, G. (2011, October). *When the nurse wants to be called doctor.* Retrieved October 29, 2011, from http://www.msnbc.msn.com/id/44748258/ns/health-health_care/t/when-nurse-wants-be-called-doctor/#.TqzJ4mBUOX4

Institute of Medicine (IOM). (2011). *The future of nursing: Leading change, advancing health.* Washington, DC: US Government Printing Office.

Meleis, A. I., & Dracup, K. (2005). The case against the DNP: History, timing, substance and marginalization. *Online Journal of Issues in Nursing, 10.*

National Council of State Boards of Nursing (NCSBN). (2011). *Regulation of advanced practice nursing.* Retrieved November 6, 2011, from https://www.ncsbn.org/2011_Regulation_of_Advanced_Practice_Nursing.pdf

National Organization of Nurse Practitioner Faculties (NONPF). (2006, October). *Statement on the practice doctorate in nursing: Response to recommendations on clinical hours and degree title.* Retrieved October 29, 2011, from http://www.nonpf.com/displaycommon.cfm?an=1&subarticlenbr=16

National Organization of Nurse Practitioner Faculties (NONPF). (2007). *NONPF recommended criteria for NP scholarly projects in the practice doctorate program.* Retrieved October 29, 2011, from http://www.nonpf.com/displaycommon.cfm?an=1&subarticlenbr=16

Neilheisel, M. B., & Kaplan, L. (2011). DNP student's clinical practice hours. *The Nurse Practitioner, 36,* 9.

Sneed, N. V., Edlund, B. J., Allred, C. A., Hickey, M., Heriot, C. S., Haight, B., & Hoffman, B. (1995). Appointment, promotion and tenure criteria to meet changing perspectives in healthcare. *Nurse Educator, 20,* 23–28.

Towers, J. (2009, September–October). *National organizations: Exploring roles for DNPs.* Paper presented at the Fourth National Doctors of Nursing Practice Conference on Exemplars of DNPs in Practice and Education: Defining Ourselves, Miami, FL.

CHAPTER 17

# Health Care Economics and Policy: Obstacles and Opportunities for Advanced Practice

Nancy C. O'Rourke, Margaret Ackerman, and Leah McKinnon-Howe

---

The introduction of the Doctor of Nursing Practice (DNP) degree has been both innovative and controversial. Challenging traditional pathways of nursing education, the DNP has the potential to better prepare nurses engaged in advanced practice for their current roles given the complexity of a changing health care system and further offer solutions to the nursing faculty shortage. The supporters of the DNP movement believe this degree will bring research and policy to the clinical realm and provide practice leadership roles in a variety of settings, including nursing executives, quality managers, clinical program directors, and nursing faculty positions.

As a result of the changing health care system, the doctorally prepared nurse must be equipped to impact health care delivery, design, and policy through education and advocacy efforts. This chapter examines the economic drivers of health care reform and its impact on the role of the DNP through discussion of legislative, regulatory, and policy barriers as well as opportunities for activism, which can assist in shaping the future role of nursing. To this end, the goal of this chapter is to familiarize the doctorally prepared nurse with the current climate of health care and suggest avenues for advancing the professional practice of nursing.

## ■ HEALTH CARE ECONOMICS

### Background

The United States leads the world in health care spending, with 16.2% of the Gross Domestic Product (GDP) going toward health care, which has contributed to an economic crisis in our country (CMS, 2010a). With more dollars being spent on acute care and only 3% being spent on public health, the health care system in the United States is disproportionate and dysfunctional. As a result, the country is ranked by the World Health Organization as 37th in quality and fairness of national health care systems (CMS 2010b; World Health 2000).

Medicare, which was established in 1966 to provide insurance coverage for the elderly, is dependent on supply-sensitive care. Supply-sensitive care refers to services where the supply of a specific resource has a major influence on its utilization rates (Wenneberg, Fisher, Goodman, & Skinner, 2008). Physician visits, specialty referrals, hospitalizations, diagnostic testing, and intensive care unit stays are examples of supply sensitive care, and such services may also result in significant regional variation in quality and expense. Spending for Medicare recipients has been highest at end of life, with 32% of all Medicare dollars being spent on patients with chronic illness with an anticipated life expectancy of less than 2 years. As such, chronic illness and longevity have led to exorbitant Medicare spending, the majority of which is allocated toward physician and hospital fees (Wenneberg et al., 2008). In 2006, a small Texas community was documented to be the second most expensive health care market in the country. In that community, Medicare spending was almost twice the national average, reportedly $15,000 per enrollee (Gawande, 2009). Physicians owned hospitals as well as expensive imaging equipment. Rates of surgery were higher than in other demographic areas, creating a lucrative environment for physician investors, since under the Medicare fee for service (FFS) reimbursement structure volume generates income (Gawande). This experience highlights the problems with the current FFS payment system, which incentivizes volume rather than quality of care or healthy outcomes.

Despite the millions of dollars being spent on health care and the near bankruptcy of the federal government, clinical outcomes are poor. In fact, in comparing health outcomes to other nations statistically, the United States ranks lower with respect to basic measures, including infant mortality and the management of chronic disease. A 2008 report by the Commonwealth Fund, *Death Before Age 75 from Conditions That Are at Least Partially Modifiable with Effective Medical Care*, concluded that the United States is the worst of nineteen wealthy countries. The number of adults age seventy five or below who die from curable illness was almost twice as high in the United States as compared to countries that do the best on this measure (Commonwealth Fund, 2008). Most shocking of all, of the 23 wealthiest countries, the American health care system ranks last in infant mortality (Table 17.1), with rates doubling those of Japan and Sweden (Reid, 2007).

In addition to rising Medicare costs, private health insurance premiums, as well as unemployment rates, have risen, leading many to lose health benefits and creating socioeconomic disparity in our health care system. Increasing numbers of Americans are without basic health care, while others have state-of-the-art care for the same conditions. High insurance

**TABLE 17.1  Infant Mortality Rates, 2005**

| Country | Deaths per 1,000 Births |
| --- | --- |
| Sweden | 2.4 |
| Japan | 2.8 |
| Norway | 3.1 |
| France | 3.6 |
| Germany | 3.9 |
| Switzerland | 4.2 |
| United Kingdom | 5.1 |
| Canada | 5.3 |
| Poland | 6.4 |
| United States | 6.8 |

*Source:* OECD, Health at a Glance, 2007.

co-payments and medication costs have resulted in some not seeking care for chronic illnesses (Himmelstein, Warren, & Woolhandler, 2009). End-of-life care is especially impacted by health care trends, as preventable but untreated medical conditions correlate with increased acute care hospitalizations and the treatment of chronic illnesses in the hospital setting. The public's perception that health care spending is responsible for large and ultimately unsustainable deficits in the federal budget has forced the government to take corrective action to address a crumbling system (Dodaro, 2008).

### Reform Initiatives: The Affordable Care Act

After 20 years of political debate and disagreement over a national health plan, the Affordable Care Act (ACA) was passed in 2010. The passage of this legislation indicates the urgency to reform the U.S. health care system. The ACA will provide insurance for an additional 32 million Americans, but millions will still lack coverage (CBO, 2010). A shortage of primary care providers coupled with a lack of providers who are accepting new patients is likely to contribute to longer wait for primary care appointments and ultimately create decreased access to care. Even with coverage, the deductibles, copayments, and medication expenses will continue to increase out of consumers' pocket costs, again leading patients to choose not to seek out the services for chronic conditions (Doty, Edward, & Holmgren, 2005; Himmelstein et.al., 2009).

The ACA recognizes the need for increased access and changes to reimbursement structures that shift from traditional fee for service, rewarding volume and services, to a global payment system that focuses on prevention, quality of care, and outcome data. Funding for this new health insurance entitlement program, one that will insure 30 million people beginning in 2014, must come entirely from lowering Medicare payment expenses (Master, 2011a).

Finally, economic development, job creation, and an end to decades of wage suppression caused in part by unsustainable increases in employer health care costs depend on a leap in efficiency and quality that both depends on, and is necessary for, Medicare and Medicaid savings (Master). This has taken a very long time; however, there is now an emerging consensus that in order to achieve these substantial savings, there must be a laser beam focus on those Medicare and Medicaid beneficiaries who historically have had the greatest needs, poorest quality of service and, as a result, are creating the highest cost to the system. These beneficiaries are referred to as the *12/60* population; the identifiable 12% of beneficiaries, who account for 60% of public payer expenditures (Master, 2011b).

### ■ OPPORTUNITIES

Legislation and regulations that will change the shape of health care are agressively being developed and, in some instances, nurses may not be included in the dialogue. Looking toward the future and providing health insurance to all, the Institute of Medicine (IOM) report in 2009 has advocated for the removal of regulations and statutes that create barriers to nursing practice and further has supported the development of regional nursing coalitions to address education and utilization of the nursing workforce nationally (IOM, 2009). Across the country, nursing leadership coalitions are forming to respond to the recommendations of the IOM report. Regional Action Committees (RACs) representing the full spectrum of nursing specialties are supported by the Robert Wood Johnson Foundation, and are uniting around this work nationally. The potential for all nurses to advance their professional practice has never been greater. The numbers of nurses and advanced practice nurses is the largest in history and as we gain political capitol and momentum, change is inevitable. The economic downturn in health care and the passage of the ACA has had a huge impact on the nursing profession. The cohort of Americans who do not have health insurance on any given day numbers 45 million—approximately 15% of the U.S. population (Reid, 2009). As a result, many Americans do not get elective care because of copays. In hospitals, patients have shorter lengths of stay and higher acuity. All this has resulted in beds closing and fewer jobs for nurses in acute care hospitals. The shortage of primary care physicians in the United States is expected to worsen (Bodenheimer & Pham 2010). Chronic conditions also pose a major challenge to the sustainability of the health care system. According to Dartmouth Atlas of Health Care, the majority of care for people with chronic illness is given in the inpatient setting, resulting in significant cost burden (Wenneberg et al., 2008). This increased number of hospitalizations and specialty visits has resulted in fragmentation of care, which leads to poor clinical outcomes and higher costs. Better care coordination has been shown to result in lower costs and improved outcomes (Robinson, 2010). However, primary care is so difficult to access that one in five patients urgently seek care in the emergency department (IOM, 2009). There are currently less than 287 thousand primary care physicians in the United States. The number of nurse practitioners and physician assistants is rising, with 83 thousand nurse practitioner and 23 thousand physician assistants providing one fourth of the primary care coverage in the United States (Naylor & Kurtzmass, 2010). Countries with better primary care access have better clinical outcomes (Starfield et al., 2005), so in the United States, unless the number change with respect to access to care, we can expect to see a further decline in clinical outcomes.

Advanced practice nurses are faced with the biggest challenge of all, as health care reform is written that excludes nurse practitioners and clinical specialists as primary care providers from participating as equals in the new business models such as the Accountable Care Organizations (ACOs) and Medical Homes. In 1997, the Balanced Budget Act supported Care Coordination as a means to reduce the cost of health care (Robinson). Demonstration projects using care coordination models supported decreased Medicare expenditures or increased quality of care for health care services and beneficiary satisfaction. Nurses have taken a central role in care coordination for decades, focusing on patient education, prevention, and self-management of chronic disease. Further, Care Coordination has clearly been shown to benefit those who have numerous contacts with health care systems (Robinson).

As the ACA will shift from a fee for service structure to a global payment structure, greater focus will likely be placed on community based care for people with chronic illnesses. Community health nurses presently play a major role in managing patients with chronic illnesses in the community and in health centers. However of late, changing homecare regulations have resulted in fewer reimbursable visits for homecare nursing and higher unemployment in that specialty. There will be many opportunities for nurses to impact health care as Patient-Centered Home Care Models and ACOs are developed. Effective lobbying and passage of legislation and recognizing and reimbursing the care provided by nursing in these community models should be a focus of policymakers and nursing advocates. In this area, DNPs can use their leadership skills and advocate for change, as well as developing innovative programs to meet the needs of a changing heath care system.

The ACA also has expanded Title VIII of the Public Health Service Act, which is an expansion of the loan repayment and scholarship program. Under the expansion of Title VIII, there are increased monies available to nursing students and more repayment options (Webb & Marshall, 2010). The ACA provided a 50 million dollar grant through the department of Health and Human Services to fund Nurse Managed Health Clinics and also established 45 commissions, committees, boards, and advisory panels to advise the Secretary of Health and Human Services and Congress on a number of issues, including the role of nursing in health care delivery (Webb & Marshall, 2010). Nursing education must shift focus from hospital based patient care to care management of patients in other settings and focus on being an integral part of an interdisciplinary team in ACOs.

Nursing administrators have felt the economic impact on nursing as they struggle to staff a changing paradigm. Hospital staffing ratios are changing with new laws that require safe staffing ratios, while hospital admissions are down. Quality measures to evaluate the impact of nursing interventions on patient outcomes are being incorporated. In Canada, a system called Health Outcomes for Better Information and Care is used. This standardized approach for collecting and organizing data and information on health outcomes allows administrators to guide allocation of care. DNPs bringing theory and clinical innovations to nursing practice are well positioned to be leaders in the evaluation and collection of nursing quality outcome data.

These escalating health care costs and increasing demands for health care services, driven in large part by the movement toward universal health care, continue to force policy makers to examine through public policy, changes that can be made to control costs and maintain quality. The passage of the Affordable Care Act presents us with the first meaningful opportunity to change health care since public insurance was introduced in the early 1900s. Under the ACA, the opportunities for DNPs to take leadership roles and direct the future of nursing are endless. Be it the development of innovative models of care, changing bedside practice, educating future nurses, producing quality outcome data, or leading organizations through the change, DNPs have a clear role in transforming nursing and with their educational preparation and skill sets, are well prepared to accept this challenge.

## ■ OBSTACLES

The enactment of the Affordable Care Act is predicted to attract millions of patients, previously uninsured, into the already ailing U.S. health care system. Access to care is now at critical mass. Increased demand, a shortage of primary care providers, and legislation that mandates health care for all have created numerous opportunities for APRN roles to develop and flourish. Much of the discussion of universal health care focuses on the costs of providing care and reimbursement to providers. In 2009, the IOM commissioned the Robert Wood Johnson Foundation (RWJF) to bring together a group of stakeholders including nurses, physicians, corporate representatives, academics, and innovators of health care change who outlined the need for regulations and statutes that create barriers to NP to be removed. The report, *The Future of Nursing*, speaks to the role nurses should play in health care reform and is a compelling statement of how nurses should be engaged to meet the health needs of the nation (IOM, 2011).

Accordingly, advanced practice nurses have made great legislative strides in this era of health care reform. A key example is the role of nurse practitioners in Massachusetts. In 2006, under tremendous pressure from the federal government to channel uncompensated care funds toward preventative care rather than acute care, Massachusetts led the country in health care reform efforts by enacting Chapter 58, a law that mandates health coverage for all Massachusetts residents. This was the most ambitious health reform legislation to date and laid the foundation for the Affordable Care Act (ACA). The enactment of this Chapter 58 in

Massachusetts brought 500,000 patients, previously uninsured, into the health care system (Massachusetts Connector, 2011). The increased demand for services, particularly primary care, spurred the APRN profession to legislatively define "primary care provider," including nurse practitioners in the definition and further mandating insurers to offer their services as a reimbursable option to subscribers. With approximately 6,000 nurse practitioners in Massachusetts, this move had the potential to exponentially increase access to care.

As the reform movement spread across the states, APRN groups sought to capitalize on the opportunity to advance practice. Vermont successfully changed regulations to eliminate supervision of APRNs by physicians. New York APRNs gained a legislative victory with the passage of global signature authority and Florida APRNs were supported by the Federal Trade Commission in their longstanding battle with their respective Medical Societies over prescriptive practice (J. Elwell, personal communication, June 23, 2011; FTC, 2011). In short, the mandate of universal health care has positioned the nursing community to practice to their fullest extent and to be active participants in health care reform.

Despite a political and legislative climate ripe for change, many advanced practice nurses still experience significant barriers to practice because of outdated state statutes and regulations and insurer policies regarding reimbursement of nursing practice. Certified Registered Nurse Anesthetists (CRNAs) continue to have significant opposition from the Anesthesiologists in obtaining prescriptive privileges. Despite the clear need for behavioral health services, clinical psychiatric specialists (CNSs) and psychiatric nurse practitioners have great difficulty in states where collaboration and supervision are required, as the numbers of psychiatrists willing to work with them is declining. Given the implementation of the ACA and the current need to redesign health care, APRNs are well positioned to overcome some of these barriers.

The National Nursing Centers Consortium (NNCC), an organization comprised of nurse managed non-profit health centers, recognized an opportunity and began an advocacy campaign to support and sustain the financially embattled nurse managed health centers. As a direct result of their work, the Pennsylvania Department of Public Welfare (PDPW) examined the use of nurses in their network. The request for proposal from PDPW asked organizations to describe their policy on the use of all health care providers and specifically cited using nurses and nurse practitioners to the "fullest extent of their education and training." Because of NNCC's grassroots campaign and advocacy, Medicaid managed care plans sought to partner with nursing and APRNs for a more efficient and effective delivery of health care (Ritter, 2010).

Much of the discussion of universal health care focuses on the costs of providing care and reimbursement to providers. In this vein, states began to develop alternative payment models that would promote quality and, it is hoped, decrease costs, while providing better access to health care for all populations. Payers began to evaluate the concepts of "global payment" and "accountability," requiring both providers and payers to be transparent in their data reporting methods. The ACA proposes models that eliminate the fee for service system, using instead a global payment or capitated system (Massachusetts Health Care Quality and Cost Council Final Report, 2009). Two of these models include the Patient Centered Medical Home (PCMH) Model and the ACO. PCMH was originally designed for chronically ill pediatric patients who require most of their care in the home but has expanded to include other chronic populations, such as the elderly and the severely physically disabled. In both of these models, a "team" approach is used, and patients with complex medical issues are managed by a team of clinicians as determined by the primary care provider.

The medical community (Commonwealth Care Alliance Clinical Group), seeking a model of care that solidified the physician as the "captain of the ship," has coined the term

"Medical Home" and "Patient Centered Primary Care." The premise that only a physician could direct the team care became the mantra and it would ensure that medicine had a strong foothold in primary care. Other health care providers such as nurse practitioners and physician assistants could remain part of the team, but the proposed model would clearly relegate them to a subordinate role. Both of the aforementioned models are physician-led, and in this capacity the MD functions as the primary care provider. In many states, nurse practitioners have been excluded from the panel of primary care providers. Nursing, in general, has been relegated to the role of "care management," coordinating and overseeing the care of medically complex patients and those with chronic diseases such as hypertension and diabetes. Data reporting of quality and outcomes would occur at the aggregate practice level, making nursing's contributions once again the "invisible" in the outcome measures.

At Commonwealth Care Alliance Clinical Group in Boston, Massachusetts, an innovative Medicaid managed Senior Care Options program for fragile geriatric patient care is coordinated and delivered by advanced practice nurses. Advanced practice nurses partner with primary care physicians and manage care for very complex fragile elders living in the community. Over 70% of the patients they care for have been designated by Commonwealth of Massachusetts standards as nursing home certifiable, but all but 1% are living in the community with the support of enhanced primary care and care coordination provided by an interdisciplanary team at Commonwealth Care Clinical Group (CCCG). In this program, the NPs assume a dual role as direct care provider and insurance care manager, providing the lead on the delivery of primary care in the home, managing hospitalizations and skilled nursing facility stays, co-coordinating home services, and further authorizing all necessary durable medical equipment, specialty appointments, and transportation for a range of needs. Leaders of the inter-disciplinary team, the nurse practitioners arrange for in-home podiatry, behavioral health, physical therapy, palliative care, point of care testing, and a host of other services. The members and their families enjoy a higher quality of life and have 55% of hospitalizations than that predicted by Medicare risk scores (Lewin, 2009).

Rehospitalization rates are 86% of that found in the general far more healthy national Medicare population (Master, 2011b). The NPs are the anchor of the primary care team, but because of the legislative barriers in some states, they are precluded from being designated the primary care provider of record.

Although the state of Massachusetts recognized the NP as a primary care provider, it was not until recently, that the National Council on Quality Assurance (NCQA) recognized PCMH models led by nurses. As such, advanced practice nurses at the Commonwealth Care Alliance who were serving in a primary care provider role were relegated to the status of "care manager" and unable to qualify for reimbursement as PCPs. As the concept of ACOs becomes the reality, the premise that only a physician can direct the team has been challenged. National NP organizations lobbied strongly for provider neutral language, inclusion in legislation, and regulation and acceptance by accrediting bodies like NCQA, Joint Commission on Accreditation of Healthcare Organizations, and Utilization Review Accreditation Committee. Despite gaining such recognition, the number of NP led PCMH models and nurse managed health centers is small. However, across the country, nurse managed clinics and NP-led private practices are successful models of care and are producing the types of quality outcomes demanded by ACOs, demonstrating that cost effectiveness and quality of care could be achieved without a physician at the helm. Outdated state laws restricted advanced nursing practice but without clear rationale for doing so. Studies clearly show that patient care does not decline in states with less regulation on advanced practice, and a growing body of evidence supports the quality of care provided by advanced practice nurses (Bauer, 2010).

Looking toward restructuring the business of health care, the Center for Medicaid and Medicare Services (CMS) proposed a model that theoretically would save money and has become a major focal point for health reform. They had been monitoring health care systems that were shifting the way they provided primary care. Experts like Dr. Elliot Fisher at Dartmouth proposed a model of team care, in which prevention and quality should produce savings. And if savings were realized, the insurers, the health care system, and the individual providers would share in the profits. If there were no savings, then of course, they would all share in the losses as well (Fisher, Goodman, Skinner, & Bronner, 2009).

ACOs are legally defined entities consisting of groups of a primary care providers affiliated with hospitals or another business entity that oversees payments from insurers under the proposed global payment system. Each patient would represent a dollar payment per month or per year to the ACO. The ACO would be the fiduciary body that dispensed the health care monies to physicians or practices based on quality care at fixed reimbursement rates (Fisher et al., 2009). This model was first developed as a response to the universal problem of poor quality, waste, and high costs in fragmented fee for service care to Medicare beneficiaries with chronic illnesses. Recognizing that FFS is the way most Medicare beneficiaries will receive care in the United States for the foreseeable future, Section 3022 of the ACA established a Medicare Shared Savings Program for hospital and related physician practices, if they come together as "ACOs" as a way to achieve the *accountability* and the focus to improve care and reduce costs. The ACO does not recognize the nurse practitioner as a primary care provider, but leaves it to the discretion of the physician whether a nurse practitioner should be included on the team.

Independent Provider Organizations (IPOs) and hospital corporations directed the discussion of how to shift to global payment and vertically integrate the flow of health care reimbursement dollars. The structure of payment needed to be more transparent, equitable, and based in the quality movement, and the development of a payment model that controls reimbursement through data and outcome measures seemed desirable. The concept of "ACOs" began to take shape.

Nurses have the ability to influence health policy but must first recognize opportunities for actions that create momentum toward wider spread change. Individual action and involvement with coalitions made up of nursing and non-nursing organizations can have widespread influence in the health policy discussion. Further, the identification of statutory, regulatory, and organizational practice barriers that devalue or undervalue the care that nurses provide represents significant opportunities to educate and influence legislators and policy makers, as well as consumers.

Barriers to practice occur on many levels and range from inadequate knowledge of state and federal nursing regulations by the nursing community to consumer perceptions of nursing practice. Nursing is making progress in the political arena. Every patient encounter presents an opportunity to educate the consumer about the uniqueness of nursing education and training, and the ability of the nurse to provide high-quality patient-centered health care across the care continuum. There is tremendous confusion among consumers regarding the various roles, titles, and credentials held by professional nurses. Measures that increase nursing visibility are key to garnering consumer recognition and support of the various nursing roles. Over the past few years the professional nursing community has partnered with Johnson and Johnson in a publicity campaign to increase the public's awareness of the nursing profession. Patient experience surveys support the perception that the public views nurses as more trustworthy and caring than physicians; however, the consumer is still not aware of all the roles that nurses play in health care. Nurses at the bedside, nurse educators, and nurses serving in a leadership capacity should be advocating for the profession by educating the public during every encounter.

In addition to consumer misconceptions regarding nursing care, there are variations in nurse practice acts from state to state, and the advanced practice registered nurses (APRNs) are often restricted by the policies of third party payers and the organizations that employ them. Such policies are unnecessarily restrictive and limit patients' access to care. Lower rates of reimbursement for the care provided by APRNs and refusal to reimburse for care management services provided by nurses are two examples of policies that negatively affect the consumer's ability to access care and manage chronic disease effectively.

Understanding the policies employed by third party payers and organizations that employ nurses and their impact on patient care would allow nurses from the bedside to the boardroom to be proactive in effecting policy change. Nursing leaders, educators, and administrators who are actively engaged in policy and program development may have the greatest ability to change institutional policies during this pivotal time in health care reform. Educating the nursing community around the legislative and policy process is integral to creating an environment that supports nursing practice. To date, there are three nurses serving in the U.S. Congress. Dr. Mary Wakefield, RN, is the new administrator of Health Resources and Service Administration and is a strong advocate of advanced practice nurses (Hahn, 2010). However, we must recognize that we still have much work to do within our own ranks, if we hope to be as proficient and effective as our physician colleagues in the policy and lobbying arenas.

There is significant variability among the statutes and regulations that govern advanced nursing practice from state to state and are a result of structural flaws in the U.S. health care system (IOM, 2011, p. 96). The laws and regulations that govern nursing practice have not kept up with the growth of the nursing profession. As a result, today's nursing competency extends far beyond its limited scope of practice and authority (IOM, 2011, p. 97). Restrictions on nursing's scope of practice may limit or prohibit the advanced practice nurses from practicing independently, requiring them to be supervised by or linked to a physician in some capacity, such as for prescribing medications, admitting patients to hospitals, ordering and interpreting diagnostic tests, performing certain exams, and ordering and authorizing home care and hospice services.

In the IOM's report on the Future of Nursing, Barbara Safreit points out that:

> because all states base their licensure on the underlying principle that the practice of medicine encompasses both the ability and the legal authority to treat all human conditions, the scope of practice for APRNs (and other health professionals) are exercises in legislative exception making, a "carving out" of small, politically achievable spheres of practice authority from the universal domain of medicine. (IOM, 2011, p. 97)

As the contributions of the nursing community to health care reform have become more evident, so has the opposition to the expansion of scope of practice regulations that would increase access to primary care services. Some members of the medical community have viewed APRNs as competitors, with increased tension surrounding professional practice boundaries. The issue is not limited to physicians and nurses; it encompasses many disciplines including psychiatry, dentistry, and physical therapy (IOM, 2011, p. 107).

Across the nation, state Boards of Registration in Medicine (BORM) have begun to seek changes in BORM regulations that impact these other disciplines, in an attempt to further carve out areas of practice solely relegated to physicians. This has raised issues regarding violations of restraint of trade laws, with involvement of the Federal Trade Commission to settle these disputes. The ability of nursing to recognize and respond to these assaults on practice remains limited. As the nation moves forward with health care reform and competition increases among all health care provider groups, the nursing profession will need to be familiar with all regulatory and statutory language affecting nursing practice in order to protect the nurse's ability to practice to the fullest extent of his or her education and training.

The Consensus Model document on advanced practice regulation exemplifies how the nursing regulatory community has come together to provide a stronger, more unified platform from which nursing can argue that they should be included in health reform decisions and solutions. The aforementioned are based on the premise of practicing nursing to the fullest extent of the education and training (Stanley, Werner, & Apple, 2009).

The Concensus Model document establishes guidelines for licensing, accreditation, certification, and education for the four advanced practice roles: CRNAs, CNSs, certified nurse practitioners, and certified nurse midwives. It further clarifies the scope and role of advanced practice nursing, which will help consumers and policy makers to better understand the pivotal role that these providers can play as the demand for qualified providers of care increases, in a newly reformed health care system (Stanley et al.). The challenge that lies before us is the widespread implementation of the model, which will become the responsibility of nursing leaders and individual organizations and put nursing in a position to achieve the goals of health care reform (Stanley et al.).

The nursing community, through the IOM report and the development of Regional Action Coalitions supported by the RWJF, is identifying policies and practices that have sought to break down barriers to nursing practice. It is now developing strategies that are clinically relevant, rooted in practice, and transformative in nature to address the need for change to state nurse practice acts that are outdated and restrictive. In order to realize the goals of health care reform, nursing leaders must work with individual state organizations, regulatory and licensing boards, and policy makers to clearly define nursing practice and eliminate outdated language in statutes and regulation that creates unnecessary restrictions on nursing at all levels of practice. The formation of these coalitions is the first step in nursing coming together as a political force, and the realization that our greatest strength lies in our ability to reach consensus and speak as one voice.

The nursing community continues to face enormous challenges as it responds to the well-funded, organized, and experienced American Medical Association (AMA). The IOM report on the future of nursing cited the example of the AMA-sponsored Scope of Practice Partnership (SOPP), which was jointly formed in 2006 with six other medical specialty organizations to defeat proposed legislation in several states that would expand scope of practice for allied health professionals, including nurses (IOM, 2011, p. 110). Distributed by the AMA, resolutions, position papers, and petitions that seek to limit scope of practice of all health care providers other than physicians have been prolific and deliberate in the past 5 years. To that end, the AMA created and released a set of 10 documents entitled the AMA Scope of Practice Data Series (2009) with the intent of using the material to educate policy makers and others on the "qualifications of particular limited licensure health care professions," including audiologists, dentists, naturopaths, nurse anesthetists, nurse practitioners, optometrists, pharmacists, physical therapists, podiatrists, and psychologists. The purpose of these reports was to "provide the background information necessary to challenge the state and national advocacy campaigns of limited licensure health care providers who seek unwarranted scope-of-practice expansions that may endanger the health and safety of patients" (AMA, 2009, p. 4).

In response to the AMA's campaign and SOPP documents, several nursing and non-nursing organizations have formed working coalitions to help to protect the role of nursing and other health providers. Thirty-five organizations came together in 2006 to form the Coalition for Patient Rights (n.d.). This advocacy group represents a diverse group of health care professionals, including advanced practice and registered nurses, audiologists, chiropractors, foot and ankle surgeons, naturopathic doctors, occupational therapists, physical therapists, and psychologists and has been a vocal advocate for consumer access to health care services and choice of health care providers. Their rebuttal position statement entitled *Health Care Professionals Urge Cooperative Patient Care; Oppose SOPP & AMA Resolution 814* highlights the need for the SOPP member organizations to cease their divisive efforts and work with other groups of health care providers to improve access to a wide variety of health care professionals who deliver affordable, effective health care to patients.

Given the clear need for change in our health care system, framed in significant opposition from the AMA, nursing must be prepared to measure and articulate the value of the care they provide through quality data collection and the use of health information technology.

In order for the nursing profession to fully realize its potential as full partners in the health care reform process, its members must develop the leadership skills and competencies that allow them to serve as patient advocates, clinicians, researchers, nurse educators, nurse administrators and executives, nurse informaticisits, and health policy experts. There are common competencies shared by the various nursing and ARPN roles, which serve as the foundation for an array of leadership opportunities including knowledge of the care delivery system. Other competencies can be tailored to the particular nursing role, context, place, or time (IOM, 2011, p. 224). These skills provide a broad base of support for grass roots activism, which is needed to monitor and respond to the wave of policy initiatives created by the aforementioned resolutions and partnerships within the larger health care community. That being said, the strength in any organization lies in the support of its individual members.

Nursing professionals can further develop leadership skills in a variety of ways including advanced education and training in formal leadership programs, mentorship, and involvement in the health policy process. The American Organization of Nurse Executives (AONE) competencies illustrate that communication, relationship building, knowledge of the health care environment, foundational thinking skills, personal journey disciplines, systems thinking, succession planning, change management, and business skills are important areas of development for the nursing community (AONE, 2011). These traits and skills are not inherent in all nurses and need to be developed much like the clinical skills that were acquired early in a nurse's education. The foundation for much of this work is experiential and requires further education and training (see the Appendix at the end of this chapter).

## ■ CONCLUSION

The impact of spiraling health care costs in the United States has contributed to an economic recession and the passage of the first meaningful health reform legislation—the Affordable Care Act (ACA)—since 1965. The ACA has many implications for nursing and provides opportunities for the DNP to have a major impact on health care in the arenas of advanced practice, education, administration, research, and policy. Advanced practice nurses need to advocate for legislation that will enable independent practice legislation. Nursing leadership must note emerging trends and develop polices and standards that measure outcomes. Nursing educators must make curriculum revisions that focus on roles that will prepare student nurses for the future, such as interdisciplinary teamwork, community based nursing, and care management. Policy initiatives should be integrated into the curricula of all nursing schools to develop a better understanding of the implications of legislation and policy on nursing practice. We must seize the opportunity to collaborate effectively within and across disciplines, work in teams, and be effective patient advocates. While nursing practice is grounded in the basic tenets of ethical care, we must have leaders who develop theories of innovation, expand the foundations for quality and safety improvements, and seek out opportunities to contribute to ongoing discussion of heath care policy and reform efforts (IOM, 2011, p. 224). The opportunity for the nursing profession to come into its own has never been more timely. Developing well-prepared nurse leaders and a sufficient workforce that is able to respond to the health care needs of the nation is the key to our future success.

We are at a "tipping point" not only in effecting significant reform to our health care system, but in the contributions and direction of nursing in the future. As a profession, nursing must organize and speak with one voice and one purpose. With the impetus of the IOM report and the development of Regional Action Coalitions, this work has begun both at the state and national levels. However, nursing leaders and organizations will need to focus on having a strong presence in all of these legislative and policy initiatives. We must move forward the development of policy and advocacy efforts and not allow health care reform to obliterate the professional advances made by nursing over the last 30 years. We should heed the words of Florence Nightingale: "Unless we are making progress in our nursing every year, every month, every week, take my word for it we are going back" (Nightingale, 1914).

# ■ REFERENCES

American Medical Association. (2009, October). *AMA scope of practice data series: Nurse practitioners.* Chicago, IL: American Medical Association.

*AONE nurse executive competencies (nurse executive competencies).* (2011). Retrieved from http://www.aone.org/resources/leadership%20tools/PDFs/AONE_NEC.pdf

Bauer, J. C. (2010). Nurse practitioners as an underutilized resource for health reform: Evidence-based demonstrations of cost-effectiveness. *JAANP, 22*(4), 228–231.

*Best on Board.* Retrieved August 5, 2011, from www.bestonboard.org/website/home.html

Bodenheimer, T., & Pham, H. (2010). Primary care: current problems and proposed solutions. *Health Affairs, 29*(5), 893–899.

*Coalition of patient rights* (CPR). (n.d.). Retrieved from http://www.patientsrightscoalition.org/

CBO. (2010). *Cost estimates for the 111th congress: H.R. 4872, Reconciliation Act of 2010 (final healthcare legislation).* Retrieved June 28, 2010, from http://www.cbo.gov/costestimates/CEbrowse.cfm

CMS (centers for Medicare and Medicaid Services). (2010a*). National health expenditure data: Historical.* Retrieved July 18, 2011, from http://www.cms.gov/nationalhealthexpenditure-data/o2_nationalhealthaccountshistorical.asp#top

CMS. (2010b). *Table 2. National health expenditures aggregate amounts and average annual percent change by type of expenditure: Selected calendar years 1960–2008.* Retrieved July 18, 2011, from National Health Accounts Historical.asp# top of page.

Dodaro, G. (2008). *Long-term fiscal challenge driven primarily by health care.* Washington, DC: GAO.

Doty, M. M., Edwards, J. N., & Holmgren, A. L. (2005). *Seeing red: Americans driven into debt by medical bills: results from a national survey.* New York, NY: The Commonwealth Fund.

Federal Trade Commission. (2011). *Letter to Daphne Campbell, House of Representatives. Florida, March 22, 2011.* Retrieved April 18, 2012, from www.ftc.gov/os/2011/03/V110004campbell-florida.pdf

Fischer, E., Goodman, D., Skinner, J., & Bronner, K. (2009). *Health care spending, quality and outcomes: more isn't always better. A Dartmouth Atlas project brief.* Hanover, NH: The Dartmouth atlas. Retrieved from http://www.bing.com/search?q=dartmouth+atlas+data&src=IE- SearchBox&FORM=IE8SRC

Gawande, A. (2009). The cost conundrum: what a Texas town can teach about health care. *The New Yorker,* June 1, 86–104.

Hahn, J. (2010). Integrating professionalism and political awareness into the curriculum. *Nurse Educator, 3*(35), 110–113.

Himmelstein, D., Thorne, D., Warren, E., & Woolhandler, S. (2009). Medical bankruptcy in the United States, 2007: Results of a national study. *American Journal of Medicine, 122*(8), 742–746.

*H-160.947 Physician Assistants and Nurse Practitioners (AMA resolution).* (n.d.). Retrieved from https://ssl3.ama-assn.org/apps/ecomm/ PolicyFinderForm.pl?site=www.amaassn.org&uri=%2fresources%2fdoc%2fPolicyFinder%2fpolicy files%2fHnE%2 fH-160.947. HTM

Institute of Medicine. (2009). *Distinguished nurse scholar-in-residence.* Retrieved August 5, 2011, from www.iom.edu/ Activities/Education/NurseScholar.aspx.

Institute of Medicine. (2011). *The future of nursing-leading change, advancing health.* Washington, DC: The National Academies Press.

Lewin, D. (2009). Associates study 2009/SNP Alliance, study done at Commonwealth Care Alliance.

Massachusetts Health Care Quality and Cost Council Final Report. (2009). *Roadmap to cost containment.* Retrieved from http://www.mass.gov/Ihqcc/docs/roadmap_to_cost_containment_nov-2009.pdf

Massachusetts Connector. (2011). Retrieved from https://www.mahealthconnector.org/portal/site/connector/menuitem.ab426e09b06869c2dbef6f47d7468a0c

Master, R. J. (2011). *Update on a rapidly changing policy environment and its relationship to us.* Scripts from the Doc. 87: January 28, 2011.

Master, R. J. (2011). *Some numbers to share.* Scripts from the Doc. 101: August 12, 2011.

Naylor, M., & Kurtzmass, E. T. (2010). The role of nurse practitioners in reinventing primary care. *Health Affairs (Millwood), 29*(5), 893–899. Retrieved July 18, 2011, from http://www.ncbi.nlm.nih.gov/pubmed/20439877

Nightingale, F. (1914) Retrieved from http://allnurses.com/general-nursing-discussion/ideas-nursing-quotes-124448.html

Reid, T. R. (2009). *The healing of America: A global quest for better, cheaper and fairer health care.* New York, NY: Penguin Press.

Ritter, A. (2010). *Community-based health centers: nurse practitioners contributing to access* (pp. 305–316). New York, NY: Springer.

Robert Wood Johnson foundation (Scholars, fellows, and leadership programs). Retrieved August 5, 2011, from http://www.rwjfleaders.org/programs/robert-wood-johnson-foundation-executive-nurse-fellows-program

Robert Wood Johnson foundation (Health policy fellows). Retrieved August 5, 2011, from http://www.healthpolicyfellows.org/fellowship_info.php

Robert Wood Johnson foundation (Investigator awards in health policy and research). Retrieved August 5, 2011, from http://www.investigatorawards.org/

Robinson, K. (2010). Care co-ordination: A priority for health reform. *Public Politics and Nursing Practice, 11*(4), 266–274. Retrieved August 7, 2011, from ppn.sagepub.com at Univ Massachusetts Boston

Sigma Theta Tau International (Nurse Faculty Leadership Acadamy). Retrieved August 5, 2011, from http://www.nursingsociety.org/leadershipinstitute/nursefaculty/Pages/default.aspx

Stanley, J. M., Werner, K. E., & Apple, K. (2009). Positioning advanced practice registered nurses for health care reform: Consensus on APRN regulation. *Journal of Professional Nursing, 25*(6), 340 doi:10.1016/j.profnurs.2009.10.001

Starfield, B., Shi, L., Grover, A., & Macinko, J. (2005). The effects of specialist supply on populations' health: Assessing the evidence. *Health Affairs, 24*, 97–107 (published online March 15, 2005; 10.1377/hlthaff.w4.184).

The Wharton School, University of Pennsylvania (Wharton Nursing Leaders Program). Retrieved August 5, 2011, from http://executiveeducation.wharton.upenn.edu/open-enrollment/health-care-programs/Fellows-Program-Management-Nurse-Executives.cfm

The Commonwealth Fund, Multinational Comparisons of Health Systems Data. (November 2006). Retrieved from www.commonwealthfund.org

Webb, J., & Marshall, D. (2010). Healthcare reform and nursing: What does it mean? Guest editoral. *Journal of Nursing Administration, 40*(9), 345–347. Retrieved July 31, 2010, from http://ovidsp.tx.ovid.com.ezproxy.lib.umb.edu/sp-

Wenneberg, J. E., Fisher, E. S., Goodman, D. C., & Skinner, J. S. (2008). *Tracking the care of patients with severe chronic illness: The Dartmouth atlas of health care 2008*. Lebanon, NH: The Dartmouth Institute for Health Policy and clinical Practice Center for health Policy Research, Dartmouth Medical School.

World Health Organization (WHO). (2000). *World Health Report, 2000* [Annex Table 8], Geneva, Switzerland: Author, p. 195.

■ APPENDIX

There are a many leadership programs available to the APRN that are designed to enhance leadership skills across the health care continuum. A number of examples follow with links to their respective websites:

Robert Wood Johnson Foundation Executive Nurse Fellows Program
http://www.rwjfleaders.org/programs/robert-wood-johnson-foundation-executive-nurse-fellows-program

Robert Wood Johnson Foundation Health Policy Fellows and Investigator Awards Programs
http://www.healthpolicyfellows.org/fellowship_info.php
http://www.investigatorawards.org/

Best on Board
http://www.bestonboard.org/website/home.html

Wharton Nursing Leaders Program
http://executiveeducation.wharton.upenn.edu/open-enrollment/health-care-programs/nursing-leaders-program.cfm

Wharton's Fellows Program in Management for Nurse Executives
http://executiveeducation.wharton.upenn.edu/open-enrollment/health-care-programs/Fellows-Program-Management-Nurse-Executives.cfm

Nurse Faculty Leadership Academy (NFLA) (through Sigma Theta Tau International)
http://www.nursingsociety.org/leadershipinstitute/nursefaculty/Pages/default.aspx

Distinguished Nurse Scholar-in-Residence http://www.iom.edu/Activities/Education/NurseScholar.aspx.

CHAPTER 18

# The Critical Need for Global Nursing Leadership

Sheila M. Davis, Inge Corless, and Patrice Nicholas

Global: of, relating to, or involving the entire earth; worldwide.
—*American Heritage Dictionary*, n.d.

There are numerous challenges in global health. These challenges are perpetuated as global leaders fail to recognize the critical role that nurses play in this area. Nurse leaders must therefore fill the global health leadership void and those with a practice doctorate are poised to embrace this challenge. In this chapter, we will examine some of the challenges in global health and the role the Doctor of Nursing Practice (DNP) can play in addressing these issues.

Global health is becoming much more integrated into national and public health discussions across various disciplines. Both nursing and medical schools have content related to global health as part of their curricula, and many students entering the health professions do so with an early commitment aimed at participation in global health activities. Many students are drawn to health care delivery in resource-limited settings, and although discussions of global health are often limited to "other" places, it is critical that a more inclusive view of global health be incorporated. While the term "resource-limited" is often reserved for discussions regarding the developing world, it is also an accurate description of many parts of the United States and therefore it is vital that we incorporate U.S. resource-limited settings in global endeavors.

The United States is considered a "developed" or "resource-rich" country, yet stark health disparities exist and resources are not equally shared among various demographic groups. The United States ranked 30th in infant mortality in 2005, a measure often used to evaluate the quality of health care for a nation (MacDorman et al., 2005). Despite having the highest health expenditure per person in the world, measures of health indicate that the United States lags in the health of segments of our population. There are many potential explanations for this discrepancy between poor health outcomes and higher expenditure per person in the global and public health arena, which are beyond the scope of this chapter. However, such startling statistics help focus on the importance of bidirectional global exchange and how "resource-rich" states fail to deliver care to many populations. Lessons learned from other areas of the world can and should be applied to many health care delivery models domestically.

Insisting on a more inclusive view of global health serves many critical functions. This shared accountability acknowledges the interconnectedness of our world. Booming industry, social conditions, and modernity have garnered increased international mobility for both people and pathogens. Transmission of infectious diseases across continents is now a reality while the devastating effects of noncommunicable diseases are also felt through our mutual interconnectedness. No nation can effectively remove itself from this responsibility of addressing global health, nor is it in their best interest.

There are an estimated 100 million health care workers worldwide with a projected shortage of more than 4 million workers. Sub-Saharan Africa, which has 33% of the global burden of illness and the deaths of mothers and children, has only 2.8% of world's health workforce (Global Health Workforce Alliance, 2010). In 17 countries in sub-Saharan Africa, there are 50 or fewer nurses per 100,000 people—below the recommended 100 nurses per 100,000 people (The Global Fund, n.d.). There is not only an unequal distribution of health care workers between continents but also unequal distribution among rural versus urban areas and among the distribution of different cadres of health care workers. Having the lowest distribution of health care workers and congruently the highest disease burden creates the "perfect storm" in global health care delivery.

## ■ MILLENNIUM DEVELOPMENT GOALS

In September 2000, a vision for the future of the world was established with the millennium development goals (MDG). The eight goals addressed were: "eradicating extreme poverty and hunger, achieving universal primary education, promoting gender equality and empowering women, reducing child mortality, improving maternal health, combating HIV/AIDS, malaria, and other diseases, ensuring environmental sustainability, and a global partnership for development" (United Nations, 2011).

The target year for achieving these improvements in health is 2015, but unfortunately health trends are not promising. Even in a setting of increased awareness of health disparities and greater commitments from richer nations to global health campaigns, needs far outweigh efforts. The World Health Organization (WHO) identifies the gaps in achieving the goals as gaps in social justice, responsibility, implementation, and knowledge (WHO, 2006). There are no quick or easy "fixes" for the gaps identified by WHO. Viewing global health as a shared responsibility continues to be difficult in settings of financial stressors and the changing dynamic of the economic and political strife in many countries in the world. Implementation of effective health programs that have measurable outcomes to assess overall impact on the individual and community level remain less of a priority for funders. The silo approach to global health, for example funding HIV/AIDS programs to prevent transmission from mother to child of the virus, and ignoring critical issues such as other methods of HIV transmission or concurrent medical challenges such as TB, have proven to be expensive, duplicative, and often disruptive to the public sector of health care. Many donor initiatives that utilize the silo approach are born of good intentions yet fail to attain the level of cultural congruency needed for effective change.

Human rights are central to the achievement of the MDGs and perhaps the missing link in many siloed humanitarian efforts. A more comprehensive view of health that includes a reduction in poverty; adequate access to food, water, and education; and economic opportunities has remained elusive in most global health efforts. The cause and effect relationship of poverty and disease and acknowledgment of the impact of structural violence on health mandate a new paradigm for global health delivery. The utilization of a human rights approach to health framework can provide guidance to expand the scope of interventions to address the root causes of poor health.

## ■ HUMAN RIGHTS APPROACH TO HEALTH

Applying a human rights approach to health has begun to infiltrate the global health literature and vernacular.

> In a human rights framework, health is a matter of justice—a product of social relations as much as biological or behavioral factors. It is the inequities in these social, and inherently power, relations for which the state (and sometimes other actors) can and should be held accountable from a human rights perspective. (Yamin, 2008, p. 46)

The concept of right to health first gained traction after the atrocities of World War II, and in 1948 the Universal Declaration of Human Rights was ratified (WHO, 1948). Although simple in concept, there has been no consensus by political or global leaders about the prioritization of health in many nations of the developed or developing worlds. In the United States, health is viewed by policy makers as a privilege not a right, and health as a human right has not been formally recognized. Once the debate of who deserves health is resolved with the acknowledgment of health as a fundamental human right, attention can be directed to addressing the critical issues of access and global health delivery.

## ■ CURRENT STATE OF GLOBAL NURSING

Nurses are the foundation of health care globally. Thirty-five million nurses are integral to health care delivery in every country of the world, but this critical cadre of health care professionals is often absent from decision making in global health delivery. Inherent in any discussion of global nursing and midwifery is the acknowledgment of the lack of consistency of education, clinical preparation, and status within the health care system and countries as a whole, factors that add to the ambiguity surrounding the impact and importance of the nursing profession (WHO, 2009). Global scope and standards of nursing practice remain elusive and the discussion is further complicated by a lack of consistency in midwifery preparation and its inclusion or exclusion from the realm of nursing. There is little information available on nurse-sensitive indicators in global health delivery although, interestingly, vaccination coverage is directly linked to the density of nurses and is almost entirely independent of physicians (Global Health Council, n.d). It is essential that we articulate the value of nurses in global health delivery by employing explicit evaluation methods to show improved patient outcomes with quality nursing care.

Virtually voiceless in higher level global health leadership, a momentum is growing to demand nursing representation. In May of 2011 expressing extreme concern at the lack of nursing policy presence within the WHO structures, an emergency resolution was passed by the governing body of the International Council of Nurses (ICN) at its biennial meeting held in Valetta, Malta. The official representatives of ICN member national nurses associations voted unanimously to demand that the WHO Director

General empower and finance nursing leadership positions throughout the organization (ICN, 2011). This effort by ICN drew attention within the global nursing community but did not appear to have any impact thus far on changing the current leadership structures.

## ■ INTERNAL AND EXTERNAL NURSE MIGRATION

Discussions of global nursing often revolve around issues of international nurse migration. Aiken and colleagues (2004) discuss the "push" and "pull" factors of nurse migration. Factors that push nurses to leave their home include poor wages, economic instability, dysfunctional health systems, risk and burden of AIDS, and personal safety concerns. The pull to developed countries includes higher wages, better living, improved working conditions, and educational opportunities for advancement, all of which contribute to the allure of migration. Thus the "brain-drain" phenomenon results in resource-limited settings being further deprived of vital human resources.

Other factors critical to the migration discussion include the migration from rural to urban areas, movement from employment in the public sector to the private sector, and leaving the nursing profession for better paying and/or less stressful work environments. Although criticism of the aggressive recruitment by the developed world for nurses from resource-poor settings is problematic and pointless to argue, complexities arise when individual rights of nurses to migrate are ignored. Remittance income (money being sent home by the nurse employed elsewhere) can be a substantial factor in a struggling economy of a developing country and is encouraged by a number of countries as one mechanism to infuse hard currency into their system.

Blanket resolutions forbidding nurse migration are limited in vision and do not address the core issues of a dysfunctional health system in home countries or countries that recruit nurses. Solving their own issues of nursing shortages, the developed world needs to examine new approaches to invest in nursing and avoid the "quick fix" of mass importation of nurses. A majority of nurses would prefer not to leave their homes and would prefer to be part of the solution if given the opportunity to receive better wages, improved working conditions, and career advancement opportunities. Restricting a person's choice and limiting the migration of nurses who choose to exercise their human right of mobility are complex issues that require further examination.

Adhering to the shared commitment to improve global health, donors and developed nations need to invest in public sector infrastructure to strengthen capacity in developing countries health systems. Funneling global aid to the public sector is a more sustainable strategy to minimize reliance on global aid. Restructuring aid to focus on improved long-term outcomes of health systems and building of local economies will begin to address the push and pull of nurse migration.

## ■ DEVELOPMENT OF GLOBAL NURSE LEADERS: A PRACTICE DOCTORATE

Acknowledging the importance of nursing leadership at all levels of international development, the creation of nurse leaders globally is critical. The lack of progress in achieving many of the MDGs is disappointing and due in large measure to the absence of nursing leadership in influencing health in resource-limited countries. Ketefian (2008) discusses the need for doctorally prepared nurses as part of this solution and advocates for a movement toward preparation of nurses at the doctoral level. She suggests that "the most important goal of nursing doctoral education is to prepare leaders who can use their expertise to guide and lead country and international efforts to address health, education, and policy needs" (p. 1401). Although relatively new to the global landscape, nurses with clinical/practice doctorates can provide much needed leadership and advance nurses at the forefront in developing new models of care delivery.

Globally, academic nursing continues to evolve. For example, in Rwanda, a total restructuring of the Rwandan nursing educational system is currently occurring with an emphasis on upgrading the nursing profession by investing in the educational pathways for nursing. A nationwide program is underway to upgrade A2 level nurses to the A1 level that will move entry level for nurses from a high school level to a 3-year postsecondary school diploma. In addition, strengthening the small but growing bachelor and master's level programs in nursing is preparing the next cadre of nurse educators and clinical leaders. Currently, the advanced practice/nurse practitioner role is emerging, but thus far remains limited in many resource-limited settings including Rwanda. The International Council of Nursing (ICN) established an advanced practice/nurse practitioner network in 2000. This network estimates that there are nearly 40 countries that have established or are in the process of developing advanced practice nursing roles (Cross, n.d.). With an overwhelming health care worker shortage globally, producing a more efficient, competent, and critical thinker in nursing is in the best interest of the population as a whole.

Rolfe and Davies (2009) trace the history of doctoral education in nursing from its beginnings in the 1930s in the United States and in Europe in the 1990s. Although there are PhD prepared nurses working globally, there are few nurses from the developing world who have had access to doctoral education. Rolfe and Davies (2009) join Ellis and Lee (2005) in seeing the value of a clinical doctorate for nurses in global health delivery: "application to practice is at the philosophical core of the professional doctorates" (Ellis & Lee, 2005, p. 2). The emphasis of the clinical doctorate on systems approaches to practice-oriented problems, quality improvement, and real time application support the important roles that nurses with clinical doctorates could offer in advancing nursing practice globally.

Distinguishing between types of doctoral education (traditional PhD and practice/clinical doctorate) is important. Making the distinction between Mode 1 (empirical/scientific discovery) and Mode 2 (generation of knowledge from practice), Rolfe and Davies (2009) advocate for the clinical doctorate as "the production of knowledge in the context of the situation to which it will ultimately be applied rather than the context of the laboratory or the academic research study" (p. 1272). Involving individuals who are in the specific context is important. Such key informants include clinicians, patients, managers, community members, and others as indicated by the situation.

This approach differs widely from the traditional scientific approach to new knowledge or scientific discovery. One simple example to illustrate between Mode 1 and Mode 2 approaches is the evaluation of a new patient registration system in a rural clinic in a resource-limited setting that is described in the following scenario. Utilizing a Mode 1 approach, researchers may administer a survey to incoming patients and assess how many patients attend each clinic session in addition to other key pieces of data. In application of the scientific rigor of a Mode 1 approach, the researchers would interpret the results at predetermined time periods in the study and would not alter the environment or setting in order to maintain a consistent environment. In our example, 3 months after opening the clinic, health care providers at the clinic note that patients are avoiding the clinic and going to the mobile clinic in order to bypass the registration process.

Regardless of obvious dissatisfaction of the patients and community with the registration system, in order to maintain the study protocol, no changes to the system could be made until all data had been collected without jeopardizing the integrity of the study. Obviously, such a response is dependent on the research question and study design. The example of a data safety monitoring board stopping a placebo controlled pharmaceutical study where one of the arms of the study is demonstrably receiving inferior care could be emulated in the previous example.

Applying a Mode 2 approach, if the clinicians noted the dissatisfaction with the system at the 3-month interval, community meetings could be held to identify what in the system is not acceptable to the patients. Strategic changes in the registration process could be made immediately to the system, thereby utilizing a more real-time feedback loop. This type of approach is one that expert clinicians would be likely to grasp with advanced education in nursing.

This obviously oversimplified example, is meant to illustrate the opposite ends of the spectrum of approaches, Both Mode 1 and Mode 2 applications are important to global health delivery, but the emphasis and evaluation is different. "The validity or 'truthfulness' of Mode 2 knowledge-production is measured according to its contribution to tangible improvements to practice rather than whether it generates 'pure' decontextualised theoretical knowledge" (Rolfe & Davies, 2009, p. 1271). In global health delivery efforts, knowledge generated through practice should be prioritized with the utilization of the scientific discovery methodology reserved for areas where acquisition of this information would influence care delivery and/or improve patient outcomes. Investigation that highlights disparities, concerns about adherence, symptom management, and stigma also contribute to improving patient care. Generation of new knowledge if only for academic pursuits, although interesting for some, may contribute to the inefficiencies in global health delivery, funding, and priorities.

The debate whether nurses with clinical or professional doctorates are capable of conducting scientific research is destructive and nonproductive—a debate that has distracted the nursing profession from much more critical dialogues and issues. Curricula differ among DNP programs, with some more heavily focused on research than others, and some graduates obtaining additional education in these areas. A much more productive dialogue would include advocating for the assessment of an individual's competency in research design and statistical analysis rather than a blanket moratorium on the involvement of DNP professionals in scientific generation of knowledge. Dreher and Glasgow (2009) discuss the role of the practice doctorate, "discouraging the conduct of empirical research in any doctorate is an alarming direction, particularly for a discipline that requires ongoing evidence-based and practice-based knowledge development for both professional, advanced, and now doctoral advanced nursing practice" (p. 406).

## ■ INTERDISCIPLINARY, MULTIDISCIPLINARY, AND TRANSDISCIPLINARY GLOBAL HEALTH CARE DELIVERY

Nowhere is the importance of a team approach to care delivery more applicable than in global health. Commonly used in educational settings, the term "multidisciplinary" may be defined as the teaching of common material to people from different disciplines, while the term "interdisciplinary" curriculum implies learning between students sharing their experiences and unique perspective with those from different disciplines. Less familiar to most in health care, "transdisciplinarity entails not only a transcendence of disciplinary boundaries, but to some extent the transcendence of the very idea of disciplines" (Rolfe and Davies, 2009, p. 1270). Reluctance to embrace collaborative models of care delivery is an unfortunate reality in the resource-rich and resource-poor worlds. Although there is an increasing rhetoric in health care about the need for multiple disciplines to be part of care delivery, rarely does this move beyond mission statements or task forces. Fostering mutual respect and acknowledgment of different but important contributions to health delivery is an ongoing process and emerging models of common content being taught for nursing and medical students as a combined class may be part of the solution. This would require an overhaul of nursing and medical education. "Transprofessional education might be as important as interprofessional education. An examination of the skill mix in selected countries of sub-Saharan African underscores the importance of professionals learning to work with nonprofessionals in health teams" (Frenk, 2010, p. 1948). Ability to work with transprofessional teams is of critical importance and is rarely taught or stressed at all in health provider education.

Task shifting has become a necessary part of global health but is sometimes threatening to different cadres of health care workers. Voiced concerns of nurses include the creation of new cadres of health care workers, lack of supervision and training of auxiliary workers, and lack of involvement of health professions in decision making about task shifting (World Health Professional Alliance, 2008). A shift in language to *task-sharing* may better embody the intent of a team approach to health care delivery. All members of the team, regardless of position in the health care system, should have accountability to the patient with a feedback loop to continually assess patient outcomes. For example, if a task formally done by nurses is shifted to a community health worker (medication delivery), the nurse is still accountable to that patient and health system to uphold the highest quality of patient care possible. Similarly, shifting of the management of antiretroviral medications for patients with HIV from a physician to a nurse does not dissolve the responsibility of the government entities (including a physician in leadership role) to provide adequate staff and training to the nurses now tasked to deliver high quality HIV treatment and monitoring.

Frenk and colleagues (2010) discuss their vision for health professionals for a new century. "Individual professions might have distinctive and complementary skills that could be considered the core of their special niche. But there is an imperative for bringing such expertise together into teams for effective patient-centered and population-based health work" (p. 1951). Competency-based curriculum and team learning are critical for preparing the next generation of health professionals. This method of education is more easily adapted to a changing global health environment and can include measurement of the impact on the health delivery system. As Frenk continues to urge, the priority for education evaluators must be attainment of specific competencies, and not "turf protection" (p. 1951).

## ■ DNPs IN GLOBAL HEALTH

The converging realities of the current health care worker shortage, lack of global nursing leadership, grim achievements in improvements in MDGs, and a call for a new model of global health care delivery that is based on competencies and transprofessional teams require a shift in the global nursing paradigm. The DNP, the terminal practice degree in nursing, is well positioned to play a major role in the transformation needed in global health.

The DNP essentials adopted in 2005 would benefit from updating but core elements of DNP education prepare future global health nursing leaders. As previously discussed, Rolf and Davies' (2009) call for doctoral education in the practice generated knowledge model of discovery correlates well with the preparation and intent of the DNP degree.

All eight essentials are important and pertain to the global arena but only essentials two, three, five, six, and seven will be discussed in more detail. The second essential, *organizational and systems leadership for quality improvement and systems thinking*, addresses health care disparities and a systems approach to care. "These graduates are distinguished by their abilities to conceptualize new care delivery models that are based in contemporary nursing science and that are feasible within current organizational, political, cultural, and economic perspectives" (AACN, 2006). In the context of current and future global health needs, new care delivery models will be critical to the provision of equitable, quality global health.

The convergence of the art and science of nursing is evident in third essential, *clinical scholarship and analytical methods for evidence-based practice nursing*. As new knowledge is being generated in practice settings, it will be critical that the DNP nursing leader be well versed in evidence-based practice and the application of theory to their practice setting.

Essential five, *health care policy for advocacy in health care,* is particularly critical due to the call for more global nursing leaders. Integral to effective system improvement is the political will of national and international government leaders. It is only through persistent and strategic engagement on multiple levels that there can there be sustainable and far-reaching policy change. DNPs can play a lead role in advocacy on the individual, family, community, national, and global levels. Incorporating the framework, health as a human right, can provide guidance in establishing fiscal priorities and activism for high quality, equitable, and accessible health care.

Regardless of the label used to indicate global cross-discipline and creative health care teams, Essential six, *interprofessional collaboration for improving patient and population health outcomes* will require strong leadership, a role that DNPs are qualified to fill. Maintaining a strong professional nursing identity, DNPs are well positioned to provide the key linkage between different cadres of health care workers. Advocating for patient-centered care with multiple layers of accountability will ensure that task-sharing leads to greater access and improved patient outcomes.

Rooted in a holistic approach to patient care, nursing's foundation of care has always been comprehensive. Essential seven, *clinical prevention and population health for improving the nation's health,* although specific to national health can be easily be broadened to incorporate what is more traditionally thought of as global health. Bidirectional learning acknowledges the critical knowledge exchange between health care providers in the developing and developed world. Applying successful models of global health delivery from a resource-limited setting to a setting in a resource-rich setting is a less accepted practice, but one that may contribute in very meaningful ways. Learning to provide quality care with limited resources will be very important as health care costs increase.

A good example of the transfer of models from resource-limited settings to the United States is the Prevention and Access to Care and Treatment (PACT) Project implemented by Partners In Health. As a large international nongovernmental health organization providing health care in 12 countries globally, Partners In Health has successfully applied bidirectional exchanges to enhance clinical care. Learning from the success of the community health worker (CHW) model in Haiti, a CHW-centric program was installed in Boston to provide culturally congruent support for low income patients who are the most vulnerable and least equipped to navigate the complex health system (Partners In Health, n.d.).

# ■ CONCLUSIONS

The emergence of the DNP in the United States as a practice doctorate is poised to offer significant leadership in the global health arena. Innovative approaches to care delivery, task sharing, and practice knowledge generation are needed. The call for nursing participation in policy and in global health delivery will require an infusion of nurse leaders best prepared to contribute to the allocation of resources and to the provision of a human rights-based approach to health. By partnering with nurse leaders in developing regions, DNPs can advocate for policy reform to increase nursing's visibility and to prioritize upgrading of the nursing educational system.

A radical transformation in the provision of dignified, equitable, and quality health care for the poor is desperately needed. Unfortunately it is likely that we will continue to be a world of shrinking resources and competing priorities. A fundamental shift in our shared accountability toward each other is critically important as we strive to make global health a priority. There is a Haitian Creole saying, *Tout Moun Se Moun* (we are all human beings). We all must live by this simple, but essential guiding principle.

# ■ REFERENCES

Aiken, L. H., Buchan, J., Sochalski, J., Nichols, B., & Powell, M. (2004). Trends in international nurse migration. *Health Affairs, 23*(3), 69–77.

American Association of Colleges of Nursing. (2006, October). *The essentials of doctoral education for advanced nursing practice.* Retrieved from http://www.aacn.nche.edu/dnp/pdf/essentials.pdf

Cross, S. (n.d.). *Network history-nurse practitioner/advanced practice network.* International Council of Nurses, ICN. Retrieved August 23, 2011, from http://www.icn-apnetwork.org

Dreher, H. M., & Glasgow, M. E. (2009). Global perspectives on the professional doctorate. *International Journal of Nursing Studies, 48,* 403–408.

Ellis, L., & Lee, N. (2005). The changing landscape of doctoral education: Introducing the professional doctorate for nurses. *Nurse Education Today, 25*(3), 222–229. doi: 10.1016/j.nedt.2005.01.009.

Frenk, J., Chen, L., Bhutta, Z. A., Cohen, J., Crisp, N., Evans, T., ... Garcia, P. (2010). Health professionals for a new century: Transforming education to strengthen health systems in an interdependent world. *The Lancet, 376*(9756), 1923–1958. doi: 10.1016/S0140-6736(10)61854-5

Global. (n.d.). *The American Heritage® Dictionary of the English Language, Fourth Edition.* Retrieved August 20, 2011, from http://www.thefreedictionary.com/global

Global Health Workforce Alliance. (2010). *Adding value to health-global health workforce alliance-annual report 2010.* Retrieved from http://www.who.int/workforcealliance/knowledge/resources/annualreport2010/en/index.html

International Council of Nurses (ICN). (2011). *Open letter to Dr Margaret Chan, Director General of the World Health Organization from the International Council of Nurses.* [Press release]. Retrieved from www.icn.ch/images/stories/documents/news/press_releases/2011_PR_07_Open_Letter__NursingVoiceExcluded_WHO.pdf

Ketefian, S. (2008, October). Doctoral education in the context of international development strategies. *International Journal of Nursing Studies, 45*(10), 1401–1402.

MacDorman, M. F., Martin, J. A., Mathews, T. J., Hoyert, D. L., Ventura, S. J. (2005). Explaining the 2001-02 infant mortality increase: Data from the linked birth/infant death data set. *National Vital Statistics Reports, 53*(12), 1–22.

Partners In Health. (n.d). *PACT Program.* Retrieved August 23, 2011, from http://www.pih.org/pages/usa

Rolfe, G., & Davies, R. (2009). Second generation professional doctorates in nursing. *International of Nursing Studies, 46,* 1265–1273.

The Global Fund. (n.d.). *Health system strengthening.* Retrieved April 6, 2012, from www.the-globalfund.org/en/performance/effectiveness/hss/

United Nations. (2011). *Millennium development goals report 2011.* Retrieved from http://www.un.org/millenniumgoals

World Health Organization (WHO). (2006). *Engaging in health-eleventh general programme of work 2006–2015: A global health agenda.* Retrieved from http://whqlibdoc.who.int/publications/2006/GPW_eng.pdf

World Health Organization (WHO). (1948). *Preamble-Constitution of the World Health Organization.* 2–3. Retrieved from http://whqlibdoc.who.int/hist/official_records/constitution.pdf

World Health Organization (WHO). (2009). *Global standards for the initial education of professional nurses and midwives.* Retrieved from www.who.int/hrh/nursing_midwifery/en

World Health Professionals Alliance (WHPA). (2008, March 11). *Health professions demand strong principles for task shifting* [Press Release]. Retrieved from http://www.whpa.org/pr03_08.htm

Yamin, A. (2008). Will we take suffering seriously? Reflections on what applying a human rights framework to health means and why we should care. *Health And Human Rights: An International Journal, 10*(1). Retrieved from http://www.hhrjournal.org/index.php/hhr/article/view/27/89

# *Index*